THE THERAPEUTIC STATE
Psychiatry in the Mirror of Current Events

THE THERAPEUTIC STATE

Psychiatry in the Mirror of Current Events

Thomas Szasz

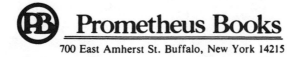

Prometheus Books

700 East Amherst St. Buffalo, New York 14215

Published in 1984 by
Prometheus Books
700 East Amherst Street
Buffalo, New York 14215

Printed in the United States of America

Library of Congress Catalog Card No. 83-63057
ISBN: 0-87975-239-4 cloth
0-87975-242-4 paper

CONTENTS

Acknowledgment

This volume comprises a collection of pieces written, for the most part, for newspapers, magazines, and book reviews. Also included are a few items originally published in professional journals and two essays not previously published. Except for minor corrections, all of the material is reprinted in its original form.

I want to take this opportunity to thank Ralph Raico for editorial assistance with the essays written for *Inquiry;* my daughter, Susan Marie Szasz, for proofreading the galleys; Cynthia Brown Dwyer for preparing the Index; and the various publishers for opening their pages to me and for permission to reprint.

PREFACE

Although mental illness is said to be an illness "like any other," and although psychiatry is said to be a medical specialty "like any other," it is obvious that neither assertion is true. Specialists in neurology, cardiology, gynecology, urology, rheumatology, hematology, immunology, and the other branches of medicine are concerned with the workings of various body parts and systems and with helping persons suffering from diseases that affect these parts or systems. But what are psychiatrists concerned with?

The answer to this question has been a matter of debate ever since psychiatrists first came on the scene of human history, about two hundred years ago. The basic reason for the controversy over the nature of psychiatry lies in, and is revealed by, the embarrassing contradiction between the ostensible and the actual practices of psychiatrists. This should not surprise us. The same has been true for every important institutionalized ideology throughout history. That it is true for psychiatry too—indeed, that it is true for psychiatry but not for, say, cardiology or neurology—can make us draw two quite different inferences: One is that psychiatry is less developed than other branches of medicine and hence more time and effort are needed to bring it up to par with its sister specialties. This is the position today not only of the leading psychiatric authorities but also of the leading opinion-makers of our society, from justices of the Supreme Court to editorial writers for the *New York Times*. Another inference is that this contradiction is an important feature of psychiatry that we must treat as a clue to its true character. This has been the position I have espoused ever since I started to write about psychiatry, more than thirty years ago.

Although the pieces assembled in this volume are as varied as the daily events of our life—each taking off from some newsmaking political event, criminal trial, or literary happening—they all share a particular point of view on psychiatry. I have stated that view in several scholarly publications and there is no need for me to restate it here. Furthermore, it is set forth—perhaps better than in my more formal works—in the editorials, essays, and reviews that follow. Let me note here, however, that there is nothing particularly original in my approach, although its application to psychiatry has been astoundingly neglected. People have always known that actions speak louder than words. This insight was given a more sophisticated form by the great American philosopher Charles Sanders Peirce, who asserted that "What a thing means is simply what habits it involves."[1]

9

So we must inquire into, and familiarize ourselves with, the habits of psychiatrists. It is not hard to do this. Of course we must not let ourselves be distracted by the psychiatrists' endless self-serving chatter about what they do or think or by their gothic tales of miraculous cures in the private spaces of their cloistered offices. Instead, we must keep our eyes on their observable performances in mental hospitals, courts of law, and other public places. By laying bare the professional habits of psychiatrists, I believe I have gone a long way in answering the questions people most often ask about the mental-health profession, such as: What is mental illness? Is psychotherapy effective? Is electroshock a treatment or a torture? Should it be banned? Does it help or harm patients to be confined in mental hospitals? Is the insanity defense necessary?

There is an obvious reason why we have so much difficulty giving satisfactory answers to these important questions. It is because, as the great English legal scholar James Fitzjames Stephen observed, "Men have an all but incurable propensity to try to prejudge all the great questions which interest them by stamping their prejudices upon their language."[2] Accordingly, to answer the questions that puzzle people about matters of so-called mental illness, we must make ourselves aware of the ways in which both psychiatrists and mental patients use language—to impose their "reality" on each other, and everyone else. Perhaps only in this way will we be able to see that two and two make four—that fraud is fraud and force is force—regardless of who deceives or coerces or of how one justifies one's behavior.

Notes

1. Charles S. Peirce, "How to Make Our Ideas Clear" (1878), in *Values in a Universe of Chance: Selected Writings of Charles S. Peirce (1839-1914),* ed., Philip P. Wiener (Garden City, N.Y.: Doubleday Anchor, 1958), p. 123.

2. James F. Stephen, *Liberty, Equality, Fraternity* (1873) (Cambridge: The University Press, 1967), p. 176.

I

"MENTAL ILLNESS"

The Myth of Mental Illness

The premise underlying theology is the existence of God. Theologians can neither define God nor demonstrate his existence; for them and their followers the existence of God is obvious, beyond need of demonstration. Those who deny the existence of God are mistaken, misguided or worse. The burden of proof is on the non-believer to prove the non-existence of God.

Now the premise underlying psychiatry is the existence of mental illness. Psychiatrists can neither define mental illness nor demonstrate its existence; for them and their followers the existence of mental illness is obvious, beyond need of demonstration. Those who deny the existence of mental illness are mistaken, misguided or worse. The burden of proof is on the critic of psychiatry to prove the non-existence of mental illness.

Psychiatry: A Pseudoscience. The proposition that mental illness is a myth—which I first advanced in a paper in 1960 and developed more fully in a book published a year later—is expressly intended to sap the pseudoscientific ground on which psychiatry rests. It insinuates the idea that just as God exists only for those who believe in imaginary beings or "powers" (religion), so mental illness exists only for those who believe in imaginary illnesses or "causes" (psychiatry).

Why is the subject matter of psychiatry believed to be mental illness? The idea of mental illness receives its main support from such phenomena as neurosyphilis (syphilis of the nervous system) and traumatic or senile dementia (degeneration of the brain). These are conditions in which disorders of behavior, or so-called psychiatric symptoms, are caused by a demonstrable disease, a "pathology." However, correctly speaking, these are diseases of the brain, not of the mind. They are diseases in the same sense that arteriosclerosis and arthritis are diseases. They are diseases of a part of the body, the brain. In short, they are literal diseases. According to most contemporary psychiatrists all mental diseases are of this type.

Where the Medical Model Fails. Revealingly, psychiatrists often speak of "medical diseases *underlying* psychiatric symptoms," but specialists in diseases of the heart, lungs, or stomach do not speak of "medical diseases underlying cardiac, pulmonary, or gastroenterological symptoms." Psychiatrists thus

---

First published as "Mental Illness: A Myth?" in *The ABC of Psychology,* ed. by Leonard Kristal (London: Michael Joseph, 1981), pp. 150-55. Reprinted with permission.

assume that a disease or defect of the nervous system, perhaps a very subtle one, will one day be discovered to be the cause and hence the explanation of all so-called mental diseases.

This view implies that human problems now classified as mental diseases are *not* the consequences of conflicting personal aspirations, *not* the outcome of moral values, social controls, and similar individual or cultural factors. Instead such problems are attributed to physiological or chemical processes yet to be discovered, and hopefully remedied, by medical scientists. In short, mental illnesses are regarded as basically similar to bodily diseases, the only difference being that the latter affect the heart, lungs and other organs, and manifest themselves as symptoms which can be directly traced to these organs, whereas the former affect the brain and manifest themselves as "mental" or "psychiatric" symptoms, symptoms which can be directly traced to the brain.

This view rests on two fundamental errors. First, to be at all analogous to a disease of the heart or kidney, a disease of the brain would have to manifest itself by neurological signs, not psychiatric symptoms; that is, it would have to be something like impaired gait or vision rather than something like depression or paranoia. Secondly, if psychiatrists believe or "know" that so-called mental patients suffer from diseases of the brain, then for the sake of clarity and honesty they ought to say that and not something else.

Calling a Spade a Spade. There are some psychiatrists, now in the minority, who believe that mental illnesses exist, but who do not consider them to be simply the symptoms of brain disease. They correctly observe that a diseased brain does not "secrete" confused speech like a diseased kidney secretes albumin-rich urine. They see mental illnesses as abnormalities or deformities of the "personality," which a person acquires or develops in a variety of ways (not necessarily through brain disease). They consider mental illness to be both a cause and a consequence of interpersonal and social conflict.

My objection to this "psychosocial" model of mental illness is again two-fold. First, it implies that countless personal, religious, legal, political and social problems can be classified as "diseases," and that life would be meaningful and peaceful if these problems were prevented or cured. This view simply replaces a biological oversimplification with a psychosocial oversimplification.

Second, whereas the advocates of the biological view classify certain brain diseases as "mental diseases," the advocates of the psychosocial view use the term "mental disease" metaphorically but nevertheless insist that it is a literal disease. Put differently, the organic psychiatrist claims that mental illness *is* a disease and then names the wrong "organ" as the seat of the malady (mind rather than brain), but the psychosocial psychiatrist claims that mental illness is a disease *like* other diseases, which conveniently obscures the differences between deviance and disease.

Toward Greater Integrity and Responsibility. In pointing out the mythical nature of mental illness I am pointing out that psychiatrists have a vested interest in manufacturing and maintaining their mythology. I am attempting, if you like, to destroy their pretensions and privileges.

Mental illnesses do not exist; indeed, they cannot exist, because the mind is not a body part or bodily organ.

Inevitably the idea of illness, whether of the mind or the body, implies deviation from a norm. In the case of physical illness, the norm is the structural and functional integrity of the human body or some part of it. In the case of mental illness, it is impossible to name a single norm which is not stated in psychological, social, moral, or legal terms—all typical psychiatric symptoms or diseases, from agoraphobia to sexual intercourse with animals, conform to and illustrate this principle.

In asserting that mental illness is a myth, I am not asserting (as some of my critics have claimed) that certain distressing phenomena do not exist. On the contrary, it is belief in the existence of mental illness that prevents us from grasping and accepting the truth about behaviors labeled "mentally diseased." In other words, just as disbelief in God does not imply disbelief in his alleged creations, so disbelief in mental illness does not imply disbelief in the myriad phenomena we now label mental illness. Personal misery and social unrest, aggression and suffering, quite unavoidably exist. But they are not diseases. We categorize them as diseases at great peril to our integrity, responsibility and liberty.

Medicine and Madness

All too often, the language in which a personal or social problem is couched subtly but inexorably supplies its solution. Nowhere is this more evident than in the field of so-called mental illness.

In earlier times, when "the problem" was witchcraft—that is, when persons who provoked punishment for certain antisocial actions, or who were scapegoated for other reasons, were said to be witches possessed by demons—the solution was exorcism and burning at the stake. Today, when "the problem" is mental illness—that is, when such persons are said to be psychiatric patients suffering from mental diseases—the solution is to imprison them in buildings called hospitals and torture them in the name of treatment. In neither case did the "solution" arise from a hardheaded examination of the difficulty. It is against this background that we must view what is now usually called "the problem of the civil rights of mental patients."

I submit that this problem is primarily linguistic. I do not, of course, mean that it is "just" a matter of semantics or words. Rather, it is a matter of how words are used to shape popular opinion and to justify legal action and political policy. The concepts and terms "mental illness" and "mental patient" combine and confuse two entirely different and, at bottom, contradictory sets of ideas and interventions: disease and cure on the one hand, and deviance and control on the other.

Cure and Control. If we take an unbiased look at the traditional, commonsense meanings of the words "ill" and "insane," we notice that they conjure up two quite different images and refer to two quite different ideas. Illness means there is something wrong with the body of the person said to be ill, whereas insanity means there is something wrong with the behavior of the person said to be insane. This is why, traditionally, the first idea has led to interventions usually called "treatments" and "cures" and the second to interventions usually called "restraints" and "controls."

Especially in contemporary free societies, there is, for all practical purposes, no such thing as the involuntary medical treatment of adults. The social act of medical treatment comes into being not so much because the patient is sick as because he wants treatment and is willing to submit to it. In short, what ultimately justifies medical treatment is not disease but consent.

Reprinted, with permission, from *The Encyclopaedia Britannica Yearbook,* 1974, pp. 454-55.

Conversely, what characterizes involuntary psychiatric diagnosis, hospitalization, and treatment is that each comes into being not because the alleged patient wants or is willing to submit to it, but because someone other than the "patient" claims that the "patient" is "mentally ill."

The present psychiatric situation cannot be understood without some appreciation of the history of psychiatry. Briefly, modern psychiatry began in the seventeenth century, with the building of insane asylums in which all sorts of troublesome and unwanted persons were incarcerated. Originally, then, psychiatry was "institutional"; it was a kind of extralegal penology. In the course of its 300-year history, and especially during the past century, immense and unceasing efforts have been directed at redefining psychiatric confinement as "hospitalization" and psychiatric control as "treatment."

Perhaps because the best efforts of the most energetic psychiatrists have been devoted to this task—from Philippe Pinel and Benjamin Rush to Sigmund Freud and Karl Menninger—this medicalization of human problems and their coercive control by means of the police power of the state has been amazingly successful. (See Szasz, *The Myth of Mental Illness* [1961]; *The Manufacture of Madness* [1970]; *The Age of Madness* [1973].) As a result, no other group in modern history has been so consistently and unrelentingly persecuted, and deprived of their human and constitutional rights, as the insane or so-called mentally ill.

Involuntary and Voluntary Mental Hospitalization. The most important deprivation of human and constitutional rights inflicted on persons said to be mentally ill is involuntary mental hospitalization; that is, the coerced confinement of the person in an institution called a mental hospital. Many thousands of persons are now so confined in the United States, and countless more in other countries. While the precise legal requirements for commitment differ from state to state and from nation to nation, the procedure, in effect, is based on and justified by the closely connected ideas of mental illness and dangerousness. This is exemplified by the traditional American legal formula for commitment, which speaks of the alleged patient as suffering from a "mental disease or disorder" and of being "dangerous to himself or others." Regardless of the legal phraseology in which commitment laws are enshrouded, their implementation depends almost entirely on the ideology that animates the psychiatrists and judges who practice this sort of "medicine." Their ideology has been, quite simply, paternalistic.

"If a man brings his daughter to me from California," a prominent psychiatrist testified before a U.S. Senate committee, "because she is in manifest danger of falling into vice or in some other way disgracing herself, he doesn't expect me to let her loose in my hometown for that same thing to happen" *(Constitutional Rights of the Mentally Ill,* Washington, D.C.: U.S. Government Printing Office, 1961, p. 71). Jurists have held the same view of the problem. In denying damages to a man who had entered a mental hospital voluntarily, was subsequently prevented from leaving, and sued, a

Connecticut appeals court judge ruled that "mental patients are often not in a condition to appreciate what is for their own best interests or what their real desires are" *(Roberts* v. *Pain,* 124 Conn. 173, 199 A. 115 [1938]).

Although most of the people committed to mental hospitals against their will are poor or old, many prominent persons have also suffered this fate, both in former times and in our own. King Ludwig II of Bavaria; Mary Todd Lincoln, President Lincoln's widow; U.S. Secretary of Defense James Forrestal; Ernest Hemingway; and the dissident intellectuals in the U.S.S.R. —these are but a few of the famous victims of psychiatric incarceration as a method of social control.

While in many cases persons committed to mental hospitals ostensibly lose only the right to leave the hospital, actually they often lose all their civil rights. They may be declared incompetent to manage their persons and assets; may lose the right to vote, drive a car, or practice their profession; may be subjected to the most brutal and injurious acts imaginable to modern man—called psychiatric treatments; and are permanently stigmatized as "ex-mental patients."

Although some mental hospitalization is nominally and semantically "voluntary," so-called voluntary mental patients incur many of the same deprivations of civil rights suffered by the involuntarily hospitalized mental patient. Indeed, because voluntary mental hospitalization is always potentially and often actually a covert form of involuntary mental hospitalization—and because this type of hospitalization now involves many more persons than does involuntary mental hospitalization—this psychiatric intervention is perhaps an even greater threat to civil liberties than is involuntary mental hospitalization. Both in fact and by law, voluntary mental patients are treated essentially the same way as involuntary mental patients. Moreover, patients hospitalized voluntarily often enter a psychiatric institution under the threat of commitment. Once confined, they cannot secure their release as can medical patients, and when they insist on release against psychiatric advice, they may be committed by their relatives and physicians. The prisoner status of such patients was openly acknowledged by a 1971 decision of the Supreme Court of Utah, in which the court held "that a voluntary patient at the [mental] hospital is as much 'confined' and has as little freedom as a mentally alert trusty in a jail or prison" (*Emery* v. *State,* 483 P. 2d, 1296).

Psychiatric interventions may be invoked against persons accused of crime at every point where the criminal process impinges on the accused. At every such point psychiatry is used to deprive the accused of freedom and dignity in the name of protecting his mental health and treating his mental illness. A person accused of a crime may thus be declared mentally unfit to stand trial and be confined in a mental hospital until he is declared to be fit. Such a person is deprived of the Sixth Amendment guarantee to a speedy and public trial, and may be imprisoned, under psychiatric auspices to be sure, without trial. Ezra Pound was so confined for 13 years. Tens of thousands of Americans have been, and continue to be, so confined, some drawing a psychiatric life sentence for a trivial offense. A defendant allowed to stand trial may plead not guilty by reason of insanity—a plea that may be entered for him by his attorney without his understanding its implications. He may, as a result, draw an indefinite sentence of psychiatric incarceration in lieu of a possible acquittal or a finite prison sentence. Finally, once in jail, a prisoner may be declared psychotic and transferred to a hospital for the criminally insane.

This brief survey does not exhaust all of the ways in which psychiatric interventions are now used as methods of social control—through legislatures and courts, through medical organizations and mental institutions, and last but not least through the personal desire to control others. Our society is shot through with the use of psychiatric incriminations and excuses, from declaring wealthy relatives mentally incompetent or their wills invalid to evading the draft and abortion laws. (See Szasz, *Law, Liberty, and Psychiatry* [1963]; *Psychiatric Justice* [1965]; *Ideology and Insanity* [1970].)

Reforms. For centuries, involuntary psychiatric interventions were regarded as things done *for* the so-called patient rather than as things done *to* him. This perspective, which is still the official psychiatric posture, precludes genuine reforms in the mental health field. In recent years, however, increasing numbers of persons, both in the mental-health professions and in public life, have come to acknowledge that involuntary psychiatric interventions are methods of social control. With this recognition, the question with respect to psychiatric reforms becomes whether we want to retain such methods and introduce certain safeguards into their use, or whether we want to abolish their use altogether. On both moral and practical grounds, I advocate the abolition of all involuntary psychiatry.

This goal could easily be attained. However, because of our intense devotion to the medical perspective on human problems, efforts to do so may prove to be, at least for the time being, unpalatable and impractical. To attain this goal, we would first have to accept that so-called mental-health problems are not medical but human—that is, economic, moral, social, and political problems. In other words, mental illnesses are metaphorical diseases.

It is impossible, of course, to understand the metaphorical nature of the concept of mental illness without coming to grips with the literal meaning of the concept of ordinary or bodily illness. When we say a person is ill, we usually mean two quite different things: first, that he believes, or his physician believes, or they both believe, that he suffers from an abnormality or malfunctioning of his body; and second, that he wants, or is at least willing to accept, medical help for his suffering. The term "illness" thus refers primarily to an abnormal biological condition, the existence of which may be claimed, truly or falsely, by patient, physician, or others. Secondarily, it refers to the social role of patient, which may be assumed or assigned.

The accepted or literal meaning of "illness" is thus an abnormal biological condition; for example, a myocardial infarction. When mere complaints—for example, a person's complaints about his body or about the bodies or behaviors of other persons—are defined as illnesses, we are faced with the metaphorical use and meaning of "illness." In short, bodily illness stands in the same relation to mental illness as a defective television set stands to a bad television program. Of course, the word "sick" is often used metaphorically. Comedians tell "sick" jokes, economies become "sick," sometimes even the whole world seems "sick." But only when we call minds "sick" do we systematically mistake and strategically misinterpret metaphor for fact and send for the doctor to "cure" the "illness." It is as if a television viewer were to send for a television repairman because he dislikes the program he sees on the screen. (Szasz, "Mental Illness as a Metaphor," *Nature,* 242:305-307, March 30, 1973.)

To attain the goal of abolishing involuntary psychiatry, we would also have to acknowledge that so-called psychiatric diagnoses, prognoses, hospitalizations, and treatments not explicitly sought by clients for their own use are coercive. In other words, compulsory psychiatry is an exercise in social control, like penology but unlike medicine. And finally, we would have to conclude that involuntary psychiatric interventions violate the protections guaranteed by the Constitution of the United States (and fly in the face of basic principles of human fairness and justice) and must therefore be abolished.

The mere act of speaking about protecting the "civil rights of mental patients" is an injury to their civil rights. To speak of the "civil rights of slaves" implicitly legitimizes the legal distinction between slaves and free men and hence deprives the former of liberties and dignities enjoyed by the latter. Today we accept that this is nonsense: that being a slave means not having any civil rights, or at least having fewer of them than free men. But we still speak of the "civil rights of mental patients." And by so doing we implicitly legitimize the legal distinction between insane patients and sane citizens and hence deprive the former of liberties and dignities that the latter group enjoys.

Not until a free people accept and demand that civil rights be independent of psychiatric criteria, just as they are now independent of religious criteria and are becoming independent of racial and sexual criteria, and not until legislators and jurists deprive physicians, and especially psychiatrists, of the power to exercise social control by means of quasi-medical sanctions, will the civil rights of persons accused of mental illness, or otherwise faced with involuntary psychiatric interventions, be protected.

What would become of psychiatry if involuntary psychiatric diagnoses, hospitalizations, and treatments were abolished? In principle, psychiatry would then become more like any other medical specialty, such as dermatology or ophthalmology—practiced only on voluntary clients. More generally, it would become like any other profession, such as accounting or architecture—contracting for the sale of certain services and products with informed buyers in a free market. In practice, psychiatry would then have to identify and define—as it never has had to before—the services it offers for sale. Clearly, such a change would spell the doom of psychiatry as we now know it. If it survived the change, which seems doubtful, psychiatry would emerge as a system, or as several systems, of applied secular ethics. Hence, its practitioners would find themselves in competition, not with clinicians, but with clerics.

Models of Madness

Psychiatrists are in solid agreement that there are two kinds of people in the world: sane and insane; and that it is the task of mental-health professionals to identify and control insane individuals. Similarly, anti-psychiatrists are in solid agreement that there are two kinds of societies in the world: sane and insane; and that it is the task of anti-psychiatrists and other radical reformers to identify and combat mad governments.

Because each of these views depends on the premise that terms such as "insane" and "mad" convey meaningful ideas, and because there is now worldwide consensus that the most characteristic instance of madness is schizophrenia, it is logical to begin an attempt to unravel the problem of madness by examining the origin, nature, and present status of the concept of schizophrenia.

In its most elementary sense, schizophrenia is, in my opinion, simply a word—a word invented by Eugen Bleuler, just as psychoanalysis is a word invented by Sigmund Freud. The idea that some people have a disease called "schizophrenia"—and some, presumably, do not—was not discovered, but was invented. To appreciate the import of this distinction, we have to review, at least briefly, our concept of disease, especially as it existed in the context of the medical culture in which Bleuler announced his invention.

Let us, therefore, project ourselves back into the minds of physicians and psychiatrists around 1900. When they spoke of disease, they meant, typically, something like syphilis. "Know syphilis in all its manifestations and relations," declared Sir William Osler, "and all things clinical will be added unto you." This is obviously no longer true today. In the United States, Osler's maxim has been replaced by another, which asserts that "mental illness is our number-one health problem." This would make schizophrenia, the most common and most disabling of the so-called mental diseases, the successor of Osler's syphilis, showing us immediately what a gulf separates us from him. For, clearly, a physician may know all there is to know about schizophrenia, and could still be totally ignorant of medicine.

The Oslerian image thus points to a lesson we forget at our own peril.

Adapted from a talk on Radio 3 in the BBC series "The State of Depth Psychology." Reprinted, with permission, from *The Listener* (London), December 1, 1977, pp. 721-23.

22

That lesson is the tacit agreement among physicians that, henceforth, they will distinguish between complaints and lesions, between being a patient and having a disease; and the resolution to regard as diseases only those processes occurring in the body which they could identify, measure, and demonstrate in an objective, physicochemical manner. Thanks to the work of numerous medical investigators around the turn of the century, physicians finally grasped that totally dissimilar biological phenomena were actually all different manifestations of the same disease process, called "syphilis." Thus, with the development of clear-cut anatomical, histological, biochemical, immunological, and clinical criteria for syphilis, it was possible to say not only that certain persons hitherto unsuspected of this disease were, in fact, syphilitics, but that others, suspected of it, were not.

These events were of the most far-reaching importance for physicians, including psychiatrists. By about 1900, European psychiatry was a well-established medical speciality. Its respectability and legitimacy, both scientifically and politically, depended wholly on the medical premise that the psychiatrist's patients, like those of the physician or surgeon, suffered from bona fide diseases. The difference, in this view, between non-psychiatric and psychiatric patients was that, whereas the diseases of the non-psychiatric patients caused them to have fevers and pains, those of the psychiatric patients caused them to have hallucinations and delusions.

Viewed against this historical background, the story of the origin of the modern concept of dementia praecox, or schizophrenia, appears in quite a different light from that in which it is usually presented. The official story is that, in the second half of the nineteenth century, medical scientists began to be able to identify the precise morphological character and the material causes of many diseases; and that this led quickly to effective methods of prevention, treatment, and cure for some of these diseases. Physicians learned to identify many of the infectious diseases and their causes: puerperal fever, tuberculosis, syphilis, gonorrhea, diphtheria; they also learned to be able to prevent and treat some of them. According to this version of the history of psychiatry, as some medical investigators discovered and identified diphtheria, so others (in particular, Bleuler) discovered and identified schizophrenia.

As I see it, this is not what happened at all. It is true that, around the turn of the last century, medical investigators discovered a host of diseases; but it is not true that psychiatric investigators discovered and identified certain other diseases—in particular, dementia praecox (schizophrenia) or other so-called functional psychoses. Psychiatrists made no discoveries according to which the people allegedly suffering from these diseases would have qualified by Virchow's criteria—which were then the only ones that counted—as having a disease. According to these criteria, known technically as the cellular-pathological model of disease, a disease of the body is a disease of the cells. The real question which the modern scientific physician puts to himself when called to treat a case is: "What cells are out of order and what can be done for them?"

Actually, Emil Kraepelin, who coined the term "dementia praecox" in 1898, and Eugen Bleuler, who coined the term "schizophrenia," thirteen years later, discovered no histopathological lesions or pathophysiological processes in their patients. Instead, they acted *as if* they had discovered such lesions or processes; named their so-called "patients" accordingly; and committed themselves and their followers to the goal of establishing the precise identification of the presumably "organic" nature and cause of these diseases. In the course of this process, Kraepelin and Bleuler, together with Freud, Jung, and the other pioneer psychopathologists and psychoanalysts, managed to bring about the great epistemological transformation in our medical age: that is to say, from histopathology to psychopathology.

Although modern psychiatry began with the study of paresis and the efforts to cure it, it soon turned into the study of psychopathology and the efforts to control it. It has now become the study of misbehavior and the efforts to manage it. And schizophrenia is its sacred symbol—the largest grab-bag of all the misbehaviors which psychiatrists, coerced by society or convinced by their own zeal, are now ready to diagnose, prognose, and therapize.

This is why I consider Kraepelin, Bleuler, and Freud the conquistadors and colonizers of the mind of man. Their society wanted them to extend the boundaries of medicine over morals and law—and they did so; it wanted them to extend the boundaries of illness from the body to behavior—and they did so; it wanted them to conceal conflict as psychopathology, and confinement as psychiatric therapy—and they did so.

One of the developments since the first publication of my book *The Myth of Mental Illness* has been the so-called "anti-psychiatry" movement. Like the movement of traditional psychiatry which it seeks to supplant, this movement, too, is centered on the concept of schizophrenia and on helping so-called schizophrenic patients. Because both I and the anti-psychiatrists oppose certain aspects of psychiatry, our views are often combined and confused. It is true, of course, that in coercive psychiatry, the anti-psychiatrists and I face the same enemy. So did, in another context, Stalin and Churchill. The old Arab proverb that "the enemy of my enemy is my friend" makes good sense, indeed, in politics and warfare. But it makes no sense at all in intellectual and moral discourse.

I reject the term "anti-psychiatry" because it is misleading and cheaply self-aggrandizing. Chemists do not characterize themselves as "anti-alchemists," nor do astronomers call themselves "anti-astrologers." If one defines psychiatry conventionally, as the medical specialty concerned with the diagnosis and treatment of mental diseases, and if one believes, as I do, that there are no mental diseases, then one is, indeed, committed to opposing psychiatry as a speciality—not of medicine, but of mythology. But since I believe that people are entitled to their own mythologies, this opposition must be clearly limited to the use of force or fraud by the mythologizers in the pursuit of their ersatz religion. This is why I have always insisted, and continue to insist, that I am against involuntary psychiatry, or the psychiatric rape of the patient by the psychiatrist—but am not against voluntary psychiatry, or psychiatric relations between consenting adults.

On the other hand, if one defines psychiatry operationally, as being whatever psychiatrists do, then it is necessary to articulate one's attitude toward each of the numerous practices psychiatrists engage in. I have tried to do this in several of my publications. As against this sort of analytical approach, the very term "anti-psychiatry" implicitly commits one to opposing everything that psychiatrists do. Moreover, anti-psychiatrists do not even clearly state whether they object only to involuntary psychiatric interventions, or also to those that are voluntary; to all involuntary psychiatric interventions, or only to those practiced by their political adversaries.

Ronald Laing began his work with the study of schizophrenic persons. The title of his first book, *The Divided Self,* is a literal English translation of the Bleularian Greek term "schizophrenia" and a virtual repetition of the classic psychiatric view of the schizophrenic as a so-called "split personality." Four years later, in 1964, with Aaron Esterson, Laing published *Sanity, Madness, and the Family.* Subtitled "Families of Schizophrenics," it is a report on the study of eleven hospitalized schizophrenic patients and their families. Nowhere in this book do the authors identify the legal status of any of the so-called "schizophrenics"—that is, whether they are voluntary or involuntary patients. There is, interestingly, also no mention of what, if any, roles Laing and Esterson played in depriving these persons of their liberty; or if they were deprived of their liberty by others, what, if any, roles Laing and Esterson played in trying to help them to regain it.

Furthermore, much of the fame of Kingsley Hall, and of its offshoots, and of the anti-psychiatrists who rule over them, rests on the claim that it offers a method of helping "schizophrenic patients" superior to those offered by other psychiatric institutions or practitioners.

I have long maintained that if there is no disease and no patient, there is nothing and no one to treat. Insofar, then, as others make the same claim, that is, that schizophrenia (and mental illness generally) is not a disease, they are compelled, in my opinion, to go further and conclude as well that there is no "treatment" for it. However, inasmuch as many persons whom psychiatrists now diagnose as schizophrenic seek help (especially if the "help" is not forced on them and if they don't have to pay for it), we are confronted with the social reality of so-called "psychotics," supposedly lacking an "insight" into their "illness," clamoring for its "treatment."

Ronald Laing accepts such persons as "residents" in his "communities," and legitimizes them as "sufferers" who, because of their very so-called "victimization," are more worthy than others. There is thus a moral-economic premise built into his system of asylum care which is inexplicit, but is all the more important for being so. It is, moreover, the same premise that animates large numbers of men and women today throughout the civilized world. Briefly put, it is the premise that it is wicked for people to purchase, for money, medical or psychiatric help, or the sort of help given at Kingsley Hall; but that it is virtuous to purchase it for suffering. In espousing this position, Laing places himself squarely midstream of the main current of contemporary thought about "health care." That current, in both communist and capitalist countries, is now fully Marxist—adopting, for "suffering situations," the famous formula: "From each according to his abilities, to each according to his needs."

Economically, Laing has thus replaced the coercion of the mental patient by psychiatry on behalf of the citizen with the coercion of the taxpayer by the government on behalf of the mental patient. Formerly, sane citizens could detain those whom they considered to be mad; now, they must maintain those who undertake to "journey through madness."

But I insist that schizophrenia is no more a journey through madness than it is a disease of the brain. Both of these statements assert literalized metaphors. Of course schizophrenia may be said to be *like* a journey or *like* a disease; but it is also *like* many other conditions or situations; for example, being childish, aimless, useless, and homeless, or being angry, obstreperous, conceited, or selfish. The point is that just as, in psychiatry, the literalized metaphor of schizophrenia as illness leads to and justifies its management by means of doctors, hospitals and drugs, so, in anti-psychiatry, the literalized metaphor of schizophrenia as a journey leads to and justifies its management by means of guides, hostels and first aid.

In short, the models of madness implicit in psychiatry and anti-psychiatry are strikingly similar. In psychiatry, the dominant image is that the schizophrenic had a "sound mind" but "lost" it. How? By destruction. Like an occupied city being burned down by a foreign invader and left in ashes, his brain is destroyed by the invading spirochaetes of syphilis or the "twisted molecules" of schizophrenia. In anti-psychiatry, the dominant image is that the schizophrenic had a "sound mind," or could have had one, but was deprived of it or was prevented from developing it. How? By plunder. Like a city being plundered by a foreign invader and left empty and barren, his personality is "emptied out" by the invading "love" of the family, society—the "oppressors."

Clearly, both of these views contain a measure of truth; how large or small that measure is depends on time, place and person. Syphilis can cause paresis. Parents, teachers, people in power can "cause" extreme human anguish and misery in those who depend on them, and do, in that sense, "drive people crazy." But what both of these models obscure are the simplest and most ancient of human truths: namely, that life is an arduous and tragic struggle; that what we call "sanity"—what we mean by "not being schizophrenic"—has a great deal to do with competence, earned by struggling for excellence; with integrity, hard won by confronting conflicts; and with modesty and patience, acquired through silence and suffering. This image, not so much of some sort of idealistic sanity or mental health, but simply of being able to endure life with decency and dignity, cannot be fitted into the paradigms of either paresis or plunder. It requires an altogether different model or perspective, something like a sculptor carving a statue out of stone.

There is no statue hidden in the stone. If a man with a piece of marble in his possession has no marble statue, it is not because his crusading enemy has smashed it, nor because it is the wrong idol, nor because his colonizing conqueror has stolen it because he wants it for himself—but because he has failed to transform the stone into a statue.

In conclusion, then, I submit that the obligation to transform oneself from infant into child, adolescent, and adult, into whatever it is we think we ought to be, and the failure to meet this obligation, all this finds no place in the theories of either psychiatry or anti-psychiatry.

A Critical Look at Psychiatry

I

A quarter of a century has passed since I began to try to clarify the core problems of psychiatry—namely, the nature of so-called mental illness and the justification for so-called involuntary mental hospitalization. My diagnosis of what ails psychiatry must have been right: during the past two decades the two most hotly debated issues in this field have been the so-called "medical model" of mental illness and the uses and abuses of mental hospitals.

II

Before scrutinizing the concept of mental illness let us examine the concept of illness itself. When we say that a person is ill, we usually mean two different things: first, that he or his physician believes that the complainant suffers from an abnormality of his body; and second, that he wants, or is at least willing to accept, medical help for his suffering. The term "illness" thus refers, on the one hand, to an abnormal biological condition and, on the other hand, to the social role of being a patient.

If a person does not suffer from an abnormal biological condition, we do not (usually) consider him to be ill. (We certainly do not consider him to be physically ill.) And if he does not voluntarily assume the role of one who is sick, he is not (usually) considered to be a medical patient. This is because the practice of modern Western medicine rests on two tacit premises—namely, that the physician's task is to diagnose and treat disorders of the human body, and that he can carry out these services only with the consent of his patient. In other words, physicians are trained to treat bodily ills—not economic, moral, racial, religious, or political "ills." And they themselves (except psychiatrists) expect, and in turn are expected by their patients, to treat bodily diseases and not the other miseries that beset man. Strictly speaking, disease or illness can affect only the body. The term "mental illness"

First published as "Ein kritischer Blick auf die Psychiatrie," *Neue Zürcher Zeitung*, February 18, 1980, pp. 17-18. Not previously published in English.

is a metaphor. Trying to cure people with "sick minds" in hospitals with drugs is therefore like trying to cleanse people with "dirty minds" in laundries with detergents. Is it any wonder that everything under the sun—from conversation to convulsion, from love to lithium—has been acclaimed and accredited as a cure for mental illness? And that, at the same time, mental illness has remained the most incurable affliction?

III

How did the metaphor of "mental illness" achieve its present status as scientific myth? The idea of mental illness arose, in part, from the fact that it is possible for a person to act and to appear as if he were sick without actually having a bodily disease. How should we react to such a person? Should we treat him as if he were ill or not ill?

Until the second half of the nineteenth century, persons who imitated illness were regarded as faking it and were called malingerers; similarly, those who imitated medical practitioners were regarded as impostors and were called quacks. As a result of the influence of Charcot, Janet, and especially Freud, this perspective was radically transformed. After the turn of the century, persons who imitated illness—for example, who had "spells"—were regarded as genuinely ill, and were called hysterics; and those who imitated physicians—for example, who "hypnotized"—were regarded as genuine healers, and were called psychotherapists. This profound conceptual transformation was both supported and reflected by an equally profound semantic transformation—one in which "spells" became "seizures," and "quacks" became "psychoanalysts."

Two quotations from Freud's early writings support these contentions. In 1893, Freud writes that "hysteria has fairly often been credited with a faculty for simulating the most various organic nervous disorders." And in 1909, although without using such direct language, Freud acknowledges that the hysteric fakes illness: ". . . [hysterical] attacks are nothing else but phantasies translated into the motor sphere, projected on to motility and portrayed in pantomine." In plain English: hysteria is the dramatic imitation of illness. Nevertheless, Freud would have us believe that hysteria is itself an illness.

The upshot of this psychiatric-psychoanalytic "revolution" is that, today, it is considered uncivilized and unscientific to treat a person who acts or appears sick as if he were not sick. We now "know" that such a person is sick: that he is mentally sick. But this view rests on the serious, albeit simple, error of confusing what is real with what is imitation; literal meaning with metaphorical meaning; medicine with morals.

IV

The phenomenon of involuntary mental hospitalization is at once independent from and interlinked with the notion of mental illness. Alexander Solzhenitsyn's protest against the "mental hospitalization" of Zhores Medvedev (in 1970) is to the point in this connection. "The incarceration of freethinking healthy people in madhouses," wrote Solzhenitsyn, "is spiritual murder. . . a variant of the gas chamber, and even more cruel." But if this is so for "healthy people" what makes it justifiable when it is imposed on "sick people"? What is there about "mental illness" that makes a "mental patient" a fit subject for "spiritual murder"? How are these procedures justified in law and how are they understood in fact?

The legitimacy of coercive psychiatry does not rest on the medical model of illness, but on the pediatric one. The mental patient is considered to be like a child, so that the psychiatrist (especially the institutional psychiatrist) must act *in loco parentis,* protecting him and providing him with treatment. Consequently there must be appropriate authorities—doctors or judges or juries—with the power to classify some adult citizens as irresponsible children (that is, as "mentally ill" persons).

Psychiatric coercion is usually invoked in response to the behavior of "irresponsible" individuals whose conduct is self-injurious or injurious to others but falls outside clear-cut categories of crime. For them the forces of psychiatry take over: the actor is no longer a moral agent but a patient; his behavior is no longer conduct for which he is responsible but a symptom of his mental illness for which he is not responsible; the police, the family, and the psychiatric profession that control him are not his adversaries but his helpers; and the institution in which he is confined is not a prison but a hospital.

V

The man of common sense is now likely to ask: But what else is there to do—should we let the suicidal person kill himself, or the homicidal person kill others? These dilemmas raise fundamental questions of ethics, law, and politics. In a society dedicated to individual freedom and responsibility, self-injurious behavior cannot justify loss of liberty. The state, the family, and the medical profession must restrict themselves to offering help; they must eschew forcing help on unwilling persons and, indeed, ought to be prevented by law from doing so. Granted, some of the increase in liberty so gained might be purchased at the cost of the impaired health or even death of some persons who make themselves ill or who want to kill themselves; but freedom must entail the right to make the "wrong" choices.

Should people also be free to be a danger to others? This problem disappears once we recognize that criminals cannot be divided into two categories—that is, persons who break the law because they choose to and persons who break it because their "mental illness" compels them to do so. All criminal behavior should be controlled by means of the criminal law, from the administration of which psychiatrists ought to be excluded.

The view that the "mentally ill" person is a "patient" helplessly in the grip of an "illness" that "causes" him to display abnormal behavior is false. Although many so-called mentally ill persons do not deliberately ("consciously") choose their "symptoms" and suffering, their behavior is, nonetheless, *conduct*. Such persons do not lack the capacity to make moral decisions; on the contrary, they exaggerate the moral dimensions of ordinary acts, displaying a caricature of decision-making behavior. "The last thing that can be said of a lunatic," wrote Gilbert K. Chesterton, "is that his actions are causeless. If any human acts may loosely be called causeless, they are the minor acts of a healthy man; whistling as he walks; slashing the grass with a stick; kicking his heels or rubbing his hand. . . . The madman is not the man who has lost his reason. The madman is the man who has lost everything except his reason."

But such an explanation is both too simple and too painful for modern man. Just as medieval man believed in religion and was offended by rational explanations demystifying theological theories and promises, modern man believes in science and is offended by commonsense explanations demystifying medical theories and promises. Unable or unwilling to bear the inexorable tragedies of the human condition, people now seek solace in the utopian claims of "scientific" psychiatry concerning the causes and cures of everything "bad" that the human heart is heir to.

Psychiatric Fraud

Perhaps because he does not have enough self-confidence, the ordinary person is likely to assume that when he cannot understand what someone in authority is saying, it is because he is too stupid or too uneducated. Authorities have always known this and have always exploited it by awing and bullying the plebes with Greek or Latin, with technical jargon, or, if need be, with gibberish.

Since psychiatry is a pseudoscience, it is not surprising that psychiatrists are especially eager to be accepted as scientific experts. Since they obviously cannot bring this about by discovering the causes and cures of mental diseases which—tragically for psychiatrists no less than for patients—do not exist, they have to do it by producing great quantities of gibberish. That is indeed the most constant and most frequent thing psychiatrists do, in speech as well as in print. George Orwell was not, but he might as well have been, writing about psychiatrists when he observed that "the great enemy of clear language is insincerity. When there is a gap between one's real and one's declared aims, one turns as if it were instinctively to long words and exhausted idioms, like a scuttlefish squirting out ink."

Although this was the furthest thing from what they had in mind, some years ago a group of mental-health educators conducted an experiment that demonstrated rather impressively the validity of my foregoing contention. The experiment consisted of the investigators' hiring a professional actor "who looked distinguished and sounded authoritative," naming him Dr. Myron L. Fox, bestowing upon him the persona of "an authority on the application of mathematics to human behavior," and coaching him to teach "charismatically and non-substantively on a topic about which he knew nothing."

"Dr. Fox" addressed a group of psychiatrists, psychologists, and social-work educators and his lecture was videotaped. The tape was then shown to another similar group and finally to a group of educators and administrators taking a graduate course in educational philosophy. In all there were 55 subjects tested. The result: "All respondents had significantly more favorable than unfavorable responses. . . . One even believed he [had] read Dr. Fox's

First published as "Learned Psychotics," *American Spectator,* April 1983, pp. 32-33. Reprinted with permission.

publications." Among the specific responses quoted by the investigators were the following: "Excellent presentation . . . Good analysis of the subject . . . Knowledgeable." That this was the idea of a group of mental-health experts about how to fake a psychiatric presentation is itself wonderfully revealing. But the best part of this experiment is, of course, that "Dr. Fox" was such a success.

"Dr. Fox's" deliberately staged gibberish was delivered in 1972. In 1982, I discovered another "Dr. Fox lecture," this time given for real by a really distinguished psychiatrist before a really distinguished audience. Since this address was published, I may quote from it, and I shall:

Recall that clinical experience and science do incrementally define the *selective* use of innovations, while policy reflexly greets innovation with prophecies of fiscal doom. In retrospect, the actual gains for health might render such poor prophets a loss! Where policy seeks formulas for determining choice and guiding treatment, science understands the fundamental basis for variability in disease and response and the method for sequentially approximating precision in the clinical process.

The author of this luminous passage, Daniel X. Freedman, is chairman of the department of psychiatry at the University of Chicago. The lines quoted are from his presidential address delivered at the American Psychiatric Association's annual meeting in May 1982.

When a prominent American psychiatrist writes such gibberish, when that psychiatrist occupies an endowned chair at one of America's great universities and is the president of the American Psychiatric Association, when the gibberish is the published text of his presidential address delivered before the American Psychiatric Association, and when the *American Journal of Psychiatry* publishes said gibberish as if it were in English and made sense—then we face a situation about which somebody ought to say something. Since no "uncontroversial psychiatrist" would dare to say that a psychiatric emperor is naked, especially when the emperor insists he is sporting the most splendid garments, I volunteer my services as a "controversial psychiatrist" (which is the least offensive diagnosis my colleagues like to pin on me) to bring this piece of psychiatric skullduggery to the attention of the public.

Freedman begins his address with these words: "I will not reprise [sic] this past active APA year, but wherever we have worked, members of APA have engaged in lively discussion and useful action on critical topics." Presumably, Freedman means that he will not review or repeat whatever it is that he is referring to.

Freedman evidently believes that "reprise" is a very serviceable word, because he uses it again, toward the middle of his address, where he writes: "The remarkable advent of pharmacotherapies has of course profoundly affected both basic science and clinical practice, and—more than I can here reprise [sic] it—complexly affected professional and public orientation to psychiatry."

That is surely an odd way of saying that the currently fashionable use of drugs in psychiatry has profoundly affected both the profession and the public. But what is it that Freedman can't "reprise" here? He says it is the "remarkable advent of pharmacotherapies." But the introduction of certain drugs into psychiatry is simply a fact or occurrence. It need not be, and indeed cannot be, reviewed.

Ever since schizophrenia—the most dreaded and mysterious of so-called mental illnesses—was invented by the great Eugen Bleuler in 1911, it was supposedly characterized, in Bleuler's own words, "by a specific type of alteration of thinking." However, since no human being can know what another thinks, this statement is necessarily false. What Bleuler meant, and said elsewhere, was that the so-called schizophrenic's "linguistic expression may show every imaginable abnormality"—for example, "poverty of ideas [and] incoherence."

Since the invention of schizophrenia, and especially since the Second World War, students of communication have been intensely interested in the language of "psychotics," which, perhaps because it is so overblown with pathetic conceit, is said to be "pathological." When so-called psychotics assert, for example, that they are the Savior or that the Russians are sending messages to their gold teeth, they lie so naively and so brazenly that their false claims are deemed to be the symptoms of madness. Ironically, the language of psychiatrists is often indistinguishable from the language of psychotics. Freedman's lecture is full of the sorts of linguistic delicts that psychiatrists regard as typical of the verbal behavior of schizophrenics.

I have already cited examples of the mumbo-jumbo Freedman passes off as professional wisdom. Here is an example of one of his pretentious claims supported by nothing more than conceit. "Clearly," Freedman declares, "all physicians attempt to enhance the individual's wishes for optimal self-regulation of functions—both physiologic and psychologic . . ." If that were true, physicians would be angels in a libertarian heaven. Since psychiatrists in general and Freedman in particular are enthusiastic supporters of psychiatric coercions and mutilations—Freedman is even eulogized by a colleague in an accompanying article for his contributions to the Yale lobotomy project—the claim about physicians' (without exception) favoring "self-regulation" is a patent falsehood.

Consistent with the magisterial style Freedman affects, he addresses the views of those with whom he disagrees in an appropriately haughty and disdainful tone. Some of those who criticize psychiatry, never named or otherwise identified, seek "simplistics as an escape from the painful exercise of judgment. Others are invested in ignoring both our science base and the real-world context for clinical decision making. They toy with the mentally ill as a metaphor for pet philosophical, political, personal, or just plain miserly bureaucratic purposes." It is difficult to be sure just what this means, though it certainly implies that Freedman is a noble person, whereas those who behave in the ways he describes are ignoble.

"One wonders," Freedman continues, "about the despairing impatience of some of our colleagues or angry residents who have written retributively silly books." Not a single reference to a "retributively silly book" is cited, however.

In short, Freedman does not "review" past events, he "reprises" them; he does not recognize writings critical of psychiatry, he regards them instead as "retributive," and "silly" as well. The paranoid talks bizarrely about unidentified "theys" plotting against him; Freedman writes presidentially about unidentified "theys" opposing the "science base" of psychiatry. But regardless of the evidence against it, we stubbornly cling to our belief that the mental patient's language is psychotic and the psychiatrist's is scientific. *Credo quia absurdum.*

The Devil's Fool

Not surprisingly, most victims of involuntary mental hospitalization are poor and powerless. However, prominent persons also manage to get committed. Why? Because "madness" often relieves people of guilt and responsibility, thus "freeing" them of the burden of having to conduct themselves competently, day in and day out.

Shadowland, by William Arnold (McGraw-Hill, 260 pp., $9.95), is the story of Frances Farmer's life, especially those parts of it that concern her encounters with psychiatry. Seemingly sharing the public's ignorance of how popular an American pastime it is to commit one's loved ones, Arnold writes as if Frances Farmer's case were unusual. Compassionate toward his subject, he even suggests that Farmer was not mad but the victim of a political conspiracy, an interpretation that prompted the *Kirkus Reviews* to dismiss the book with this revealing sentence: "All the outrage against injured innocence can't cover the stench of paranoia." Nevertheless Arnold succeeds in conveying the choreography of the *danse macabre* we call "schizophrenia-and-its-treatment" far better than do most writers on this subject, whether professionals or laymen.

Before Frances Farmer was born, her father, a passive individual, separated from his wife Lillian. A woman more than six feet tall, with strong views on everything, Lillian had campaigned for good nutrition and against Communism. In 1931, in her junior year in high school, Frances, a bright girl, wrote an essay called "God Dies," which her teacher entered in a national competition. "I wondered a little," wrote Frances, pondering the "injustices" of the world, "why God was such a useless thing. It seemed a waste of time to have Him." The essay won first prize and created a furor.

Farmer enrolled as a drama major at the University of Washington in 1935. She promptly won another contest, this one sponsored by Seattle's Communist newspaper. The prize was a VIP trip to the Soviet Union. On her return she declared: "My sympathy and support are all for Russia."

Returning to Seattle a year after leaving the university, she went out of her way to insult the dignitaries who feted her. "When one right-wing Congressman introduced himself at the reception [for her]," Arnold writes, "she called him a 'hypocrite' and calmly walked away."

Review of *Shadowland,* by William Arnold, *Inquiry,* December 25, 1978, pp. 4-5. Reprinted with permission.

Frances Farmer thus emerged from adolescence possessing a dangerous mixture of personal qualities: she was beautiful and brainy, but she was also arrogant and conceited. She exemplified the sort of person about whom it is said that she loves mankind and hates people. As a result, all her human relationships soured quickly; everyone and everything disappointed her.

Because her assets as an actress were more readily apparent than her liabilities as a person, her career was a series of quick successes that led nowhere. Within a year of her Soviet tour she was a Hollywood star.

After two years in Hollywood, she was fed up. She could "see nothing but shallowness and deceit." Again she began to speak out for left-wing causes. In 1937, she left for Broadway. Another quick success. Then an affair with a famous director, which, like her earlier marriage, soon broke up. Embracing "worthy" left-wing causes but rejecting individuals as unworthy, Farmer became increasingly isolated and lonely. She took to amphetamines and alcohol.

Frances Farmer's career was now visibly disintegrating. But her arrogance and nastiness knew no bounds. In an argument, she knocked a studio hairdresser down, dislocating her jaw. The woman filed charges. When the police discovered that Farmer had not paid an earlier fine for a drunken driving arrest, they went to her hotel. She tried, clumsily, to flee. Taken to the Santa Monica jail, she gave her occupation, in Arnold's words, "as such an unorthodox one (presumably 'cocksucker') that it caused the police booking officer to jump when he read it." Arraigned in court, this is how she dealt with the judge:

Judge: Have you driven a car since you were placed on probation?
Farmer: No, I haven't, but only because I couldn't get my hands on one.
Judge: Have you reported to your probation officer as directed?
Farmer: No, I never saw him. Why didn't he show up?
Judge (incredulously): Did you expect him to look you up?
Farmer: I expected him to be around so I could get a look at his face.

Farce? Of course! Folly? That depends on how severely those in power want to punish the person who so deliberately dishonors them. Amid giggling spectators, the judge sentenced Frances Farmer to serve the 180 days of her previously suspended sentence. She then asked to make a phone call. When the matron refused to give permission for it, she knocked her down, flooring another officer in the process. To the booking sergeant she gave her occupation as "vagrant vagabond."

Why did such a hugely successful actress—she made more than a million dollars, after taxes, in the six years prior to her arrest (and first psychiatric commitment)—say that she was a "vagrant vagabond"? Among other reasons, because she had given away all of her money. Every penny of it. To Communist causes, to Spanish Civil War groups, to migrant workers, to members of her own family. As a result, when the long-smoldering hostilities between her and her antagonists—familial, judicial, psychiatric—erupted into open warfare, she was destitute, defenseless. "The madman," as Gilbert Chesterton astutely observed, "is not the man who has lost his reason. The madman is the man who has lost everything except his reason." Frances Farmer had indeed lost, or thrown away, everything except her reason. Such a person is ready, in an imagery Chesterton would have heartily approved of, to make a pact with the Devil. Which Frances Farmer proceeded to do.

I will not give away the rest of the story. Suffice it to say that Frances Farmer spends many years in a mental hospital, is drugged, electroshocked, perhaps even lobotomized (no one seems to know for sure). Her degradation and humiliation at the hands of psychiatrists are well described and fully documented. Finally, she is released, a shell—indeed, a mockery—of her former self.

What shall we make of *Shadowland* as a critique of psychiatry? Aside from several minor "technical" errors (such as calling hydrotherapy "a primitive form of shock treatment"), the book is a moving indictment of mad-doctoring. So what? There have been many such indictments over the past two hundred years—to no avail. That is to be expected. Vested interest, prejudice, and fashion are more powerful molders of opinion than is evidence. But that does not diminish the need to document such depravities.

The main value of Arnold's book lies in letting us see Frances Farmer and the people most responsible for her psychiatric damnation, especially her mother, as human beings. Horrible human beings, but human beings nonetheless. Especially in this respect Arnold's book is vastly superior to the countless contemporary accounts of the commitments of Very Important Persons. Arnold confronts what others who write about psychiatric incarceration avoid. He reveals what others conceal. Perhaps because he is rather naive about both psychiatry and psychiatric criticism, and perhaps because he is an honest man who writes well, his book offers a much better lesson in the anatomy of madness and mad-doctoring than other similar stories.

What, finally, should we think of Frances Farmer? In a letter to William Dean Howells, Mark Twain once called himself "God's fool." That he was: loving, compassionate, considerate—and, above all, humorous. If the Devil has fools, too, Frances Farmer was surely one of them: unloving, arrogant, inconsiderate—and above all, humorless. But this is not the way we are supposed to think about "mental illness" and "mental treatment." Befogged by the vapors of a fake science, our vision of the tragicomedy that is modern psychiatry is obscured. Arnold's book is a shaft of light stabbing through the darkness.

Was Virginia Woolf Mad?

All That Summer She Was Mad by Stephen Trombley (Continuum, 1982) is a well-intentioned, but rather inept, critique of those who would diagnose, and thus diminish, the celebrated writer Virginia Woolf as mad. The principle underlying Trombley's argument is that if there is method in madness, then it is not madness. He applies this formula to Virginia Woolf's life and, presto, Virginia is no longer mad. But, then, who is?

If one looks at human existence commonsensically, it is clear that we all go through life coping with our particular problems as each of us sees fit. Virginia Woolf was no exception. She had many grave handicaps to overcome, among them the loss of both parents before reaching maturity and an emphatically female identity in a male-dominated culture. The upshot was that she developed into what is commonly considered to be a "mad artist." That is to say, she was not only a superb writer (and an important feminist, in the best sense of the word), but also a chronic mental patient. Repeatedly, she tried to kill herself. Repeatedly, she starved herself, to the point of becoming emaciated and at times ceasing to menstruate.

How should we regard such patterns of behavior? This is not the place to set forth my own answer to this crucial question. What is important for us to remember is that for the past 200 years or more, educated persons in the West have regarded such behavior as literally the manifestation of a diseased mind. That is how Virginia Woolf regarded her own (mis)behavior, writing to her husband just before her death: "I feel certain I am going mad again. . . . And I shan't recover this time." A long entry on her in the *Encyclopedia Britannica* (1973 edition) concludes with this sentence, as if it stated the most obvious thing in the world: "In a recurrence of mental illness, after finishing *Between the Acts,* she drowned herself near her Sussex home on March 28, 1941."

Stephen Trombley, an expatriate upstate New Yorker now living in London and editing the journal *Books & Issues,* begins his work by asking, "Was Virginia Woolf mad?" He then continues: "Many critics, including her biographer, Quentin Bell, and her husband, Leonard, have said that she was." Against them and others who share that view, Trombley argues "there is no

---

Review of *All That Summer She Was Mad. Virginia Woolf: Female Victim of Male Medicine,* by Stephen Trombley, *Inquiry,* December, 1982, pp. 44-45. Reprinted with permission.

real medical evidence to suggest that this is the case. . . . To my knowledge, no one has made a truly scientific medical study of Virginia Woolf. Until concrete evidence is produced, it is irresponsible to speak of her as having been mad."

These remarks imply that Trombley believes madness is an objective *medical* condition that "exists" in nature which Virginia Woolf did not "have." He does not examine or question the concept of madness and seems oblivious to the many obvious strategic uses to which it is put, not only by psychiatrists but by laymen and "patients" as well. He simply sets out to demonstrate that Virginia Woolf was not mad. Because he bypasses the question of what madness is or what people mean when they call themselves or others mentally ill, Trombley's analysis of her so-called symptoms is often naive and even irritating. For example, in connection with her refusal of food, Trombley notes that this behavior is now considered a typical symptom of anorexia nervosa, and then he comments: "But to accept this diagnosis would be to confuse the issue. *In Virginia's case,* the significance of the problem is existential, sexual, ontological" (emphasis added). Trombley seems not to understand that we call self-starvation anorexia nervosa, a hunger strike, a suicide attempt, or some other name, depending on how we want to respond, and that this is true of any so-called psychiatric symptom, whether displayed by Virginia Woolf or anyone else.

Nearly half of Trombley's book is devoted to a critical examination of the views of four of the psychiatrists in Virginia Woolf's life. There is a good deal of material here that is of interest to the student of psychiatric history. Indeed, I consider this to be the most valuable part of the book. But even the lessons of this history seem to be lost on Trombley. He is rightly indignant that psychiatrists use the term "mad" to debase and denigrate their opponents, but then he engages in the same psychiatric mudslinging. He writes: "Hyslop [one of Virginia's doctors] is zealous in his ascription of lunacy to broad social movements with which he disagrees; but, considering his views . . . we really must pause and ask, who is mad?" Obviously, not the patient but the doctor. If this sounds like R. D. Laing, it is because Trombley bases his argument on Laing's writings. Not surprisingly, he concludes that Woolf was not mad but was the blameless "female victim" of malevolent operators identified as "male medicine." Certainly, Virginia Woolf was victimized by her doctors, just as she was victimized by her husband. But that is only one side of this story. The other side, which Trombley misses completely, is the whys and ways in which Virginia and Leonard Woolf used psychiatry and psychiatrists to orchestrate their own lives, as madwoman-wife-writer and as nurse-husband-manager.

The sort of psychiatric rehabilitation of Virginia Woolf in which Trombley engages is not only so biased and incomplete as to vitiate its own important truth, it is also counterproductive. One of Trombley's aims in writing this book is to criticize psychiatry, particularly in its historical enmity toward women. But that cannot be done by selective interpretation. The fact is Virginia Woolf collaborated and colluded with the appropriate authorities of society in creating her dual identity as a madwoman and artist, in much the same way as, say, Joan of Arc collaborated and colluded in creating her dual identity as witch and soldier. Converting a martyred apostate into a saint does not hold the Church up to the obloquy it deserves, nor does converting a person diagnosed as mad into one certified as sane hold psychiatry up to the obloquy is deserves. Instead of weakening the authority of religion and psychiatry, this tactic, by adhering to their imagery and language, serves only to enforce their authority. It seems to me more accurate to argue that there is no witchcraft and no mental illness than to consecrate Joan as a saint and pronounce Virginia sane.

Pilgrim's Regress

In 1964, David Cooper and R. D. Laing, the founding fathers of "anti-psychiatry," coauthored *Reason and Violence*. In 1967, Laing contributed a chapter to Cooper's *Dialectics of Liberation*. Since then, their paths have seemingly diverged. I say seemingly, because actually they haven't: each has continued to write about the one thing he loves—namely, himself. However, each has demonstrated his love in different ways.

Cooper's style is cant in almost pure culture. For special effect, he uses oxymorons, such as the farewell in his previous book, *The Grammar of Living*. "My next book," he wrote there, "will be different. It will not be by me." I am sorry to have to report that his new book, *The Language of Madness*, is still by him.

At heart, Cooper is a naive Rousseauean. *Au fond*, human beings are rich, creative, courageous, loving, good, you name it. What's wrong with the world is that all these "goodies" have been stolen from us. I am not simplifying what Cooper is saying; I am only summarizing it. "To act politically," he asserts, "means simply regaining what has been stolen from us, starting with our consciousness of our oppression within the capitalist system." According to Cooper, everything that most of us think is bad is really good, and vice versa. Systematically inverting values is Cooper's idea of explaining social phenomena and rectifying their defects. For example: "Madness is a common social property that has been stolen from us, like the reality of our dreams and our deaths: we have to get these things back politically so that they become creativity and spontaneity in a transformed society."

Nevertheless, Cooper's work has certain redeeming qualities that deserve recognition, even respect. He does not hide where he stands—on politics, economics, or anything else. Primarily, Cooper is against the free market and individualism. "Fruit dies on the trees," he explains, "because peasant farmers can't deal with a parasitic market structure which stops the fruit that they gather meeting the mouths of other workers who supply them in turn—by their work." He praises Marx "who learnt about money and then learnt how to hate it, how to hate the market place of exchange value . . ."

Conversely, Cooper is for Communism, victims, and the prefix "anti."

Review of *The Language of Madness,* by David Cooper, and *Conversations with Children,* by R. D. Laing, *Spectator* (London), September 23, 1978, pp. 72-73. Reprinted with permission.

Anti-psychiatry was merely his first flirtation parleying a prefix into a career, as the following examples illustrate: "Anti-definition . . . is a way of opening up the definiendum. . . . Anti-classificaton means seeking and stating existing differences as opposed to enclosing entities in boxes . . ." His new antis amplify his earlier ones, such as "anti-aesthetics," eulogized in *The Grammar of Living* thus: "We have passed the last day of the 'great' one-name works of art and have entered the time of communal creation. Henceforth there will be no more Beethovens, no more Rembrandts, no more Tolstoys. . . . We shall create the quotidian Dada, an anti-aesthetics of everyday life." Enough? Not for Cooper. He has a seemingly inexhaustible supply of things and ideas he wants to invert. The clitoris is a "stunted penis" said Freud; for Cooper it's a super-phallus: "Some psycho-technicians find it incomprehensible when I say that women—*physiologically* speaking [Cooper's emphasis]—have bigger phalluses than men." For Freud, the dream was the "royal road to the unconscious"; for Cooper, "the dream is the anti-psychoanalysis."

Although there is an occasional well-turned phrase or well-observed human predicament in this book, *The Language of Madness* (an utterly misleading title, of course) is a pitiful piece of work. Even as Communist propaganda, it is primitive. "There are," writes Cooper, articulating his recommendation for social change, "two things to be done: firstly, the final extinguishing of capitalism and the entire mystifying ethos of private property; secondly, the social evolution that . . . will produce the classless society."

Why Cooper believes what he believes is his business. His personal affairs concern us only insofar as he tells us of them, which he does in embarrassing detail. For example, he tells us that he has "no secretary or fixed address"; that "there are no examples to follow, certainly not mine"; that "I was mad briefly, but for enough weeks to begin to know a little . . ."; and that "one might argue that the incapacity for homosexual experience is an 'illness' in need of 'treatment.'" Such self-disclosures don't enhance Cooper's dignity. But, then, Cooper seems to want to shame himself in public. He is a religious fanatic who wants to expiate his guilt—for what, I don't know, and if I did I would keep the information to myself. Cooper himself offers some clues. "One of the critical experiences of my life," he writes, about his favorite subject, "was when at the age of four, at a circus in Cape Town, I burst into tears because I thought the clown had been really hurt by the wicked ring master. I could not be consoled until the clown came into the audience to tell me that the hurt was an illusion, make-believe." He is still weeping, and is proud of it.

As Cooper's distinctive stylistic flourish is the prefix "anti," so Laing's is the blank page of paper. I think it's in *The Politics of Experience*, in 1967, that he first alludes to his interest in "empty white sheet(s) of paper": "Few books today are forgivable. Black on the canvas, silence on the screen, an empty white sheet of paper, are perhaps feasible." His recent books, such as *Facts of Life, Do You Move Me?* and *Conversations with Children*, contain lots of "empty white sheets." Unfortunately, not all of the pages of his most recent books are clean sheets; some are soiled by printer's ink.

According to Laing, *Conversations with Children* is an "anthology" of his conversations with his own children, which he considers important because "no similar anthology of dialogues with children has been published." He claims that the "anthology" is authentic and accurate. Since it's a record of conversations, the implication is that it is a verbatim, or near verbatim, account of what was said by each speaker. "I have added nothing," says Laing. "I am responsible for deletions, and I suppose, inevitably, some inadvertent omissions. But I have made no additions, no embellishments." How, then, did Laing obtain such a faithful record? "No tape recorder was ever used," he hastens to explain. "The conversations in this anthology were written down by me from memory over a six-year period as part of a journal I keep. They are all recorded from memory." Well, either Laing has a fantastic memory or his claim concerning the absolute authenticity of these conversations is a lie.

How does Laing justify publishing such an ostensibly intimate diary of his children's babblings (or babblings he attributes to them), thus making a part of their private world public? He knows, of course, that doing so constitutes an invasion of their privacy. But publishing such "intimacies [of] family life" was permissible, he tells us, because it "is done with the full accord of my wife—and the children." That self-justification reveals the full measure of Laing's utter contempt for an ethic of respect for persons grounded in contract. The children on whom he so generously bestows the right to contract range in age between three and eight. If a father took sexual liberties with children of that age and then told us that they (and their mother!) consented to it, we would regard his self-justification as adding insult to injury.

Why did Laing write this book? Having written several books about the unhappy communications characteristic of other people's families, Laing felt ready, he says, to present "the other side of the story . . . the language of the happy dialogue of intelligent beings . . ." Where was he going to find such "beings"? In his own family, where else? "It is," he writes gravely, "a great pleasure and relief for me to present these dialogues which express so much light-heartedness and serious delight . . . in the following pages, we are able to observe the emotional and cognitive development of two children with unimpaired faculties unfold within the interlace and interweave of relations with adults whom they do not fear and whom they like as they are liked."

The entries in the book range from the trivial to the offensive. Many entries are simply empty; for example, a third of a page is occupied by this one: "December 1973: Natasha wants sellotape for Xmas." Among the entries I consider offensive is this one: "Daddy: What was the first thing you saw when you came out of mummy's tummy? Natasha: Mummy's pussa, that's the first thing I saw when I came out of mummy's tummy."

The entry I like best (which also takes up a third of a page) reads: "Natasha [aged six]: Did you write this book? [*Do You Love Me?*]. Daddy: Yes, Natasha: They've printed it very well (turning the pages) there's not much on the paper. Look, there's hardly anything on that page. Or that page. There's the littlest I've ever seen. I think this is the silliest book I've ever seen."

What are we to make of *Conversations with Children?* It's not really a book; it only looks like one. Therein, perhaps, lies the answer to the question I posed. The book is a joke, a put-on. Intoxicated with himself, Laing is playing not only before his audience but also with it. His seemingly multi-faceted personality has now fused into a single role—namely, that of clown. Peter Mezan, who knows Laing personally, has actually characterized Laing in such a way: "In the mind's eye, under the magical sign of the caduceus, stands a gaunt, pixielike man in the garb of prophet—acid at his right hand, revolution at his left, his head haloed with the clear light of an Oriental paradise, his eyes intimating madness—crushing beneath his avenging foot the serpent of the Western rationalist tradition. . . . In a single evening I have seen him run the gamut of emotions, taking on one distinct person after another, even changing sex, and in each one appearing to be wholly himself."

How ironic, but how fitting. Laing, the clown, the Marcel Marceau of psychiatry. Cooper, the violated "madman," the vulnerable, frightened child. The fooler and the fooled. What a perfect pantomime of madness and mad-doctoring! Cooper has a big heart that bleeds for victims, especially of his own imaginings. His compassion has become cancerous and has all but destroyed him. Laing, on the other hand, has a good nose for business—in particular, for selling his dramatized impersonations of himself. So far he has sold himself as student of schizophrenia, theoretician of anti-psychiatry, charismatic healer of madness, existential philosopher, New Leftist social critic, guru of LSD, Buddhist monk, and radical critic of the family. Now he is posing as devoted paterfamilias, basking in "happy" communications with his children. Cooper is often wrong-headed, but he is honest. Laing is often level-headed, but is he ever honest?

Freud

On the wall of Freud's study hung an engraving of Pierre Brouillet's famous painting which shows Charcot demonstrating a case of "grand hysteria" to a distinguished audience. In Ronald W. Clark's *Freud: The Man and the Cause,* the author tells us, "Anna would often ask her father what was wrong with the woman who appeared to be fainting, and he would always give the same reply: that the lady was 'zu fest geschnürt [too tightly laced] . . ."

But the woman (she was no lady!) depicted in that picture was neither sick, as Charcot claimed, nor too tightly laced, as Freud told Anna. She was malingering—pretending to be sick, playing patient. In 1899, about six years after Charcot's death, Georges Guillain, a physician and biographer of Charcot, tells us, "I saw as a young intern at the Salpêtrière the old patients of Charcot who were still hospitalised. Many of the women, who were excellent comedians, when they were offered a slight pecuniary remuneration imitated perfectly the major hysteric crises of former times."

In this superb, meticulously researched and well-written biography, Ronald Clark retraces the saga of Freud's ostensible struggle to discover the nature of the disease that afflicts such a "patient" as that depicted in Brouillet's famous painting, and to find a "cure" for it. For its accuracy, near-completeness and good taste, Clark's effort could not be praised too highly. If he had only displayed the same interest in the actual subject matter of psychoanalysis as he displayed in its history, Clark would have written a more important book. As it is, he has merely produced the best biography of Freud that we possess. Still, it is a biography that holds no surprises, either in the way of new facts or new interpretations, and one whose value is impaired by being too complex for those unfamiliar with the story, and too dispassionate for those familiar with it.

Reading this story, I was struck once again by two things: first, by the prominent place that the ever-recurring pattern of pretending to be sick or playing patient (and playing doctor too) occupies in it; and, second, by the consistency and crudity with which Freud used psychopathological diagnoses as invectives and how the scientific world let him get away with it. Charcot's hysterics threw fits, as they were trained. Freud's produced memories of

First published as "Diagnostician or Accusor?" Review of *Freud: The Man and the Cause.* by Ronald W. Clark, *Spectator* (London), September 13, 1980, pp. 20-22. Reprinted with permission.

childhood sexual seductions, as they were expected. These persons were sick not because they had objectively demonstrable diseases (physical or "mental"), but rather because they were patients. This explains why it was so important for Freud and his followers to treat others as sick patients, and themselves as healthy healers (about which more in a moment).

Pretended insanity has, of course, always been a vexing problem in psychiatry, and it still is. This is because the notion of insanity and the structure of our language imply that while some people *pretend* to be insane, others *are* insane—leaving the riddle of insanity securely mystified. But it turns out that pretending to be a psychoanalyst is no harder than pretending to be a psychotic—the boundary between pretense and reality, between *playing* Hamlet and *being* Hamlet being easily befogged even by an amateur actor.

Clark himself relates two incidents, one in America, another in England, where ordinary persons successfully impersonated psychoanalysts. In 1921, an architecture student at Cornell University, represented as a friend and pupil of Freud's, lectured to a packed City Hall audience in Ithaca. The evening ended, Clark tells us, "with a member of the university faculty thanking the speaker."

In the same year, an undergraduate at Oxford pulled the same stunt. This man, according to Ernest Jones, "gave a quite nonsensical lecture, which was not detected and led to a discussion." It shows, explained Jones to Freud, "the state of ignorance at Oxford, for several professors were also present and were also taken in." That is not necessarily what this incident shows. What it shows is a very important matter which Clark does not adequately explore. Let me add here two more examples of the ease with which such impersonations can be carried out.

The first is related by the German psychiatrist Albert Moll in his autobiography, and is retold by Henri Ellenberger in his encyclopaedic *Discovery of the Unconscious*. At the beginning of World War I, a secret agent came to see Moll requesting that Moll teach him how to impersonate the role of a physician. "Moll told the man," writes Ellenberger, "that this was impossible, but that he could show him how to impersonate a psychoanalyst. He thus taught him the rudiments and the jargon of the profession in a few days and the man actually served his country throughout the war by 'exercising' his new skill."

In 1972, a Los Angeles psychiatrist and university professor hired a professional actor who looked distinguished and sounded authoritative, named him Dr. Myron L. Fox, bestowed upon him the persona of an "authority in the application of mathematics to human behavior . . . and coached him to lecture charismatically and non-substantively on a topic about which he knew nothing." Several groups of psychiatrists, psychologists, and other mental-health professionals were not only taken in by Dr. Fox but were enthusiastic about him. One respondent believed that he had read Dr.

Fox's publications. Another opined: "Excellent presentation . . . Good analysis of the subject . . . Knowledgeable."

What is fascinating about all this is that we can now look back on a whole century of psychiatry and psychoanalysis and observe a scene littered with both pseudopatients and pseudotherapists. It is revealing, moreover, that "researchers" (such as David Rosenhan and his colleagues) who pose as patients are considered to be "pseudopatients"—but ordinary men and women who pose as patients are considered to be "real patients." This phenomenon is not unconnected with a remarkable pattern concerning the incidence of psychiatric illness, as such illness was perceived and diagnosed by the undisputed master of psychodiagnostics, namely, Sigmund Freud.

The phenomenon to which I refer, which Mr. Clark notes but whose significance he obscures rather than elucidates, is that many of the pioneer psychoanalysts were not only psychiatrists but also psychotics. According to Freud, Alfred Adler was "paranoid" and Carl Jung was "crazy." According to Jones, Otto Rank was "psychotic . . . [suffering from] cyclothymia," while Sándor Ferenczi had "latent psychotic trends" and became "paranoid." Clark obscures the significance of this pattern by remarking that "the *accusation* of mental derangement . . . was to become almost endemic when certain analysts were decribing those who disagreed with them" (italics added).

But why does Mr. Clark call these psychodiagnostic acts of Freud's and Jones's "accusations"? Why doesn't he assume that Freud and Jones acted in good faith (whatever that might mean in this connection), and made bona fide "diagnoses" of "mental diseases" which afflicted these unfortunate "patients"? There is, after all, more than a chance similarity between Freud and Jones diagnosing dissenters from the psychoanalytic dogma as psychotics, and contemporary Soviet psychiatrists diagnosing dissenters from the Communist dogma as schizophrenics. That Freud found Leonardo da Vinci, Dostoievsky, and Woodrow Wilson also to be suffering from mental diseases highlights the inadequacy of dismissing his diagnoses of his colleagues as "accusations." For if those were accusations and hence false, then how can we be certain that his other diagnoses were not equally foolish and fraudulent? Indeed, if Adler and Jung were sick because they loved freedom more than Freud, then what faith can we put in Freud's case histories attempting to demonstrate the benefits of psychoanalysis? These are questions of the first importance, and it is indeed regrettable that Clark did not apply his considerable erudition, and especially his familiarity with the history of modern science, to a more searching analysis of the issues they raise.

This is not the occasion further to belabor the point that a scrutiny of how Freud treated a person—that is, as a normal colleague or as a crazy patient—is an issue absolutely indispensable for understanding what psychoanalysis is all about. But the fact that Freud was systematically mendacious about this issue—an illustration of which follows—supports the view that it played a crucial role in his work.

In 1907, Freud writes to Jung: "I beg of you . . . don't deviate too far from me . . . My inclination is to treat those colleagues who offer resistance exactly as we treat patients . . ." In 1912, Jung writes to Freud, objecting to this behavior: "I would, however, point out that your technique of treating your pupils like patients is a *blunder.*" To which Freud replies: "Your allegation that I treat my followers like patients is demonstrably untrue." That the subsequent course of psychoanalysis was based on the "training" analyses of would-be analysts—compelling them, one and all, to be involuntary patients as a condition for becoming analysts—propels Freud's denial of this strategy into center stage.

While Clark's *Freud* has received the high critical acclaim it deserves, it is, I am sorry to conclude, not quite as satisfying as some other great biographies—for example, Troyat's *Tolstoy.* The reason is simple. The greatest strength of this *Freud* is also its greatest weakness: Clark has renounced a passionate participation in the story he tells in favor of a dispassionate presentation of events, facts, and opinions. The result is that all we get to know is Freud the work-horse, the fanatical fighter for his "cause"—a figure with whom we are familiar enough already. Amazingly, despite the endless outpouring of words about Freud, his real biography is still to be written.

Shooting the Shrink

For generations, psychiatric masters ruled over their slaves and were acclaimed by the world as saviors. Now, some of the slaves seem to be revolting, and, apparently with increasing frequency, are murdering the meddling medicos.

Why should psychiatrists be assaulted and killed by their patients? For two obvious reasons, both of which the psychiatrists and the public steadfastly deny. One reason is that psychiatrists often deal with violent persons (whose behavior the psychiatrists categorize as mental illness); the other is that these persons are regularly subjected to psychiatric counterviolence (which the psychiatrists categorize as mental hospitalization and treatment).

A report on "The Dangerous Patient" in the February 1 issue of *Frontiers of Psychiatry,* published by the Roche pharmaceutical company, illustrates the currently fashionable psychiatric dogma equating violence with mental illness. The report describes the work of Drs. Stuart L. Brown and Joe P. Tupin, two University of California psychiatrists who have been trying to develop a "clinical model for the violent patient." Among the "populations" examined by these doctors were "people already proven violent," such as "multiple-time murderers, one-time murderers [and] repeatedly violent mental hospital patients." Unexamined, and unexaminable, was the premise of this sort of "research": that such persons are mad, not bad.

What do Brown and Tupin recommend to their fellow psychiatrists as the best way to "treat" such "patients"? Subduing them by brute force and brain-damaging chemicals. Tupin, we are told, "considers the use of restraints and seclusion . . . the most effective measures for treating violent patients." He "believes that restrained patients should be sedated immediately. . . . 'We give them sedatives as soon as we can, even if it's on the floor through their clothes,' he said."

To psychiatrists that may seem like therapy, but to patients it is likely to seem like assault. The stubborn fact is that violence is violence, regardless of whether it is called psychiatric illness or psychiatric treatment.

Many of the articles now appearing in the psychiatric literature emphasize the violence of "psychotic" patients and the psychiatric efforts to control

---

Reprinted, with permission, from the *New Republic,* June 16, 1982, pp. 11-15.

it with "anti-psychotic" drugs. This seems to go hand in hand with the psychotics increasing their attacks on the psychiatrists. For example, the January 15 issue of *Psychiatric News,* the American Psychiatric Association's biweekly newspaper, ran a feature article titled, "When a Psychiatrist Is Murdered." The story begins with an account of a single three-week period in 1981 in which three psychiatrists were murdered by patients. "Assaults on psychiatrists in this country," we learn, "are more frequent than is usually assumed." Revealingly, the writer adds that such attacks are frequent "even among 'low-risk' therapists who are in private practice and do not have to make decisions regarding incarceration, continued incarceration, or commitment of volatile patients." Note that a feature article in an official publication of the American Psychiatric Association now uses the term "incarceration" to identify a practice that until recently psychiatrists insisted on calling "mental hospitalization." The writer's implicit acknowledgment that people incarcerated by psychiatrists might have a grievance against their jailers is another new (and possibly hopeful) devleopment in the doctrinal literature of psychiatry.

How often do so-called psychiatric patients attack their psychiatrists? A recent study reported in the *American Journal of Psychiatry,* also published by the American Psychiatric Association, revealed that of 101 psychiatrists surveyed, about 25 percent had been attacked by a patient during a single year, and that almost 75 percent of the respondents had been attacked by a patient at some time during their careers.

Similar data abound. *Psychiatric News* refers to unpublished information from the Veterans Administration, according to which there were 12,000 patient assaults on hospital staff during a recent five-year period. In the opinion of Dr. John R. Lion, who is a member of the department of psychiatry at the University of Maryland School of Medicine, "assaults are underreported." In an actual study of assaults at a state hospital, staff reported 40 such occurrences, but when the investigators examined daily ward reports, they discovered an additional 237 assaults. "Gathering statistics about assaults is quite difficult," says Lion, "because nobody takes much interest in the subject."

But it's not quite so simple. Psychiatrists now suffer from their own success as rhetoricians: they have insisted on classifying assaults committed by mental patients as mental symptoms—and the public is increasingly inclined to view violence committed by mental patients not as violence but as "illness." Indeed, John Lion mentions that he "recently spoke to officials at OSHA [the Occupational Safety and Health Administration] and found they couldn't care less about getting involved with unsafe conditions in mental hospitals for staff due to patient assaults. They said it's not their responsibility, they take care of mechanical conditions related to on-the-job safety."

This is exactly where the medicalization of violence must lead, and it serves the psychiatrists right that they too should suffer from the mischief they have wrought. Psychiatrists have maintained that when a "mental patient" is violent, his violence is but a symptom, like the cough of a patient with tuberculosis. Ergo, if patients are not held responsible for injuring their doctors by giving them tuberculosis, why should they be held responsible for injuring them by giving them a black eye?

The popular acceptance of the view that assaults committed by mental patients are, ipso facto, the symptoms of mental illness, best "treated" with "anti-psychotic" drugs, is reflected by the way reports of such violence, in the media and in the publications of mental-health groups, refract and thus subtly reinterpret the phenomena at hand. A pamphlet published in March by the "Alliance for the Mentally Ill of Greater Milwaukee" is typical. It is devoted to pleading for less restrictive civil commitment laws—in particular, for not hampering parents in their efforts to incarcerate psychiatrically their adult children. To support this argument, the Milwaukee group's president cites two case histories. The first story begins as follows: "Mr. D. had a long history of *mental illness* and adamantly refused voluntary treatment. His parents tried the 3 party petition after a particularly *violent* episode" (emphasis added). The second story echoes the same theme. "Mr. D. H. suffered from severe *mental illness*. After *attacking* and injuring his mother, his parents initiated a 3 party petition" (emphasis added). The writer concludes by affirming her faith that the "reforms" she proposes would "save the County a great deal of money, keep the mentally ill out of the jails and court system, greatly reduce recidivism, and enable more mentally ill people to return to productive, fulfilled lives."

But the persons described in the above document are not patients but criminals, most of whom cannot "return" to "productive" and "fulfilled" lives—if for no other reason than that they never had such lives.

One more example of the frequency with which psychiatric violence now appears as a featured subject in the psychiatric literature should suffice. In the February issue of the *American Journal of Psychiatry,* three articles are devoted to this subject. One of them "Assaultive Behavior Among Chronic Inpatients," is the report of a study of five thousand patients who had resided for longer than one month in one of two large state hospitals in New York State. The authors found that "7 percent [of those patients] were assaultive toward other persons in the hospital at least once in the three months preceding the survey." To anyone familiar with madhouses, the news that such "hospitals" are not exactly places of safety for patients or staff will hardly come as a surprise. If anything about any of this is surprising, it is that psychiatrists—perhaps because they are becoming worried about their own safety—are now discussing patient violence in a way they never did in the past. "This major finding," the authors conclude, "suggests that assault is a serious problem in hospitals . . . we hope that our findings will alert the staff of psychiatric hospitals to the need to develop expertise in the psychological and physical management of assaultive patients."

Another of the articles is a report on "Case Detection of Abused Elderly Patients." It discusses several new diseases afflicting Americans, such as the "battered elder syndrome," the "battered parent syndrome," "grandparent abuse," and "granny bashing." The ugliness of these psychiatric labels reflects the ugliness of the thinking, if one can call such childish conceits thinking, that lies behind them. The beating, chaining, burning, and robbing of parents and grandparents is here categorized as "geriatric abuse" which, according to the authors, points to the need "to define and evaluate services that the abused elderly and their families require." To the theologians of mental hygiene, every new atrocity is a fresh opportunity for professional self-aggrandizement and personal gain: "The mental health fields need to teach personnel the communication and observational skills required to deal with the hostility and denial likely to be encountered in the homes of abused elderly."

The third article on psychiatric violence inveighs against court-ordered restraints on doctors with respect to the involuntary drugging of mental hospital patients. Its author, an attorney, presents several admonitory tales about the dire consequences of complying with the committed patient's wish not to be drugged. The first such tale concerns "Mr. A," who was admitted "in an acutely psychotic state . . . refused anti-psychotic medication and was not forcibly medicated . . . [He] deteriorated to the point that he violently attacked an attendant, fracturing his facial bone. Later he attacked another attendant, injuring his cervical spine."

During the 1960s, psychiatrists indulged in a veritable orgy of self-congratulation, celebrating their newly won therapeutic powers acquired through the alleged miraculous effects of "anti-psychotic" drugs. These drugs, so the public was told, transformed the odious snake pits of yesterday, where the insane were abused, into the peaceful mental hospitals of today, where the "truly sick" are humanely cared for. But those are merely flattering and mellifluous words. The brutal and ugly facts behind them won't go away. Psychiatric violence remains pervasive: mental hospital patients continue to assault each other, their relatives, and the hospital staff, and the psychiatrists continue to assault the patients. Almost in spite of themselves, it seems, psychiatrists are beginning to realize that their pseudo-medical categories are inadequate to describe the violence attendant upon their work—especially when that violence is directed against the members of their own profession. It will no doubt take longer for psychiatrists to be equally honest about their own violence. Sooner or later, though, both psychiatrists and the public will have to understand that the handling of violence of any kind cannot forever be kept away from the system society has evolved to deal with violence—that is, the legal system, with its insistence on individual responsibility and its web of rights, trials, judgments, and punishments. In the meantime, one can only hope that the escalation of this *danse macabre* of psychiatric violence—and the psychiatrists' stubborn mystifications of its elements as constituting, respectively, psychiatric illness and psychiatric treatment—will, perhaps, at last expose the Potemkin villages of psychiatry for the shams they are.

II

MENTAL HEALTH POLICY

Involuntary Psychiatry

In its recent decision in O'Connor v. Donaldson, the United States Supreme Court held for the respondent on the ground that he was compulsorily confined in a mental hospital even though he was not dangerous and was not given treatment. Was this a good decision?

Let us try to approach this question by way of an analogy. Suppose that in 1855 there had come before the Supreme Court the case of a slave named Donaldson who, having escaped from the South to one of the free states, was suing his former master, O'Connor, for damages for illegal imprisonment.

Suppose, further, that the court had decided the case "narrowly"—that is, without addressing itself to the issue of slavery—saying something like this: Since Donaldson was not chattel, and, since as a slave he was deprived of work and kept in idleness, there was no justification for holding him in bondage. Would this have been a good decision? The answer depends on one's point of view.

If one believed that Negroes should be enslaved only because they are chattel, and only in order to make them work, then one would have wholeheartedly endorsed the decision.

If one believed that Negroes should be enslaved because they are black, and because slavery is a glorious institution indispensable for the integrity of our nation, then one would have opposed the decision.

Finally, if one believed that Negroes should not be enslaved at all—indeed, that no one should be—because there can be no slavery in a free society, then one would have regarded the decision ambivalently: good, because it diminishes, albeit ever so slightly, the power of the institution of slavery; and bad, because it legitimizes the existence of this institution, which is incompatible with the moral principles on which our society rests.

The same reasoning and conclusions apply to the Donaldson case. Replace involuntary servitude with involuntary psychiatry, negritude with schizophrenia, being "chattel" with being "dangerous," work with treatment—and, *mutatis mutandis,* you have the same situation.

By deciding the case as it did, the Court simultaneously weakened psychiatric slavery and strengthened it.

First published as "On Involuntary Psychiatry," *New York Times* (Op-Ed), August 4, 1975, p. 19. Reprinted with permission.

It weakened it by holding, explicitly, that if the patient/slave is non-dangerous/non-chattel, and is not receiving treatment/is not working, then he may not be confined/enslaved.

It strengthened it by holding, implicitly, that if the patient/slave is dangerous/chattel, and is receiving treatment/is working, then he may be confined/enslaved.

Perhaps some will object to this analogy on the ground that "dangerousness" and "chattel" are not analogous terms. But, from the point of view of whether a person should or should not be enslaved, they are analogous: Both are strategic ascriptions to justify depriving the person so classified of liberty.

People do not come into the world labeled "chattel" and "not chattel," "schizophrenic" and "not schizophrenic," "dangerous" and "not dangerous." We—slave traders and plantation owners, psychiatrists and judges—so label them.

To be sure, some people *are* dangerous. We in America—especially if we live in the big cities—need hardly to be reminded of this painful fact. But in American law, dangerousness is not supposed to be an abstract psychological condition attributed to a person; instead, it is supposed to be an inference drawn from the fact that a person has committed a violent act that is illegal, has been charged with it, tried for it, and found guilty of it. In which case, he should be punished, not "treated"—in a jail, not in a hospital.

But I touch here precisely on the issue that the Court avoided or evaded. "We need not decide," said the justices in a unanimous opinion, "whether, when, or by what procedures, a mentally ill person may be confined by the state on any of the grounds which, under contemporary statutes, are generally advanced to justify involuntary confinement of such a person. . . ."

The crucial question thus remains unanswered: On what grounds, if any, may an individual be deprived of liberty by being incarcerated in a mental hospital?

The Donaldson ruling implies, and my impression is that it is already widely interpreted as meaning, that the Supreme Court has upheld, once more, the constitutionality of involuntary mental hospitalization for "patients" alleged to be "dangerous" because of "mental illness."

But even if we grant (not that we should) that some sort of psychiatrically identifiable but legally unprovable kind of dangerousness exists, and that society should take some sort of notice of it, it does not follow, logically or legally, that involuntary psychiatric confinement is the proper response to it.

For such "dangerousness," I maintain, is but a form of secular heresy; and, like heresy, it cannot, in the United States, be the ground for depriving a person of any human right, especially of liberty. Perhaps the Supreme Court will yet so rule.

The ACLU's
Mental Illness Cop-Out

George Orwell's *Animal Farm* was rejected by a dozen publishers, mainly because it made Stalin look bad. Since the watchword among modern liberals, especially in Europe, had long been *"Pas d'ennemis a gauche"* ("There are no enemies on the left"), this was simply not done. In a hitherto unpublished preface to *Animal Farm,* Orwell flailed against this hypocrisy, and concluded with this ringing denunciation: ". . . it is the liberals who fear liberty and the intellectuals who want to do dirt on the intellect: it is to draw attention to that fact that I have written this preface."[1]

Orwell's criticism was directed against England, not the United States, where the situation is, indeed, somewhat different, especially today. Although liberals here too see the mote on the right through a microscope and the beam on the left through inverted opera glasses, the object of their greatest hypocrisy is not Communism but Psychiatry. Thus, civil libertarians, and especially the ACLU, refuse to confront the attack upon liberty by institutional psychiatry, and hence cannot take a clear stand against it. The upshot is that they hedge and fudge and, in the end, come down squarely *against* liberty and *for* psychiatry.

My purpose here is to present a brief history of the American Civil Liberties Union's betrayal of civil liberties. This betrayal is prompted, in my opinion, by a stubborn effort to avoid direct confrontation and conflict with the psychiatric ideology and industry.

The Cop-Out

During the first few decades of its existence, the ACLU took no notice of psychiatry and involuntary mental hospitalization. Once it did, however, it was love at first sight: the Union's immediate response to psychiatric incarceration was to embrace it as a heaven-sent—nay, science-sent—answer to the problem of social deviance and social control.

In his official history of the ACLU, Charles Markmann relates, with unconcealed pride, how, toward the end of the Second World War, "The Union . . . began to draft model statutes for the commitment of the insane. . . . Twenty years after the first Union draft of a model bill for commitments to mental hospitals, Congress enacted for the District of Columbia a law

---

Reprinted, with permission, from *Reason*, January, 1974, 1974, pp. 4-9.

closely following the Union's proposals."[2]

In short, the Union has a fairly long and unqualifiedly disastrous history of uncritically accepting the concept of "mental illness," whose "treatment," by imprisonment, is then casually delegated to the psychiatric profession.

There were, of course, many reasons for this cop-out then, and why it continues, in attenuated form, now. The popularity and scientific legitimacy of psychiatric principles and practices is one. The lure of a paternalistic approach to troublemakers, which sees the psychiatric as against the penological approach to law enforcement as "humane" and "progressive," is another. The third, the one to which I want to call attention here, is more personal. We know, after all, that organizations do not move by themselves. They are moved, this way or that, by individuals who have strong convictions and the will to see their convictions prevail. Two persons who meet these criteria are Dr. Karl Menninger and Mr. Ramsey Clark. These men are not merely defenders, but enthusiastic advocates, of involuntary mental hospitalization. Dr. Menninger has long been, and Mr. Clark now is, prominent in the ACLU. Their established positions on commitment, and the historic position of the ACLU on this issue, are, however, now coming into ever sharper conflict with the opinion of those members of the Union who are no longer afraid to recognize psychiatry's threat to civil liberties.

Karl Menninger's Views

Dr. Karl Menninger is generally recognized professionally as the most respected and politically as the most influential psychiatrist of our time. He is a founder of the famed Menninger Clinic and Foundation, a former president of the American Psychoanalytic Association, the recipient of countless psychiatric awards and honors—*and* he has long been a vice-chairman of the National Committee of the ACLU.

I summarize below, in the form of paradigmatic citations, Menninger's views on mental illness, crime, justice, and involuntary mental hospitalization.

> We insist that there are conditions best described as mental illness. . . . All people have mental illness of different degrees at different times, and sometimes some are much worse, or better.[3]
>
> From the standpoint of the psychiatrist, both homosexuality and prostitution—and add to this the use of prostitutes—constitute evidence of immature sexuality and either arrested psychological development or regression. Whatever it may be called by the public, there is no question in the minds of psychiatrists regarding the abnormality of such behavior.[4]
>
> The very word *justice* irritates scientists. No surgeon expects to be asked if an operation for cancer is just or not. . . . Behavioral scientists regard it as equally absurd to invoke the question of justice in deciding what to do with a woman who cannot resist her propensity to shoplift,

or with a man who cannot repress an impulse to assault somebody. This sort of behavior has to be controlled; it has to be discouraged; it has to be *stopped*. This (to the scientist) is a matter of public safety and amicable co-existence, not of justice.[5]

Eliminating one offender who happens to get caught *weakens* public security by creating a false sense of diminished danger through a definite remedial measure. Actually, it does not remedy anything, and it bypasses completely the real and unsolved problem of *how to identify, detect, and detain potentially dangerous citizens.*[6]

[In a society properly informed by 'behavioral science',] indeterminate sentences will be taken for granted, and preoccupation with punishment as the penalty of the law would have yielded to a concern for the best measure to insure public safety, with rehabilitation of the offender if possible, and as economically as possible.[7]

When the community begins to look upon the expression of aggressive violence as the symptom of an illness or as indicative of illness, it will be because it believes doctors can do something to correct such a condition. At present, some better-informed individuals do believe and expect this.[8]

Do I believe there is effective treatment for offenders. . . .? *Most certainly and definitely I do.* Not all cases, to be sure. . . . Some provision has to be made for incurables—pending new knowledge—and these will include some offenders. But I believe the majority of them would prove to be curable. . . . The willfulness and the viciousness of offenders are part of the thing for which they have to be treated. They must not thwart our therapeutic attitude. . . . It is simply not true that most of them are "fully aware" of what they are doing, nor is it true that they want no help from anyone, although some of them say so.[9]

Some mental patients must be detained for a time even against their wishes, and the same is true of offenders.[10]

As these passages show, Menninger divides social sanctions imposed on offenders or alleged offenders into two types: "punishments" administered with "hostile intentions," and "treatments" administered with "therapeutic intentions." The former are bad and should therefore be abolished; the latter are good and should therefore be used as widely as possible. Menninger thus urges that we abandon the legal and penological system with its limited and prescribed sanctions called "punishments," and replace it with a medical and therapeutic system with unlimited and discretionary sanctions called "treatments." In short, he proposes the destruction of law and justice—in the name of science and therapy.

In a recent article in the *New York Times Magazine,* entitled "A Model Clockwork-Orange Prison," Phil Stanford reported on the Patuxent Institution in Maryland, an institution which combines the most repressive, anti-civil-liberties aspects of both prison and mental hospital—the sort of thing Dr. Karl Menninger has advocated throughout his entire professional life. Menninger knows Patuxent, and he knows what he likes. "Dr. Karl Menninger, perhaps the country's most honored psychiatrist, thinks Patuxent is a 'great idea'," writes Stanford. "He [Menninger] says, 'It's the only one of its kind. . . . Patuxent is a progressive step forward.'"[11]

Ramsey Clark's Position

The other prominent civil libertarian and a leading figure in the ACLU to whose views on psychiatry I wish to call attention is Ramsey Clark. Mr. Clark is a former attorney general of the United States, and the chairman of the National Advisory Council of the ACLU. I list below a few passages from his best-selling book, *Crime in America,* which illustrate his views on crime, mental illness, the indeterminate sentence, and involuntary mental hospitalization.

Most people who commit serious crimes have a mental health problem.[12]

Poor mental health, alcoholism and drug addiction are present in most crime. . . . It finally has become clear to the public that alcoholism is a health problem. . . . Drug addiction is an illness. Medical science can discover cures and provide care. . . . Drug users should be placed in correctional programs that cure and provide the opportunity to stay cured. The user's crime, until it causes him to commit other crimes, is against himself. When an individual is first found to be a user, criminal sanctions are neither necessary nor desirable. Where commitment is necessary, civil commitment of a contractual nature offers the opportunity for physical control over the addict without the stigma of a conviction for crime—and therefore the best chance for rehabilitation. Voluntary participation, which is the basis for civil commitment, creates an attitude helpful in achieving a cure.[13]

Punishment as an end in itself is itself a crime in our time. The crime of punishment, as Karl Menninger has shown through his works, is suffered by all society. . . . The use of prisons to punish only causes crime.[14]

If rehabilitation is the goal, only the indeterminate sentence will be used. . . . The sentence to a fixed term of years injures beyond its irrationality. . . . Indeterminate sentencing affords the public the protection of potentially long confinement without the necessity that long sentences be served. . . . The day of the indeterminate sentence is coming. . . . If we release persons who have the capacity for further crime, only temporary safety has been afforded.[15]

Behavioral scientists can tell us how to condition violence from our personal capability. Psychiatry, psychology, anthropology, and sociology hold the key. . . . We can do this. It is more important than the ABM system to our personal safety.[16]

Malnutrition, brain damage, retardation, mental illness, high death rates, infant mortality, addiction, alcoholism—these are the principal causes of crime.[17]

In my opinion, these passages constitute some of the purest and most concentrated extracts of mistake, misinformation, and just plain bunk that the reader is likely to find in the literature on crime and mental illness! However, it does not really matter whether the reader agrees with me that these passages constitute Mr. Clark's genuflections before the altar of modern institutional psychiatry, or whether he regards them as true facts and sound judgments. What matters is that we recognize Mr. Clark's enthusiastic endorsement of involuntary psychiatric interventions, and especially involuntary mental hospitalization; that we face the fact of his unqualified support of indeterminate sentences as "rational" sanctions, and of his uncompromising opposition to fixed sentences as "irrational" sanctions; and that we not deceive ourselves about his utter neglect of the deprivations of civil liberties inherent in the kinds of confinements he advocates. In short, in a conflict between civil liberty and mental health, Mr. Clark comes down squarely on the side of mental health—that is, on the side of psychiatric totalitarianism.

Addiction

The ACLU's position on "alcoholism" and "drug addiction"—these terms being themselves misleading metaphors, implying that the self-determined uses of certain substances are, by their very nature, diseases requiring diagnosis and treatment by physicians!—is still another act in the drama of the Union's systematic sellout of liberty for "health."

When it first encountered alcoholism, the Union thought it had met the devil; however, it soon "recognized" that alcoholism was not really an "evil," but an "illness." "In the preoccupation with loftier matters that characterized its first decade," writes Markmann, "the ACLU hardly noticed the daily violations of civil liberties and law by which Prohibition was enforced. It has been suggested that in part this blind spot might well have arisen out of the fact that so many of the Union's early leaders were social workers, clergymen, and reformers to whom, at least in the abstract, Prohibition seemed genuinely desirable because of the manifold evils of drink."[18]

This is *justifying* the ACLU's position on Prohibition, not *explaining* it. It might be well to recall, in this connection, that while the ACLU tacitly supported Prohibition, many others—for example, that "arch-reactionary," H. L. Mencken—valiantly opposed it.

The Union's position on what it calls the problem of drug addiction— but what I think civil libertarians should call the right to self-medication— leaves one no option but to conclude that the ALCU has never been, and is not now, primarily concerned with civil liberties at all; but that it seeks instead, under the banner of civil liberties, to transform our relatively open society into one that is completely closed—that is, into a Therapeutic State.

A landmark decision regarding addiction, supported by one of the most admired civil libertarians in America, and hailed by the ACLU with unrestrained enthusiasm, is *Robinson* v. *California* (1962): The United States Supreme Court here ruled that addiction is a disease, whose proper cure is imprisonment in a mental hospital.[19] In his concurring opinion, Justice William O. Douglas asserted that

> The addict is a sick person. He may, of course, be confined for treatment or for the protection of society. Cruel and unusual punishment results not from confinement, but from convicting the addict of a crime. . . . A prosecution for addiction, with its resulting stigma and irreparable damage to the good name of the accused, cannot be justified as a means of protecting society where a civil commitment would do as well. . . . If addicts can be punished for their addiction then the insane can also be punished for their insanity. Each has a disease and each must be treated as a sick person.[20]

Evidently neither Justice Douglas nor the ACLU is willing to consider the possibility that neither the "addict" nor the "insane" is sick, and that—especially from the point of view of civil liberties—the best way to "treat" them would be by leaving them alone. Furthermore, neither Justice Douglas nor the ACLU is willing to face the inconsistency inherent in their prescription—namely, that if the addict and the insane are sick, then the proper remedy is to *offer* treatment to them, rather than to *impose* it on them. For surely Douglas and the ACLU must know, as nearly everyone knows, that persons with cancer and heart disease—and even with gonorrhea and syphilis! —cannot be forced to submit to treatment they do not want. How, then, does the mere *claim* of some "civil libertarians" that certain persons are sick justify their *further claim* that these persons should be detained against their will? and their *still further claim* that the persons so incarcerated should be forced to submit to interventions which they call treatments but which the "patients" call tortures?

The sad tale of the ACLU's support of health, as defined by medical authorities and the society they serve—rather than its support of civil liberty, as defined by those deprived of it and by common sense—goes on and on and shows no signs of abating. Summarizing the ACLU's stand on alcoholism, Markmann concludes, in 1965, as follows:

> Having made an initial inroad on entrenched ignorance by the overthrow of the California law making narcotics addiction a crime [referring here to the *Robinson* decision], the Union, however belatedly, has begun a similar campaign against the parallel callousness that treats the alcoholic as the criminal he is not rather than as the sick man he is. . . . The Union will attempt to bring the law abreast of medicine and justice. Individual judges in considerable number have long recognized that alcoholism is a disease, but they have been hobbled not only by the prevailing lack of facilities for its treatment but particularly by

the middle-class stupidity that keeps on the statute books laws that require men of good will on the bench either to violate their oaths by ignoring evidence or to behave, against all their principles, like Puritan witch-hunters.[21]

This, then, is some of the evidence that makes me conclude that the ACLU is actually an ideological, and perhaps in part also an economic, captive of the "liberal" medical-psychiatric establishment, rather than an independent defender of civil liberties. In other words, the ACLU is, in effect, a lobby for the American Medical Association and the American Psychiatric Association: it is in the interests of these medical guilds that ever-more human conditions and problems be defined and treated as diseases—and it is this interest that the ACLU serves. As such a lobby, it is hardly surprising that the ACLU cannot recognize, much less fight, the enemies of civil liberties who wear not brown shirts but white coats—who are members not of the Ku Klux Klan, but of the American Psychoanalytic Association.

The Alabama Case

The latest incident in this brief account of the history of the betrayal of liberty for lunacy by the ACLU which I want to mention is a suit in which the ACLU and Dr. Menninger met in court.

In the fall of 1970, following the dismissal of a group of employees from an Alabama mental institution, the dismissed workers and the guardians of the patients sued the State, contending that the staff reduction made effective treatment impossible. This suit has become something of a *cause célèbre* in legal-psychiatric circles, many civil libertarians celebrating, I think once again quite mistakenly, the court's support for their claim that hospitalized mental patients have a "right to treatment." I mention this case here, however, only because it brought together Dr. Karl Menninger and the ACLU in court—testifying against each other! This scene—and the boundless confusion and hypocrisy concerning psychiatry in the top echelons of the ACLU which it signifies—deserve, I think, more public exposure than they have received.

The case was tried in the Federal District Court in Montgomery, Alabama, in 1971. The ACLU Foundation was authorized by the Court to participate as *amicus curiae* to the same extent as the plaintiffs and defendants, and thus played a major role in all aspects of the case, including oral arguments. The State of Alabama, the defendant in the case, invited several experts to testify in its behalf, among them Dr. Karl Menninger. Although Menninger must have known that the ACLU was supporting the plaintiffs, he chose to testify for the defendants. Here is how his participation is described in *Civil Liberties,* the official organ of the ACLU:

> Menninger appeared as a witness for Alabama. "I am very much in disagreement with computer medicine," he announced. "Boy scouts can give treatment," Menninger claimed. "Patients need love more than psychotherapy." He

said he would rather have "more clergymen than psychiatrists and psychologists."

On cross-examination, Attorney Dean revealed that at the Menninger Clinic in Topeka, there is one psychiatrist for every eight patients. Menninger justified this by the difference in "economic base," the difference in type of patients and the difference in services offered. Nobody asked him why persons who are involuntarily incarcerated in state mental institutions should get less professional care than those who decide to pay their own way in private institutions.[22]

From the same report we learn that

The ACLU Board of Directors is still polishing its policy on mental commitments. However, most of the Union's leaders appear to agree on certain minimal standards: Involuntary commitment should be the last resort to which society turns in dealing with the mentally impaired. Before commitment there must be clear demonstration that the individual is a danger to himself or to others. . . . And there must be assurance that the individual who is committed will, in fact, be treated adequately.[23]

In other words, while the victims of institutional psychiatry are perishing, the ACLU is "polishing." How reassuring. And how very reassuring that the ACLU no longer refers to mental *illness* or mental *patients!* But if there is no illness—and none is mentioned in the paragraph I here excerpted—then what is there to *treat?* And how much more reassuring still that the ACLU insists on "adequate treatment"—for *involuntary* patients! Would electroshock do? Or is that inadequate, and would nothing less than lobotomy satisfy the "minimal standards" of the ACLU?

I say: Enough! If the ACLU is *still* unprepared to defend the *civil liberties* of Americans accused of "mental illness," the least it could do is get out of the way—that is, stop justifying and supporting involuntary mental hospitalization—and let others, not so confused or corrupted or both, defend the victims. If it doesn't, then its acronym should be clearly understood to stand for the American Civil Lunacy Association—an association for the defense of lunacy, the privileged territory of the psychiatric mafia.

The masthead of the September 1972 issue of *Civil Liberties,* from which I quoted above, perhaps explains further the ACLU's consistently confused position on psychiatric matters and its subtly hostile attitude towards the victims of institutional psychiatry. Among the officers of the ACLU listed on this masthead, the first is its Chairman of the Board of Directors; and the second is its chairman of the National Advisory Council: Ramsey Clark.[24]

Creative Paranoia

Zola accused the General Staff of the French Army of deliberately incriminating an innocent Jew as a traitor. Dreyfus's enemies were, of course, in a bind: since they knew that Dreyfus was innocent, they could be fair to him only by admitting that they were guilty.

The same considerations hold for the American Civil Liberties Union's relationship to the involuntary mental patient. Since civil libertarians believe that, within the bounds of the criminal law, people should be legally free to behave as they like, the Union could be fair to the mental patient only by admitting that it has been wrong or wicked or both.

The moral is that the enemies of civil liberties are to the right—and yes, to the left, also—and above and below, and before and behind. They are everywhere. Psychiatrists call such fear for liberty paranoia. Those who love liberty call it eternal vigilance.

Notes

1. George Orwell, "The Freedom of the Press," *New York Times Magazine,* October 8, 1972, p. 76.

2. Charles L. Markmann, *The Noblest Cry: A History of the American Civil Liberties Union* (St. Martin's Press, 1965), pp. 400-01.

3. Karl Menninger, *The Vital Balance: The Life Process in Mental Health and Illness* (Viking, 1963), p. 32.

4. Karl Menninger, "Introduction," in *The Wolfenden Report: Report of the Committee on Homosexual Offenses and Prostitution* (Stein & Day, 1964), p. 6.

5. Karl Menninger, *Man Against Himself* (Harcourt, Brace, 1938), p. 69.

6. Karl Menninger, *The Crime of Punishment* (Viking, 1968), p. 17.

7. Ibid., p. 108.

8. Ibid., p. 207.

9. Ibid., pp. 260-61.

10. Ibid., pp. 265.

11. Phil Stanford, "A Model Clockwork-Orange Prison," *New York Times Magazine,* Sept. 24, 1972, p. 71.

12. Ramsey Clark, *Crime in America: Observations on Its Nature, Causes, Prevention, and Control* (Simon and Schuster, 1970; Pocket Books, 1971; page numbers refer to Pocket Books edition), p. 43.

13. Ibid., pp. 75-76.

14. Ibid., p. 199.

15. Ibid., pp. 202-05.

16. Ibid., pp. 245.

17. Ibid., p. 322.

18. Markmann, op. cit., p. 348.

19. *Robinson* v. *California,* 370 U.S. 660 (1962).

20. Ibid., p. 674.

21. Markmann, op. cit., p. 406.

22. "The First Landmark: Mental Patients' Rights," *Civil Liberties,* No. 289, Sept. 1972, pp. 5-6.

23. Ibid., p. 5.

24. Ibid., p. 4.

The ACLU and Involuntary Mental Hospitalization

In "The ACLU's Mental Illness Cop-Out," I wrote that the ACLU has supported, and continues to support, involuntary mental hospitalization. I did not write that every one of the 80 members of the ACLU's Board of Directors, or that Mr. Neier himself, personally support psychiatric incarceration. By asserting that some members of this Board and that Mr. Neier himself oppose such incarceration, Mr. Neier makes it appear as if I were wrong and "reckless." By this sort of reasoning, one could equally well assert that the American Psychiatric Association opposes involuntary mental hospitalization—when in fact it does not—because some of its members oppose it.

Further examples of my "recklessness" are that I failed to mention that the ACLU is seeking "more precise criteria for commitment" and believes that psychiatric incarceration should be used only as "a last resort." Seeking criteria for commitment implies that commitment is a morally and legally valid imposition of loss of liberty. As to advocating commitment only as a "last resort," the American Psychiatric Association also advocates it only as a last resort. I don't know anyone who advocates it as a first resort. Here, then, Mr. Neier himself supplies the most damaging evidence in support of the thesis of my article—namely, that the ACLU is intimately wedded to the prevailing psychiatric ideology which seeks to legitimize and regulate procedures for depriving persons of liberty who have been neither charged with nor convicted of any offense whatsoever.

What I have called the ACLU's "betrayal of civil liberties for mental health" is further illustrated by Mr. Neier's attempt to justify the ACLU's support of civil commitment in *Wyatt* v. *Stickney* on the grounds that the victims of psychiatric incarceration "should at least get showers, decent food" and so forth. No decent person can oppose such amenities for the victims of any kind of oppression. But Mr. Neier is working and writing for the American Civil Liberties Union, not the American Red Cross! I can only regret that Mr. Neier and the ACLU cannot see or do not agree that when a person is unjustly deprived of his liberty, the moral mandate of an organiza-

---

First published as "The ACLU and Involuntary Commitment," a reply to Aryeh Neier, *Reason,* April 1974, p. 29. Reprinted with permission.

tion ostensibly devoted to the protection of civil liberties is to fight for his release from captivity, rather than for his comfort in it; and that when it fights over the conditions of his confinement, it inevitably authenticates the validity of that confinement. When Japanese-Americans were confined in "relocation camps," was it the duty of the ACLU to fight for their freedom, or for their showers?

Perhaps it would have been more accurate if I had described *The Noblest Cry* not as an "official history" of the ACLU, but as an "adulatory history" of it. However, the facts I have quoted from this book are not in dispute. Is this, then, "recklessness" on my part, or is Mr. Neier's mentioning it—not to mention his mentioning my support of Mr. Nixon in 1972—an attempt to discredit me when he cannot dispute my evidence?

Mr. Neier also cites my claim that "the ACLU is actually an ideological, and perhaps in part also an economic, captive of the 'liberal' medical-psychiatric establishment," and says that he "cannot imagine" what I mean by it. Had he read the next sentence, he would have seen just what I mean by it. It reads: "In other words, the ACLU is, in effect, a lobby for the American Medical Association and the American Psychiatric Association: it is in the interests of these medical guilds that ever-more human conditions and problems be defined and treated as diseases—and it is this interest that the ACLU serves." This, then, is what Mr. Neier's rhetoric of "recklessness" comes down to: I am reckless toward the ACLU in making this perfectly valid charge against it, but he is not reckless towards me in calling the first half of my criticism meaningless, omitting the second half, and topping it off with a gratuitous slur on my character.

Repeatedly, Mr. Neier refers to what he thinks and what he did. But my essay was about the ACLU, not about Mr. Neier. I am glad that Mr. Neier's views on psychiatry and civil liberties are closer to mine than to the ACLU's. This hardly invalidates my criticism of the ACLU. But it raises a question: Why does Mr. Neier write this letter for the ACLU?

It seems to me, in short, that what I have written about the ACLU is not reckless but embarrassing. The ACLU has no hesitation in publicizing embarrassing facts about persons whose political policies it opposes; I have none in publicizing embarrassing facts about the ACLU whose psychiatric policies I oppose. Is this recklessness on my part, or evidence that the ACLU can dish it out but can't take it?

Condoning Psychiatric Slavery

The American Civil Liberties Union has a long history of uncritically accepting the concept of mental illness and of casually delegating to the psychiatric profession the "treatment" of this "illness" by imprisonment. The chairman of the ACLU's National Advisory Council is Ramsey Clark. His view on civil commitment epitomizes the organization's approach to the problem: "Where commitment is necessary, civil commitment of a contractual nature offers the opportunity for physical control . . . without the stigma of a conviction for crime. Voluntary participation, which is the basis for civil commitment, creates an attitude helpful in achieving a cure."

The fact that psychiatric imprisonment is called "civil commitment" is, of course, simply a part of the linguistic deception characteristic of the mental-health system. Since civil commitment results in the loss of liberty, and subjects the victim to health hazards at the hands of medical criminals whose ostensible healing function is legitimized by the state, it entails far greater deprivation of rights than does incarceration in prison, a penalty carefully circumscribed by constitutional guarantees and judicial safeguards.

After the New York Civil Liberties Union's adoption of an anticommitment resolution in 1969, the board of directors of the national ACLU engaged in some soul-searching concerning the pros and cons of commitment. Thus, the ACLU arrived at its present policy on psychiatric coercion after having thoroughly familiarized itself with the medical, moral, and legal parameters of the problem. Its 1976 policy statement represents a well-considered position and is the more important for being so. I shall first quote and comment on the most important parts of this policy statement and then conclude with a general assessment of the ACLU's continued support of psychiatric imprisonment and torture.

The ACLU's *1976 Policy Guide* devotes three pages to what it calls "The Mentally Ill." "Policy #236" is entitled "Civil Commitment." The fact that the ACLU begins its presentation of the rights of persons threatened with psychiatric deprivations of their constitutional rights by adhering without any qualification whatever to the conventional psychiatric terminology, foreshadows its conclusions. According to the ACLU, some persons are "mentally ill," or have a "mental illness." At the same time, involuntary mental

---

Reprinted, with permission, from *Inquiry,* March 6, 1978, pp. 3-4.

hospitalization is not imprisonment; it is "civil commitment."

"The individual should not be incarcerated prior to a hearing, except in an emergency. . . ." Being psychiatrically incarcerated *after* a hearing is, in this view, sufficient protection for persons accused of mental illness.

"During such periods of emergency commitment, no action should be taken on the person which might have a permanent effect, and the use of drugs should be limited solely to those deemed by the attending physician to be medically essential to reasonable custody prior to the hearing." Do physicians ever admit to using drugs that are not "medically essential"? The question the ACLU should be confronting here is not only what to do with the person accused of mental illness, but also who defines that person as mentally ill and who defines what constitutes a "medically essential" psychiatric intervention. Note that at the beginning of the above paragraph the victim of psychiatry is identified as a "person"; in the sentence following the one quoted above, however, he is called a "patient." It is precisely this involuntary transformation of a human being from person to patient that the ACLU ought to scrutinize and oppose. How can one be a patient if one has no disease? Why should one be a patient if one does not want to be (even if one has a disease)? The ACLU assiduously avoids these questions.

Moreover, by specifying that "the use of drugs should be limited . . . to [those] essential for reasonable custody . . ." the ACLU endorses the use of drugs as chemical straitjackets. In so supporting the use of chemical agents under pseudomedical auspices for "custodial" purposes—that is, for the forcible control of individuals innocent of crime—the ACLU comes down squarely in support of some of the most odious psychiatric methods of social control (now widely used in the Sovient Union and righteously denounced in the West).

"Persons being held pending judicial commitment proceedings . . . must have full opportunity to prepare for the commitment proceeding and make an informed defense." In the courtroom, one can defend oneself only against an accusation. But the ACLU bases its policy on the premise that mental illness is not a legal accusation but a medical abnormality. It never calls the victim a person "accused of mental illness."

"While the hearing in a civil commitment proceeding need not necessarily take on the physical appearance of a trial . . . the hearing should be held in an open courtroom, whether in or outside of a hospital." How can a hearing in an open courtroom not take on the physical appearance of a trial? Why should it not take on such an appearance? Note the ACLU's concern with the *physical appearance* of the hearing, rather than with its *human reality.*

"The judge should carefully instruct the jury on the relevant criteria for commitment, insuring the use of defined standards. . . ." This recommendation is completely inconsistent with the previous recommendation to avoid the appearance of a trial. Moreover, it reveals—perhaps more dramatically than any other single sentence in this dismal document—the ACLU's implacable hostility to both lunacy and liberty. Why? Because it is in the very nature of the problems that "mental illness" poses that there are no meaningful "defined standards" for commitment, nor can there be any. But let us suppose that there were such standards. Would that make strict judicial adherence to them enough to satisfy a true civil libertarian that fundamental human rights are protected? In effect, what the ACLU is saying here is that American chattel slavery is all right, so long as judges and juries make sure that only blacks are enslaved; or that Nazi genocide is all right, so long as judges and juries make sure that only Jews are gassed. Instead of scrutinizing and opposing the judicial procedures used to imprison and torture "lunatics," the ACLU strengthens still further the forces of the dominant social ethic by making its persecutory practices conform to the highest procedural standards of the law.

"The individual shall be present at the hearing. . . . If the hearing is held in a hospital, the individual should not appear in hospital attire, as this might prejudice the jury against his or her case." Holding the commitment hearing in a madhouse does not prejudice the jury; seeing the victim garbed as a madman does!

"The state must probe beyond a reasonable doubt the need for commitment and the absence of less drastic alternatives with an equal chance of correcting the individual's alleged malady." By thus linking "the need for commitment" to a "malady," the ACLU here takes the position that the purpose of involuntary mental hospitalization is curing the patient's mental illness. It then immediately contradicts this position, as we shall see in a moment, by endorsing the protection of others from the danger the "patient" poses as an equally legitimate ground for his involuntary psychiatric treatment.

"The state is obligated to finance treatment in noncoercive settings before it invokes involuntary commitment proceedings." Although this whole document is highly revealing of the ACLU's prejudices about mental patients, this sentence is perhaps the most revealing. Commitment is really a new version of the white man's burden: Ensconced in plush offices, supported by many of the financial and legal pillars of society, the board of directors of the ACLU views everyone threatened with psychiatric incarceration as poor! Why else should the state pay for the treatment of everyone who becomes a candidate for commitment? Marilyn Monroe was committed. Ernest Hem-

ingway was committed. Countless rich people have been, and continue to be, committed. Doesn't the ACLU know that?

Moreover, not only does the foregoing sentence reek of a condescending charity toward putative poor psychotics, it is also irrelevant to the issue under consideration—the fate of persons who resist being categorized as mentally ill and the consequences of being so labeled. Undeterred by that simple fact, the ACLU pontificates about the state financing "treatment in noncoercive settings" for such persons. But how do you provide such a service when the thing its recipient wants most is not to get the service? Never mind. I am being too literal. Obviously, the ACLU is here supporting the offering of ostensibly noncoercive "treatment" before the uncooperative subject is really given the treatment.

"The individual should be allowed to refuse any treatment for mental illness, except such treatment as may be required to prevent the patient from being a danger to others. . . ." Many of the ACLU's recommendations concerning civil commitment imply that the purpose of psychiatric confinement is to provide psychiatric treatment. But if the "patient" is allowed to reject treatment, why is he not allowed to reject hospitalization? If he is competent to make the one judgment, why not the other?

The ACLU here not only accuses the "mental patient" of threatening the safety of others, it also re-endorses the use of coerced psychiatric "treatment" for a frankly nontherapeutic purpose—that is, for preventing "danger to others." In so doing, the ACLU goes beyond supporting the odious practice of preventive detention: It endorses as well the practice of pharmacologically immobilizing the innocent individual preventively detained by psychiatric "hospitalization." Mentally healthy persons have a constitutional right to be dangerous to others. The ACLU does not explain why it proposes to strip mentally sick persons of that right. This omission is especially puzzling in view of the fact that the organization is intent on preserving all of the significant civil rights of the committed mental patient:

"No person should be deprived of his or her civil rights, such as the power to control assets, make contracts, vote, engage in occupations, and control other nonmedical personal affairs, solely by the reason of commitment." Does the ACLU really mean this? Persons incarcerated in insane asylums should have the right to work as policemen, teach school, serve as senators, pilot airplanes—perhaps even practice psychiatry?

The imbecility of the ACLU's policy on insanity here approaches infinity. If the committed mental patient retains all of these civil rights, then why should he not also retain his civil duty to obey the law? In the light of the above-quoted sentence, what does the ACLU mean by referring to mental patients as "dangerous"? Persons either injure others in a manner prohibited by law or they don't. If they injure others, their offense is a matter for the criminal law. If they don't, they ought to be left alone. The ACLU sidesteps all these basic issues.

One of the most interesting things about the ACLU's 1976 policy statement on civil commitment is what it omits: dangerousness to oneself. The danger of suicide is the foremost reason that psychiatrists now advance to justify involuntary mental hospitalization and treatment. The ACLU is silent about it. Does a person have a right to kill himself? Surely this is one of the most important questions that confront any civil libertarian who tries, sincerely and seriously, to come to grips with the civil liberties aspects of psychiatric coercion. Because the ACLU avoids this issue—it does not even allude to it as a problem—I contend that its entire position on psychiatric matters is pervaded and vitiated by bad faith.

The ACLU's 1976 policy statement on "civil commitment" is an evil document: It is nothing less than an unqualified support of psychiatric slavery—of psychiatric defamation called "diagnosis," of psychiatric imprisonment called "hospitalization," and of psychiatric torture called "treatment."

It is also a linguistically debauched document: It is poorly reasoned, it is internally contradictory, and it exudes that insincerity which, as Orwell aptly observed, characterizes the totalitarian mind at work with words.

The Right to Die

By intervening in Gary Gilmore's fate against his wishes, the American Civil Liberties Union chose to assault not only freedom and dignity, but the rule of law itself. It did so by supporting the state of Utah in its efforts to break its contract with Gilmore, thus attempting to deprive him of his last tangible human right—the right to be punished as prescribed by law. By the time this is read he may have won his right.

No one, including Gilmore and the ACLU, doubted that Gilmore committed the crimes for which he was sentenced to death. Faced with that sentence, Gilmore re-enacted the famous death scene in Plato's *Phaedo*. In that scene, as may be recalled, Socrates and some of his closest friends are gathered awaiting Socrates' execution. After some conversation, Socrates says farewell and asks the executioner to bring the cup of poison. Crito interrupts him, urging that he wait and prolong his life for as long as possible.

> But Socrates, I know that other men take the poison quite late, and eat and drink heartily, and even enjoy the company of their chosen friends, after the announcement has been made. So do not hurry; there is still time.

Crito claims to be arguing on behalf of Socrates, just as the ACLU—through its executive director, Aryeh Neier—claimed to be arguing on behalf of Gilmore. (Neier's op-ed essay in the *New York Times,* November 17, was titled "'Butting In' for the Utah Slayer." It should have been titled "Butting In' against the Utah Slayer" or "for the ACLU.") But Socrates' reply to Crito exposes the fallacy—nay, the hypocrisy—of such an attack on personal autonomy and dignity:

> And those whom you speak of, Crito, naturally do so; for they think that they will be gainers by so doing. And I naturally shall not do so; for I think that I should gain nothing by drinking the poison a little later but my own contempt for so greedily saving up a life which is already spent.

The difference between Socrates' argument and Neier's highlights the dismal disjunction between the vast scientific and technical progress that we

Reprinted, with permission, from the *New Republic,* December 11, 1976, pp. 8-9.

have made during the past 2500 years, and the equally vast moral and rhetorical regression that we have undergone.

It may be argued that Neier addressed himself not to Gilmore or his predicament, but to the issue of the death penalty. Neier himself said so: "Capital punishment is barbarous. . . . Our quarrel is with the state, not with Gary Mark Gilmore." Therein, precisely, lies the most incontrovertible proof of the ACLU's betrayal of human decency—and of the rule of law. To be sure, Gilmore cannot be compared to Socrates, for Socrates was not a vicious murderer. But a human being, whether a philosopher or murderer, has certain rights and dignities that remain his as a man awaiting execution. It is those remaining rights and dignities that the ACLU, in its self-righteous fight against the death penalty, tried to deny Gilmore. There are countless cases of men sentenced to death who do not want to die. The ACLU does not need to and should not want to carry on its struggles by choosing a case in which it can do so only by depriving the victim of his last important choice in life. The ACLU has ample opportunity to carry out its program of advocacy by choosing cases where men and women ask for its help.

The drama pitting the lawmakers and law enforcers of the state of Utah against Gilmore has been both macabre and tragic. But it highlights, as such confrontations are likely to do, where people really stand when the chips are down. The ACLU, through Neier, came down squarely against individual self-determination and suicide. "I find it very difficult to disregard Gilmore's wishes," Neier remarked on his way to concluding that "ACLU attorneys are asking the courts to prevent Utah from executing Mr. Gilmore." But if Neier found it difficult to disregard Gilmore's wishes, he might best have proved that he meant it by respecting Gilmore's choice. Furthermore, the ACLU's opposition to the death penalty would, it seems to me, be strengthened if it were narrowed to those cases where the convicted criminal prefers life imprisonment to execution, rather than vice versa.

Neier's arguments against Gilmore's execution were misleading. "I hope," he wrote, "the public will recoil with horror from the prospect of official state blindings, maimings, castrations, psychosurgery—and executions." That statement implied that execution is on a par with the tortures with which he bracketed it. I believe that resuscitating a person after a suicide attempt in order to execute him is a worse brutality than granting him the right to be executed—or, better still, the right to kill himself. Here, too, history can teach us a lesson. When William the Conqueror was crowned king in 1066, in one of his first speeches he abolished the death penalty, declaring that "I forbid that any person be killed or hanged for any cause." But if naïve civil libertarians find encouragement in that outpouring of "humanitarianism," they had better take heed of William's next statement: "Let their eyes be torn out and their testicles cut off. . ." Despite Gilmore's crimes, society is in his debt for dramatizing the fact that there are fates worse than death.

In taking the stand it did, the ACLU also went against the fundamental spirit of the rule of law upon which our civil liberties rest. Put briefly and oversimply, but nevertheless accurately, the rule of law in a free society guarantees that persons who obey the law must not be molested by the police power of the state. However, it is the duty of the state not only to respect and protect the liberty of those persons who obey the law, but also to prosecute and punish those who break the law. That is where Gilmore's fundamental right to being punished came in. The state of Utah had, in effect, promised to kill him. And Gilmore simply asked that the state show more respect for its (explicit) promise to uphold the law than Gilmore had shown for his (implied) promise to obey the law.

That the principle of contracts is fundamental to both civil law and constitutional government is stating the obvious. "It is confessedly unjust," John Stuart Mill wrote in one of his celebrated passages, "to *break faith* with anyone: to violate an engagement, either express or implied, or disappoint expectations raised by our own conduct." (Emphasis in the original.)

By analogizing Gilmore's request that the state fulfill its contract and put him to death with the requests of hypothetical prisoners to be blinded, castrated or lobotomized in order to gain their freedom, Neier and the ACLU stood the case on its head. Gilmore didn't ask for his freedom. Being blinded and lobotomized are not sentences that juries can impose. In short, Neier's assertion that "the state is forcing on Mr. Gilmore" a choice between death and life imprisonment was a falsehood. The state of Utah has, subsequent to sentencing Gilmore, not forced anything on him other than his role as convicted criminal. It was Gilmore who tried to force the state to fulfill its promise to him. And it was Neier and the ACLU that tried to force the state to renege on it.

State Mental Hospitals:
Orphanages for Adults

The crisis confronting America's state-run mental institutions cannot be solved without the realization that state mental hospitals are *fake* hospitals.

Unlike medical hospitals, state mental hospitals function mainly as homes for the homeless, as asylums for those who have, for a variety of reasons, no place of their own and none where they are welcome.

In short, they are orphanages for adults. Because the "patients" in such hospitals are not really sick, they do not need doctors to care for them.

In the last two decades, and especially in the last few years, the number of inmates in state mental hospitals has declined dramatically. The cost of running state mental hospitals, however, has not decreased; it has increased.

Mental hospital administrators and psychiatrists complain bitterly of "understaffing." Illustrative is the recent threat of psychiatrists at the Napa State Hospital in California to go on strike unless more physicians are hired. Napa now has 1,850 patients and 64 doctors, for a patient-physician ratio of 30 to 1; the psychiatrists threatening to strike want it lowered to 20 to 1. But if mental illness is an "illness like any other," as psychiatric propagandists like to put it, then even a 20 to 1 patient-doctor ratio would be grossly inadequate for mental hospitals.

Real hospitals—that is, medical hospitals, especially the good ones—often have more doctors than patients! But mental hospitals are *fake* hospitals; hence, they don't need any doctors at all (except perhaps a few consultants to care for the medical needs of the otherwise medically healthy population.)

Fundamental Change

According to conventional wisdom and conventional psychiatry, persons are confined in mental hospitals because they are mentally ill and need psychiatric care. Yet the determinants behind psychiatric confinement are numerous and complex—with the foremost being the prevailing social policy concerning it.

Reprinted, with permission, from Pacific News Service (Syndicate), February 23, 1978.

Twenty-five years ago, mental hospitalization was regarded as the best method for dealing with so-called mental patients; today, dehospitalization is. Despite this obvious reversal in social policy concerning mental hospitalization, conventional psychiatry and conventional wisdom attribute the dramatic drop in the state mental hospital population to the therapeutic triumph of certain new psychopharmacological agents.

In Japan, however, where the so-called anti-psychotic drugs have been just as popular as in the United States, the number of mental hospital patients increased by more than 500 percent during the same period. This demonstrates conclusively that the decrease in hospitalized psychiatric patients in America is not due to the therapeutic effectiveness of such drugs; instead, attributing such a decrease to the use of certain drugs is a disguise and rationalization for a fundamental change in mental hospital policies.

Consider the following paradox. Twenty-five years ago, when more than 750,000 Americans were confined in mental hospitals (most of them against their will), psychiatric leaders insisted that not a single one of them was hospitalized unnecessarily. Today, when less than 250,000 Americans are confined in mental hospitals (most of them because they want to be), psychiatric leaders insist that many of them are hospitalized unnecessarily.

"After 45 years in mental hospitals and their administration," declared Dr. Windred Overholser in 1961 (he was one of the most prominent American psychiatrists at that time), "I am convinced that the basis for the belief that persons are improperly sent to mental hospitals is, for practical purposes, entirely without foundation."

Since then, most of our larger states have reduced their mental hospital population by 60 percent and more. For example, in New York state the population of state mental hospitals dropped from 90,000 in 1955 to 26,000 in 1977. Despite this dramatic change, the N.Y. State Department of Mental Hygiene's own study "showed" that "more than a fourth of the 26,000 adult patients in mental hospitals are not ill enough to be kept there."

Twenty-five years ago, state mental hospitals housing 10,000 or more patients were often staffed by a dozen or fewer physicians (many of whom spoke little or no English). Nevertheless, mental hospital administrators and psychiatrists were proud of the quality of the "medical care" they dispensed to their patients. Today, with the number of hospitalized patients sharply down, the number of hospital psychiatrists is sharply up.

Fake Illness

The dramatic transformation of American state-hospital psychiatry during the past two decades—with a 180-degree shift in policy, from forcibly warehousing society's undesirables to refusing asylum to those who beg for it—has laid bare, as perhaps never before in the modern age, the true nature of the mental "hospital" (and the "illnesses" it supposedly "treats").

"Patients" in mental hospitals do not (as a rule) suffer from bodily diseases. And there are other crucial differences between medical and mental diagnoses and hospitalizations.

The typical sequence of events leading to a medical diagnosis and hospitalization is:

—the person *develops* certain undesirable or dangerous bodily phenomena, such as bleeding from bodily orifices, fever, or convulsions;

—from such "medical symptoms" the physician infers that the patient suffers from a bodily disease;

—depending on the nature and severity of that disease, the physician may then recommend medical hospitalization.

On the other hand, the typical sequence of events leading to a mental diagnosis and hospitalization is:

—the person *commits* certain undesirable or dangerous acts, such as attacking or killing others, mutilating or trying to kill himself, or refusing to dress or speak;

—from such "psychiatric symptoms" the physician infers that the patient suffers from a mental illness;

—depending on the dangerousness of the patient toward himself or others, the physician may then recommend (or forcibly impose) mental hospitalization.

Thus, in the case of medical illness, *the patient's body is an object,* injured or impaired by micro-organisms, chemicals, tumors, or trauma; whereas in the case of mental illness, *the patient's self is an agent* injuring or impairing himself or others with guns, drugs, threats or self-neglect.

Countless current newspaper articles on "dehospitalization" reflect the unarticulated realization of this state of affairs.

"Many of those admitted to [mental] insitutions today," we read in one such account, "are re-admissions, people who have been released from their confinement and after their release want to go back. But they find it much harder nowadays to get back in. Whether it is eagerness to escape the complexities of life on the outside, or despair, loneliness, and an inability to cope with it, the mentally disturbed often have to prove they are sick enough to be readmitted."

In other words, in the case of *medical* illness—for example, a back injury or heart attack—the physician uses X-rays and electrocardiagrams to prove whether the patient needs to be hospitalized; whereas in the case of *mental* illness—for example, depression or schizophrenia—the patient uses his own behavior and especially threats to prove that he needs to be hospitalized.

The whole discipline of psychiatry rests on treating these quite dissimilar phenomena as if they were similar or even identical.

It is now up to the American people and their policy-makers to decide what to do with their state mental hospitals. Should the states (the taxpayers) continue to spend more and more money on larger medical staffs for a shrinking mental hospital population?

Or should they demedicalize mental hospitals completely—at the cost of the moral confrontation of certain human problems and the reappraisal of their proper legal management?

Therein lies the fundamental and stubborn problems that mental hospitals pose for politicians and the public alike.

``Back Wards to Back Streets''

Like hair styles and popular songs, psychiatric treatments are largely a matter of fashion. In 1938, electric-shock treatment was introduced into psychiatry and was immediately hailed as a cure for schizophrenia. But soon the question was asked, "Does it work?" It was the same story with lobotomy. The doctor who developed it even received the Nobel Prize, in 1949, for his work—the ultimate stamp of approval of our scientific age. But again, the question soon became: "Does it work?" The latest psychiatric fad is "deinstitutionalization" —a professional sounding if grotesque term referring to the policy of transferring patients from mental hospitals to other psychiatrically supervised facilities. This policy, introduced into psychiatry about 15 years ago, has also been hailed as a revolutionary advance. Now people are again asking: "Does it work?"

As an old saying has it, ask a stupid question and you get a stupid answer. Asking whether electric-shock treatment, lobotomy, or deinstitutionalization "work" is stupid because such questions assume certain things about mental illness and mental hospitalization that are, quite simply, false.

To understand the problems that the so-called deinstitutionalization of mental patients was supposed to solve—and the problems it has in turn created—we must first be clear about why and how people end up in mental hospitals. According to conventional wisdom, "patients" are admitted or committed to mental hospitals because they are mentally ill, are dangerous to themselves or others, and need psychiatric treatment. This is all bunk. Let's examine these ideas, one at a time.

Mental illness. Aside from the possibility that there may be no such thing (that is, that "mental illnesses" are merely the names we give to certain undesirable patterns of behavior), the presence of mental illness "in" a person does not explain why he or she should be in a mental hospital any more than the presence of medical illness "in" a person explains why he or she should be in a regular hospital. Most people suffering from arthritis, diabetes or hypertension are not in hospitals. Why, then, should people suffering from "mental illnesses" be in hospitals?

Dangerousness. It is widely assumed that many so-called mental patients are "dangerous to themselves and others." If by dangerousness we mean that

---

Reprinted, with permission, from *TV Guide,* May 17-23, 1980, pp. 32-36.

such persons *injure* themselves or others, then the problems they present are not medical but moral and legal. Injuring oneself—by drinking too much, ingesting toxic drugs, etc.—may, indeed, result in disease; but the behavior itself is the act of a moral agent, comparable to marrying the wrong man or woman, or investing in the wrong stock. Injuring others is, likewise, not a medical problem: It is assault, arson, murder, or some other mischief—for which the only rational remedy is punishing the offender. Just as illness is not a crime, so crime is not an illness.

Mental treatment. Although the promise of psychiatric treatment is now an acceptable justification for mental hospitalization (both with and without the patient's consent), this is a very feeble justification indeed. In the first place, if there is no mental illness (as I contend), then there can be no such thing as mental treatment (as I also contend). But even if we accept the reality of mental illnesses and treatments, why should mentally ill persons be in mental hospitals to receive mental treatment? The main forms of psychiatric treatment today are conversation ("psychotherapy") and drugs ("chemotherapy"). Neither method requires hospitalization.

So the question remains: Why are people in mental hospitals? In my opinion, the correct answer to this question is that they are there either because they have escaped from society or because they have been expelled from it. The former are the voluntary mental patients, the latter the involuntary ones.

Some persons—because they are fearful, weak, or lazy—want to drop out of society; others—because they are ineffectual, odd, or offensive—are dropped out of it. In the modern world, the mental hospital has become the natural habitat of such persons—where they quickly become even more desocialized.

In my view, the mental hospital is not a hospital at all; it's only *called* that. Unlike medical hospitals, mental hospitals are homes for the homeless—asylums for those who have, for a variety of reasons, no place of their own and none where they are welcome. In short, they are orphanages for adults. (They are also prisons for certain lawbreakers, but this function of the mental hospital cannot be considered in this brief space.) In addition, the mental hospital furnishes employment to large numbers of people with no salable skills in a free market. Satisfying the self-defined aspirations, interests and needs of so-called mental patients was never among the aims or functions of the mental-hospital system. It still isn't.

Now we are ready to take a fresh look at the "deinstitutionalizing"—or "dumping"—of mental patients. As we saw, the problems that this policy was supposed to solve were themselves wholly artificial: If doctors and lawyers—and last but not least, the relatives of so-called mental patients—had not committed hundreds of thousands of individuals to mental hospitals, there would have been no chronic "institutionalized" patients to discharge.

About 15 years ago, for a number of complex reasons, psychiatric bureaucrats and politicians decided that mental hospitals were bad places for mental patients. This is a supremely ironic idea, since it is what involuntary mental patients had been asserting for the past 200 years. But that is beside the point here. The point is that, since most people in mental hospitals are more or less socially disabled, they cannot simply be discharged. Moreover, many mental-hospital patients (even if they enter the hospital involuntarily), come to like it in the institution—which provides them not only with room and board but also with an escape from the day-to-day responsibilities of ordinary life. In short, deinstitutionalization is just another sham "reform" or "treatment"—and here are the reasons why.

Like other psychiatric "reforms" and "treatments," deinstitutionalization is supposed to be something that we—psychiatrists, sane people, society—do *for* crazy mental patients. But it's not true. Just as years ago "crazy" people were incarcerated in mental hospitals against their will—now they are evicted from them against their will. Mental-hospital patients are not given a choice between staying in the institutions that have become their homes or moving into broken-down hotels in the slums. In the name of doing something good *for* mental patients, once more something terrible is being done *to* them.

Psychiatrists, lawyers, and sane people continue to treat deinstitutionalized mental patients as they always have—as crazy, sick, irresponsible. The vicious circle generated by a psychiatry based on "mental illness" and "mental treatment" remains unbroken: the "patients" are psychiatrically supervised and medicated (whether they like it or not); are stigmatized as crazy; and are not punished when they commit crimes (after all, they are "mentally ill" and hence not responsible for their actions).

So, of course, deinstitutionalization will not "work" either. Why should it? It's another smoke screen, another evasion—by the medical and legal professions as well as by the public—of the brutal facts of the human destiny: namely, that not everyone can "make it" in life; that those who cannot are not sick; and that a free society cannot afford to regard as "insane" or "irresponsible" either those who wish to escape from their responsibilities because they find society too demanding or those whom society wishes to expel because it finds them too demanding.

Institutionalizing human beings in the name of psychiatric care was, as now nearly everyone admits, a shame. Deinstitutionalizing them in the name of psychiatric progress is a sham.

I am frequently asked: What *should* be done, then, about those we call "mentally ill"? I have addressed the implications of that deceptively simple question in some 15 books and scores of articles; it cannot be answered here in a few lines. Drugs and talk can help. But there is, in my opinion, no medical, moral or legal justification for involuntary psychiatric interventions. Thus, "mentally ill" persons residing in hospitals should not be forcibly evicted; nor should those residing in the community be forcibly hospitalized.

Life is at once an intolerable burden and an immeasurable treasure. Our task, I believe, should be to devise fresh, more civilized ways of looking at and dealing with those who shirk their burdens—a task we cannot even begin to address so long as we insist, in the name of mental health, on lifting the burden from the shoulders of those who carry it in ways that disturb us.

The Lady in the Box

More than 35,000 people in New York City are now said to make their "home" in the subway system, in doorways, in boxes on the street. Last month, one of them—a 61-year-old woman named Rebecca Smith—froze to death in her makeshift cardboard hut. Perhaps there is, in Mrs. Smith's life and death, a lesson for us all.

Learning to live competently—so that we can take care of ourselves and, perhaps, at least for a while, of others as well—is a task we are all expected to master.

This task resembles others, such as learning to speak, to cook, to comfort a child, to play tennis. A few persons excel in one or another skill. Many learn enough to get along in life—but some of them then give up the struggle. Others fail to learn how to live, because they cannot or will not learn—a distinction that is often not easy for us to make.

Everyone does not know how to cook or play tennis. Why, then, should we expect that everyone should know how to live?

We have that expectation because every educated person now "knows" that people who do not live competently ("normally") are sick—that they are suffering from the most severe form of mental illness known to psychiatric science: "schizophrenia." This idea is supposed to be helpful—for science, for society, and above all for the "patients" suffering from this alleged malady. But it is not. In fact, it is deadly. Why? Because ideas have consequences, and this particular idea has deadly consequences.

In reading a newspaper, we learned that during the best years of her life, while her daughter was growing up, Mrs. Smith was locked up in an insane asylum, with the diagnosis of schizophrenia.

For Mrs. Smith, then, the first consequence of the idea of schizophrenia was a 10-year period of incarceration in a madhouse.

Its second consequence was involuntary electric-shock "treatment."

Its third consequence was medication with psychotropic drugs.

And its fourth one was "deinstitutionalization."

"Psychotropics" and "deinstitutionalization," terms just as grotesque and misleading as "schizophrenia," thus now complement and confirm the imagery of this "illness" and its "treatment."

Reprinted, with permission, from the *New York Times* (Op-Ed), February 16, 1982, p. A-19.

The sad truth is that Mrs. Smith was a person who did not take care of herself. That is pathetic. What makes it tragic is our refusal to acknowledge this fact simply for what it is—and instead our laying the blame for her fate upon a mysterious, indeed nonexistent, disease.

Because of this displacement and mystification, we have first accepted (and still accept) that involuntary confinement in a madhouse—during which "schizophrenics" become even more desocialized than they had been—is a form of therapy.

Because of it, we now accept that after "schizophrenics" make the madhouse their home, forcibly evicting them from it is also a form of therapy. Although institutional psychiatry is shot through and through with fake doctoring and real coercion, we continue to be surprised that the would-be beneficiaries of its "help" want none of it.

After Mrs. Smith died, her daughter came to New York City to claim her mother's body. When she was making the funeral arrangments, the newspaper said, "She was shown a coffin that had a latch. She asked for another. 'I wouldn't lock my mother up like that,' she said. 'I couldn't do that.'"

But Mrs. Smith was dead. She could not be locked up any more. When Mrs. Smith was alive, someone had her locked up. This paradox illustrates our boundless mindlessness about mental illness, personal liberty, and death.

To be sure, had Mrs. Smith not been locked up when she was, she might have died even sooner. And had she not been locked up and "treated" against her will at all, she might not have become the person she became.

These are things we will never know. What I believe we do know is that loneliness and homelessness and the inability or unwillingness to make a life for oneself are not the symptoms of a disease (like cancer or diabetes).

Of course, that knowledge—assuming it is true—will not solve the problems such persons pose to themselves and others. It will, however, help us from making the problems even worse than they are.

But, then, it is a characteristic feature of the history of healing that people often prefer a cure that kills to no cure at all. Cures directed against the nonexistent disease of schizophrenia are, moreover, doubly dangerous: They not only destroy the lives of "schizophrenics" but also the nonschizophrenics' ability to see clearly what ails the "patients."

Why Do We Fear the Retarded?

On January 15, 1978, a house in Greenlawn was burned by unknown arsonists —but for a reason that everyone knew only too well: A couple planned to turn their home into a hostel for a small group of mentally retarded persons.

Is that a reason for burning down your neighbor's house? Much as we may dislike to hear it, the answer is yes. Why? Because normal, nonretarded people "know" that the retarded are dangerous maniacs. A Long Island woman, questioned by a reporter about her objection to a hostel for the retarded, explained that she was afraid "that a hostel resident might come in with a knife and rape her."

I submit that our society in general, and our mental health experts in particular, are largely responsible for people having such a "retarded" view of the mentally retarded. For decades we have segregated the retarded in concentration camps. The stigma, the fear, and the confinement are all one package, each element reinforcing and justifying the other.

It simply will not do to say now, as the director of the Nassau County chapter of the Association for the Help of Retarded Children is quoted as saying, that "Retarded citizens, like everyone else, are entitled to live outside of institutions." Of course they are. But then what have our leading mental retardation experts been doing for decades confining them? And what have the leading lawyers, legislators, and journalists been doing supporting the system of pseudomedical confinement euphemistically called the "state school"?

The image of certain disabled and disturbing persons as especially dangerous has haunted the modern mind. In addition to retarded persons, epileptics and so-called mental patients have also been systematically stigmatized, confined, and abused. Let us stop pretending that we do not know why "normal" people so persecute "abnormal" people. We know perfectly well: because they fear and loathe them! And why do they fear and loathe them? In large part because of what respected authorities teach, or have recently taught, about such persons or groups.

As Syracuse University educators Burton Blatt and Andrejs Ozolins, two exceptional people in mental retardation studies—exceptional because they consider the retarded person's dignity more important than his disability—have soberly observed: "Rarely in the literature and rhetoric of mental

Reprinted, with permission, from *Newsday*, March 16, 1978, p. 93.

retardation is there acknowledgement that but a short time ago in our history the 'leaders in the field' were advocating what is now classed as 'ignorance and superstition' or 'misguided fears.'"

Take the case of Stanford psychologist Lewis Terman, perhaps best known for his development of the IQ (intelligence quotient) tests. You may not know of his view in 1919 that the mentally retarded tended to become "delinquent and criminal." He has had many successors in this sort of foolishness.

As the World War II Allies fought against fascism and the death-camp mentality, two Temple University criminologists went so far as to suggest that, since those lowest on the IQ scale were a burden to their families and society, they should be "painlessly exterminated." And as recently as 1965, two geneticists from the University of Minnesota were recommending voluntary sterilization for the mentally retarded.

Admittedly, many retarded persons are so seriously disabled that they cannot take care of themselves. But is that a reason for *confining* them in *closed institutions?* Small children also cannot take care of themselves; but we don't use that fact to justify their confinement in institutions.

An important historical analogy presents itself in this connection. In the 19th century, the orphan asylum was the pride of western societies determined to prove how deeply they cared for homeless children. Today, there are, for practical purposes, no orphanages. What happened to these institutions of societal benevolence? Did they disappear because we discovered the chemical causes of, and pharmacological cures for, being orphaned? Of course not! Orphanages disappeared when people decided that there was no need for them or for the professionals who ruled them—because orphans could be better cared for through adoption or in foster homes.

Similarly, institutions for the retarded could disappear, and will disappear, when people decide that there is no need for them or for the professionals who rule them because, like the orphans, the retarded can be better cared for in and by the community.

Clearly, there was never any good reason—save the desire of families to expel the infirm—to confine retarded persons in institutions under the auspices of a mental health department. Mentally retarded persons—a category too elastic to allow a good definition—are not unlike other individuals, except that they are impaired in what they can *do:* The very severely impaired cannot dress or feed themselves; the less seriously impaired are just not as capable as most of us in handling facts and figures, reading and writing.

In short, retarded persons are often only unattractive or unproductive or unable to care for themselves—characteristics not limited to members of that group.

As I indicated, for decades mental health and retardation experts have maintained that the best thing for the mentally retarded was institutionalization. Why have people believed such a falsehood? Because the "experts" have promised that it is possible to care for people without experiencing the burden of care. That is the lie our culture is so eager to believe: Its implementation is institutionalized careless care (not just for the retarded but for virtually all infirm people).

The movement to deinstitutionalize mentally retarded persons has not only failed to combat this illusion, it has aggravated it by promising that "residents" in community settings will not cause trouble. But of course they will cause trouble—at least in the sense that they will be more trouble than if they were not there. We will have to trouble ourselves—with their dignity and their genuine welfare—if we are to care for them.

With the passage of time, people have learned to tolerate persons in their midst who differ from them by virtue of color or creed. The integration into the community of the mentally retarded requires a similar tolerance of human differences. In fact, only in such a setting of tolerance will individuals with such handicaps be able to fulfill whatever may be their true potential of humanness.

Surely, not every impaired person can become a Hellen Keller. But just as surely, the story of Helen Keller illustrates how very far we are from having grasped the mystery of the human condition—in which triumphant abilities can burst forth from wellsprings hidden in tragic disabilities.

The move to deinstitutionalize the mentally retarded is an important step in the right direction. But it is a step that is certain to falter and fail, unless it is accompanied by a thorough rethinking and re-evaluation of the role the helping professions are to play in dealing with the mentally retarded.

This examination must go beyond looking at what members of the helping professions can do. It must face the question of what they ought and ought not to do—and what people, as human beings, ought to do for themselves.

Basically, the mentally retarded do not need doctors, hospitals or institutions of any kind. Like all of us, only more so—often very much more so— the retarded need people who truly care *for* them. Perhaps even more, people who take care *of* them. How to do that is not taught in medical schools or graduate schools of psychology or even in schools of divinity. It is a matter of common sense and common decency.

Your Last Will
and Your Free Will

If you are not rich, are not interested in becoming rich, don't know anyone who is rich, and are not afraid of the capricious power of corrupt psychiatrists, then you may not want to read any further. For what follows is about your free will, and your last will, and about how, if you don't watch out, psychiatrists may deprive you of both.

Wealthy persons knowledgeable about the ways of the financial world are usually very careful about the arrangements they make for disposing of their assets after their deaths. They try to reduce, as far as possible, the expenses incurred in transmitting their material possessions to their heirs; and to insure, as far as possible, that these possessions will in fact go to the beneficiaries they have designated in their last will. I will not discuss or even list the numerous financial, legal, and informal-familial strategies which our legal and economic order provides for those proficient in playing the inheritance game. All I want to do here is to call attention to one strategy which wealthy testators and their advisors have often overlooked; such neglect may cost the testator dearly in the post-mortem defense of the validity of his last will, and may result in his bequests ending up in the very hands which, by his free will, he has tried to keep them out of.

The matter I refer to is the contesting of a will by disinherited natural heirs on psychiatric grounds—that is, on the grounds that when the testator executed his last will, he was mentally incompetent to execute a valid will. A hypothetical case—schematic but typical of the sorts of problems encountered with respect to the psychiatric invalidation of wills—will help us to deal with the problem concretely.

The testator, John Doe, dies in his ripe old age and leaves millions of dollars to charities. Doe has never been married and has no children, natural or adopted. But he has several brothers and sisters, nephews and nieces, who want his money and feel "entitled" to it. The "family" retains an attorney; the attorney retains a psychiatrist; the psychiatrist listens to the family's stories about the deceased and concludes that in his "professional opinion" poor John Doe "obviously" did not know who his "rightful heirs" were and was

---

Reprinted, with permission, from the *Alternative,* November 1974, pp. 10-11.

mentally incompetent to execute the Last will he signed. John Doe's lawyer or persons representing the charities inheriting his money or someone must have exercised "undue and improper influence" on him to write such a will. Lubricated by lavish fees, brokers in law and lunacy can appear amazingly sincere and righteous in assuring courts and juries that men such as John Doe did not will what they had put in their wills, but "really" willed what their disinherited relatives would have liked them to will.

What happens next in such a case is that either there is an out-of-court settlement between the contesting parties, the disinherited relatives getting paid off, or the suit goes to court and is decided by a jury. Because of the way the laws of inheritance are written, and because of the way courts interpret such contests, it is actually not easy to break a will on psychiatric grounds. The burden of proof rests on the parties trying to set aside the will. Nevertheless, there is always some risk—great or small depending on circumstances—that the court will set aside the will and award bequests to persons whom the testator wanted to disinherit. Furthermore, even if the testator's estate prevails in court, it will have to bear the costs of defending the testator's free will and upholding the legal validity of his last will—a defense into which it can always be forced by disinherited relatives.

Is there a way in which this undignified, unprofessional, and uneconomic (except for lawyers and psychiatrists) eventuality, which can be easily foreseen in certain cases, could be avoided or prevented? There is indeed, and it seems incredible that it has never, to my knowledge, been articulated.

The preamble to last wills usually begins with a phrase like the following: "I, John Doe, of the City of . . . , County of . . . , and the State of . . . , being of sound mind and memory, . . . hereby make, etc. . . . " Then follow the contents of the will, the testator's signature, the signature and seal of a notary public, and the signatures of witnesses. Unless circumstances prevent it, the will is signed by the testator and witnesses in the presence of the attorney who has prepared the document.

Clearly, there is one thing missing from last wills which would lessen the danger of their being contested on psychiatric grounds: namely, an "Attestation Clause" declaring that James Smith, M.D., a duly licensed physician specializing in psychiatry, having been retained by the testator and his attorney, has examined the testator immediately preceding the act of the testator reading his last will or having it read to him, and of his signing it, and that he finds the testator mentally competent to make a will.

Ostensibly, a contest of wills on psychiatric grounds revolves around the matter of the testator's mental competence to make a will, or his lack of it; hence the need for psychiatrists. Actually, however, it revolves around the matter of the disinherited relatives' power, or their lack of it, to overrule the testator's free will, at least after death if not in life; hence the need for lawyers, juries, and judges. Since legislators, lawyers, courts, and juries deal, and indeed must deal, with the overt rather than the covert, the formal rather than the factual aspects of controversies arising out of will contests based on the testator's mental state; and since last wills typically begin with the testator's self-proclaimed assertion of the soundness of his mind and memory; it seems logical that at least some wills should contain formal psychiatric proof of the testator's capacity to execute a valid testament.

What would happen, what might happen, if wills contained such proof? Faced with such evidence, it seems difficult to see how the courts could allow psychiatric will-contests to develop. How could a court entertain the possibility that an estimate, a mere guess, made by a psychiatrist about a dead person might be more accurate or valid than an "examination" made by a psychiatrist of the same person while he or she was alive? Of course, it could take the position—and quite rightly—that the psychiatrist who examined the testator for his last will was not impartial, that he was in fact a party to the "improper influence" on the testator claimed by the disinherited relatives. But such a claim would unmask—so decisively and dramatically as to render its concealment on future occasions virtually impossible—the boundless hypocrisy of courtroom psychiatry, namely, that the psychiatrist who examines the dead testator on behalf of the disinherited relatives is not exactly impartial either. In short, it would become clear that in such cases, what are ostensibly the expert opinions of medical specialists are actually the semantic services of psychiatric prostitutes.

The psychiatrization of the inheritance game is a dirty business, as is the psychiatrization of any and every aspect of law and life. Cleaning up institutional psychiatry—the pseudo-medical criminal organization which both capitalist and communist societies now accept as a morally and legally legitimate "profession"—will take a long time. In the meanwhile, if you know how the game is played, you can easily protect yourself from the psychiatrist by beating him to the punch.

Dishonoring
Tennessee Williams

On February 24, 1983, Tennessee Williams died in New York. On March 5, 1983, he was buried in an elaborate Roman Catholic ceremony at St. Louis Cathedral, his body laid to rest in the consecrated ground of Calvary Cemetery. "He's finally going to be in a good St. Louis neighborhood," explained Tennessee Williams' younger brother Dakin, who made the funeral arrangements. "Now he's going to be near the right people," he added, referring to General Sherman and Dr. Tom Dooley.

Although this was the funeral Dakin Williams wanted his brother to have, it was precisely the funeral his brother did not want. In his *Memoirs* (1975), Williams wrote: "A codicil to my will provides for the disposition of my body in this way. 'Sewn up in a clean white sack and dropped overboard, twelve hours north of Havana, so that my bones may rest not too far from those of Hart Crane.'"

That this is what Tennessee Williams wanted is corroborated by David Evanier's fine obituary in the *National Review* (March 18, 1983). At the end of his eulogy, Evanier quotes from Dotson Rader's 1981 celebration of his friendship with Williams: "Several years ago . . . Tennessee was talking about death, his own, and how he wanted his burial to be. He took a piece of hotel stationery and dictated a codicil to his will, describing a shipboard service that would mark his passing, and, in very great detail, leaving instructions on precisely where in the Gulf of Mexico he wished his body to be consigned to the sea. It is to be exactly the spot where Hart Crane jumped to his death." Curiously this obituary does not mention how Tennessee Williams was actually buried.

Since we refer to a funeral as paying the deceased our "last respects," and since the funeral Tennessee Williams got was not the funeral he wanted, I submit that we paid him our "last disrespects." I think it is important that we not delude ourselves about this, that we undo this indignity visited on Tennessee Williams, and that we prevent still others from being visited on him.

Our modern Western conception of personal freedom and dignity is rooted in the ethic of respect for persons. If our conduct is informed by this

Written in March 1983. Not previously published.

ethic and if a person asserts that he wants to be treated in a certain way, then we are obligated to treat him the way he has specified. On the other hand, if our conduct is informed by the ethic of paternalism, then, even if a person asserts that he wants to be treated in a certain way, we ought to treat him as we believe he would want to be treated were he able to articulate his "true" interests.

Tennessee Williams and his family seem to have been deeply mired in an unresolved conflict between the demands of these two ethical styles. Indeed, the consequences of this conflict have already affected the disposition of Tennessee Williams' bodily remains and are about to affect the disposition of his estate as well.

In his last will, Williams left the bulk of his estate, estimated at ten million dollars, to the University of the South in Sewanee, Tennessee, "for the purpose of encouraging creative writing and writers in need of financial assistance to pursue their vocation whose work is progressive, original, and preferably of an experimental nature." The will also allocates money to care for Williams' sister Rose, who was lobotomized at the age of twenty-four and has since been confined in various mental institutions. Upon her death, Dakin Williams is to receive $25,000.

On March 12, 1983, just one week after giving his brother the funeral Dakin Williams thought Tennessee should have, the *New York Times* reported that Dakin regarded the entire will as invalid. He is planning to contest the will, he said, contending "that his brother had originally planned to leave his entire estate to him, but had changed his mind because Dakin had him committed to a drug and alcoholism rehabilitation center for three months in 1969. 'He was near death and I saved him,' said Dakin Williams. 'I maintain that I feel he was mentally impaired when he decided to cut me out.'" However, in an earlier interview Dakin Williams acknowledged that his brother deeply resented being psychiatrically incarcerated. "Tennessee never forgave me," said Dakin of that episode.

Is it not perfectly reasonable for a person to disinherit a brother who has degraded and imprisoned him as insane? It certainly seems so to me. But to Dakin Williams the very fact of such lack of insight into and appreciation for his benevolent and therapeutic intentions toward Tennessee constitutes clear evidence of his brother's insanity. It remains to be seen whether Dakin Williams files suit against the University of the South, whether the case goes to court, and whether the court rules Tennessee mentally fit or unfit to know his own best interests.

Of course, Tennessee Williams had no illusions about the horrors that may be hidden behind the mask of "family love." He saw his sister being lobotomized against her will. He saw his mother incarcerated in an insane asylum against her will. He saw himself subjected to "psychiatric rehabilitation" against his will. He would hardly be surprised—could he see us now—by the self-seeking justifications and interventions employed to deny his wishes concerning his burial and possibly the use of his estate.

The grievous violations of personal autonomy implicit in involuntary psychiatric interventions are justified in America by appeals to the overriding value of protecting the "patient's" mental health and preserving his life. "He [Tennessee] would have been dead in five or six years if I hadn't acted," is the way Dakin justified committing his brother. I don't accept this, but most people do.

We live in a secular society, not in a theocracy. That is why involuntary psychiatric interventions do not violate the protections of the First Amendment, but involuntary religious interventions do. What, then, gives a Catholic priest (or any other clergyman) the right to bury a man in a religious ceremony that the deceased did not want? Even if such a priest is not guilty of breaking the law, he is guilty of violating the ethic of respect for persons. Everyone would view giving the Pope a Jewish funeral or Menachem Begin Catholic rites as obscene and disrespectful, not merely of their wishes but of who they are. Surely, Tennessee Williams deserves no less. It is one thing for Dakin Williams to try to deny his brother's autonomy, dignity, and identity. It is another thing for clergymen to cooperate in dishonoring a person under the guise of honoring him.

American journalists, intellectuals, and psychiatrists love to denounce the demeaning of Russian writers and other critics of the Soviet Union by diagnosing them as mad. Indeed, while the Russians call such persons "schizophrenics," we insist on calling them "dissidents." Sadly however, we have treated Tennessee Williams in death rather similarly. We ignored his own wishes and imposed an identity on him he did not want.

Psychiatric Self-Defense

In the past two decades there has been a widening public recognition that much of psychiatric practice rests on or involves coercion and violence. As this recognition grew, there emerged a concern, not least among former psychiatric patients, with "patient's rights," especially the right to reject psychiatric treatment.

Since politics, however, is the art of saying one thing and doing another, the mental health establishment—which is nothing if it isn't political—lost no time in co-opting the patient's rights issue. Whereas formerly the code phrase in the mental health reform business was *mental illness,* now it became *the rights of mental patients.* The phrase *the right to treatment* has become a formidable new weapon in the psychiatrists' perennial struggle to oppress and control the "mental patient."

Today, coercive psychiatrists themselves freely admit that in the past mental patients were deprived of liberty by being involuntarily "warehoused." But that is no longer true, they say. Now mental patients are guaranteed their "right to treatment," especially with so-called anti-psychotic drugs.

The enormous importance of the right-to-treatment rhetoric is illustrated by Kenneth Donaldson's famous appeal to the Supreme Court in 1975. The appeal was brought on Donaldson's behalf by a group of mental health reform lawyers on the ground that Donaldson's rights had been violated when he was deprived of treatment during incarceration in a mental institution. The appeal was supported by every major mental health group in the country, including such traditional enemies of the involuntary mental patient as the American Psychiatric Association and the American Orthopsychiatric Association.

It is important to emphasize and recognize that the mental health establishment's sudden concern with patients' rights has thus left completely untouched the age-old problem of what to do with the "mental patient" who refuses treatment. The stubborn fact is that ever since the birth of psychiatry, people have been deprived of the right to reject the ministrations of mad doctors. For 200 years or more, people were deprived of this right on the grounds that they were "insane" or "psychotic" and hence were incompetent to manage their lives. For the past 15 years or so—since the advent of the

Reprinted, with permission, from *Reason,* May 1983, pp. 41-43.

patients' rights rhetoric—people have been deprived of this right on the ground that their "true interests" require that they receive "life-saving psychiatric treatment." Although some of the legal protections provided to mental patients might have worked to their temporary advantage, I believe that, on balance, the added legal attention lavished on the so-called rights of mental patients has served only to authenticate further the legitimacy of depriving them of the only right that counts—the right to reject treatment, the right to reject being cast in the role of mental patient; in short, the right to reject psychiatric authority.

Ending the Reign of the Psychiatric Inquisition

Whenever force is an established method of resolving an ideological conflict, it is likely that the proponents and opponents of force do not speak the same language. For example, during the waning days of the Inquisition, the advocates of clerical tortures feared heresy and the imaginary terrors of eternal damnation and embraced the Inquisition as a protection against these dangers; whereas the critics of such torture feared the Inquisition and its very real terrors and embraced the ideas of the Enlightenment as a protection against these dangers. Today, the proponents of psychiatric coercion fear psychosis and the dire consequences of psychiatric neglect; whereas the opponents of such coercion fear psychiatry and the dire consequences of involuntary psychiatric interventions.

Recently, a report on "patients' rights" in *Psychiatric News,* the American Psychiatric Association's official newspaper, explained that psychiatrists no longer think "in terms of physical restrictions on freedom but of the shackles of [psychiatric] illness itself and the patient's right to freedom from this mental restraint." The report cited the views of two "experts" on patients' rights according to whom involuntary mental hospitalization and "treatment" actually increase the involuntary mental patient's freedom:

> We would submit that commitment can be justified on the grounds of enhancing the individual's freedom. If society insisted that freedom be the only purpose of commitment, commitment to achieve a real lack of unnecessary constraints from mental illness and to increase a patient's options could be justified. . . . Such an approach . . . would place psychiatry fully behind the principle that psychiatric institutions be utilized for increasing the freedom of the mentally ill.

This rhetoric of "psychiatric slavery in the name of mentally healthy freedom" explains a seeming paradox: the professional advocates of the rights of mental patients are the most determined adversaries of former mental patients' groups that are lobbying for mental patients' right to reject treatment.

Sadly, but not surprisingly, psychiatric reformers have sought and continue to seek to improve the mental health system by doing even more for the patient, for society, or for both. Thus, they have tried to protect the patient from himself or from those who might exploit or mistreat him; they have tried to protect society from the "dangerous" patient and his "illness"; and, most recently, they have tried to restore the "sick patient" to "mental health." Each of these efforts is paternalistic in principle and coercive in practice.

The individualist approach to the core problem of psychiatry—namely, coercion in the name of mental health—is radically different. Viewing psychiatric coercion as essentially similar to religious coercion, the individualist solution to it is also similar. That solution, exemplified by the founding fathers' position on clerical power, was to protect the free practice of religion but to abolish coercion in the name of God. The individualist solution to clinical coercion is the same: to protect the free practice of psychiatry but to abolish coercion in the name of mental health.

Simple? Of course. Why, then, are so few people interested in it? The answer to that question is not so simple. I shall point here to only one of the reasons for it.

When the United States went through its birth pangs, violence in the name of God was an accepted political and legal principle throughout Europe and indeed the whole world. What justified this practice? We know the answer only too well: an alliance between church and state that made the use of force in the service of God as legitimate as the use of force in the service of Caesar. The soldier protected the commonwealth from external enemies. The inquisitor protected it from internal enemies, especially heretics.

The problem of religious coercion, like the problem of psychiatric coercion, could be approached in two ways. One way would be to look to the state to protect the victims of clerical power. This would generate a rhetoric about the rights of heretics and demands for guaranteeing the heretic's right to proper (that is, orthodox) worship. The other approach would be to recognize that the source of clerical power lies in an alliance between church and state. This realization would generate (as it did in the United States) a rhetoric about the separation of church and state and demands for making worship the private affair of the worshipper.

We can easily see how the first course only aggravates the problem. By guaranteeing the absurdity of the heretic's right to embrace the true faith, it further authenticates the legitimacy of religious coercion. Similarly, psychiatric coercion, being the result of an alliance between psychiatry and the state, can be ended only by a separation of psychiatry and the state. Any other course, particularly the state's "guaranteeing" the absurd right of mental patients to receive treatment can lead only to reauthenticating the legitimacy of psychiatric coercion. The history of mental health reform in the United States during the past 15 years illustrates and supports the validity of this interpretation.

Psychiatrists, however, contend that insane persons—out of touch with reality, misinterpreting therapy as torture—cannot competently consent to or reject psychiatric interventions. And many people, perhaps the majority of the population, believe that this is true. So some special legal mechanism is necessary for realistically implementing a separation of psychiatry and the state. Such a mechanism is prefigured in procedures that people in Western societies have developed for coping with other situations in which a moral agent's capacity to act competently is diminished or destroyed. There are two typical situations of this sort: death and incapacitating terminal illness. And there are two legal instruments that have been developed to cope with them: wills (last wills and testaments) and so-called living wills. I propose that we create a third type of will—the "psychiatric will."

Securing the Right to an Unmolested Mind

Many of us are eager to exercise our desires over the distribution of our property after we die. The purpose of the last will is to assure this by extending our control into a situation in which we cannot otherwise exercise any control at all.

While the use of last wills is an ancient practice, the use of living wills, in anticipation of a lingering, painful, and expensive terminal illness, is of more recent origin. Executed while the person is not disabled by illness, a living will directs those responsible for caring for its author to abstain under certain circumstances from administering life-sustaining measures. The legal philosophy underlying this practice is illustrated by the following opinion of a Kansas court: "Anglo-American law starts with the premise of thorough-going self-determination. It follows that each man is considered to be the master of his own body, and he may, if he be of sound mind, expressly prohibit the performance of life-saving surgery."

The psychiatric will I propose rests on the same principle and seeks to extend it to "mental treatment." It asserts, in effect, that competent American adults should have a recognized right to reject ahead of time involuntary psychiatric interventions that they may be deemed to require in the future when they are considered incompetent to make decisions concerning their own welfare. My model for the psychiatric will is the so-called living will and, more specifically, the rejection by Jehovah's Witnesses of blood transfusion as a medical treatment.

A frequently cited opinion concerning the constitutionality of allowing Jehovah's Witnesses to reject blood transfusion, even when the transfusion may be lifesaving, was formulated in 1964 by Chief Justice (then U.S. Circuit Court Judge) Warren Burger. In this opinion, Burger recalled Justice Brandeis's famous words about our "right to be let alone." "The makers of our Constitution," wrote Brandeis, "sought to protect Americans in their beliefs, their thoughts, their emotions, and their sensations. They conferred, as against the Government, the right to be let alone—the most comprehensive of rights, the right most valued by civilized man." To which Burger added these (for my present purposes, decisive) words: "Nothing in this utterance suggests that Justice Brandeis thought an individual possessed these rights only as to *sensible* beliefs, *valid* thoughts, *reasonable* emotions, or *well-founded* sensations. I suggest he intended to include a great many foolish, unreasonable, and even absurd ideas which do not conform, such as refusing medical treatment even at great risk."

As we have seen, then, where the person is conscious and rational, the courts have tended to accept the principle that a person has a right to refuse medical treatment even if the result is death. "Even in an emergency situation," an article in the *Journal of Medical Ethics* recently explained, "where death would ensue if treatment were not administered, the court upheld a patient's refusal of treatment."

Since involuntary psychiatric intervention is rarely lifesaving (and even if it were, that would not be enough under the foregoing ethical-legal principles to justify its forcible imposition on unwilling clients), the *parens patriae* rationale for psychiatric coercion is fatally undermined. The psychiatric will would implement the right to reject psychiatric treatment for people deemed to be fully competent and rational at the time they made their decision. On what constitutional, moral, or political grounds could Americans be denied this right?

Establishing the Form of the Psychiatric Will

Many people (and virtually all psychiatrists and other mental health experts) fear the danger of a "nervous breakdown" or "psychotic illness." These people believe that mental illness exists, that it is like any other illness, that it is amenable to modern psychiatric treatment, and that the effectiveness and legitimacy of such treatment do not depend on the patient's consent to it. Accordingly, such people seek protection from "life-threatening" mental illness and support the use of involuntary psychiatric interventions.

On the other hand, there are other people (including a few psychiatrists and other mental health experts) who fear the danger of compulsory psychiatry or involuntary "therapy." Some of these people also believe that mental illness does *not* exist and that psychiatric coercion is torture rather than treatment. Accordingly, these people seek protection from the powers of psychiatry and advocate the abolition of involuntary psychiatric interventions.

Let us now apply the principles underlying the last testament and the living will to the psychiatric contingency some people might want to anticipate and control, such as "sudden madness" or "acute psychosis." Since involuntary psychiatric confinement is a tradition-honored custom in modern societies, people ought to anticipate the possibility of their own sudden madness managed by others by means of commitment and coerced treatment. To forestall that happening, we need a mechanism permitting anyone who has reached the age of maturity to execute a "psychiatric will" prohibiting his confinement in a mental hospital or his involuntary treatment for "mental illness." Those failing to execute such a document before an actual encounter with coercive psychiatry would, of course, have the opportunity to do so as soon as they "recovered" from their first episode of "mental illness" or otherwise regained their competence.

Since commitment entails the loss of liberty, the foregoing mechanism for its protection is relatively weak. It requires the affirmative assertion of a desire to do without involuntary psychiatric care, and in the absence of such a declaration, the person would remain a potentially defenseless victim of psychiatric coercion. So even though this kind of psychiatric will would be a great improvement over the present situation, a more powerful document could be fashioned by shifting the presumptive rights. In this stronger version, a person would be free from psychiatric coercion unless he executed a psychiatric will in advance that asserted his right to such coercion should the "need" for it arise. This arrangement would leave most of us free from psychiatric coercion, much as we are free, without having to go to such troubles, from religious coercion.

The second version of the psychiatric will is stronger and theoretically more attractive than the first. But because the paternalistic perspective on involuntary psychiatric interventions is now so prevalent, the weaker version may be more acceptable to most people and to their elected representatives. Of course, the rejection of psychiatric interventions need not be total in either version of such a will. For example, some persons might wish to authorize coerced hospitalization and to forbid treatment by drugs or electroshock, while others might wish to authorize coerced drug therapy and to forbid confinement. Only through a mechanism such as this could the responsibilities as well as the rights of the "severely mentally ill" be expanded.

The use of psychiatric wills might put an end to the dispute about involuntary psychiatric interventions. Earnestly applied, such a policy should satisfy the demands of involuntary psychiatry's proponents (the psychiatric protectionists) and its opponents (the psychiatric voluntarists). Surely, the psychiatric protectionists could not in good faith object when people who were competent to make binding decisions about their own future chose to prohibit personally unauthorized psychiatric assistance. Nor could the psychiatric abolitionists really complain when other people who were competent to make binding decisions about their future chose to permit their own temporary (or not-so-temporary) psychiatric "enslavement."

Finally, it should be noted that although the main purpose of the psychiatric will would be to protect potential patients from unwanted psychiatric interventions, such a document would also protect would-be therapists from the risks they now face in their relations with involuntary mental patients. This dual function of the psychiatric will is inherent in its being an instrument for transforming a status relationship into a contractual relationship.

As matters now stand, psychiatrists faced with the task of having to care for "seriously ill mental patients" often find themselves in a Catch-22 situation. They are in danger of being sued both for confining and for failing to confine the "patient," for using coercive treatment as well as for failing to use it. The psychiatric will, prospectively requesting or refusing involuntary psychiatric interventions, would constitute a contract between potential future psychiatric patients and their potential future psychiatrists. Hence, while it would protect the former from psychiatric coercion or psychiatric neglect (as the case may be), it would protect the latter from charges of unauthorized treatment or unprofessional neglect.

Psychosurgery: Aborting Unwanted Behavior

Dr. Peter Black's arguments in support of psychosurgery ignore my writings and my views. For example, he declares that "they [the anti-psychosurgical writers] feel that these procedures should not be used at all regardless of the supposed indications for them." That is not my position. I would drop my moral opposition to psychosurgery if its use were strictly limited to those who want it and give informed consent for it.

Throughout his essay, Dr. Black confuses disease with deviance and cure with control, in the manner characteristic of contemporary psychiatrists and psychosurgeons. For example, he asserts that "if a man murders another or attempts suicide, some kind of action seems indicated." He evidently likes to think of homicide and suicide as similar acts; and he accepts the premise that suicide, or so-called threatened suicide, is a crime or a disease, or both. Successful suicide leaves only a corpse, and I doubt that even Dr. Black would propose driving a leucotome through the deceased person's brain. Driving a stake through his body (which used to be the punishment for suicide in England), though surgically less sophisticated, ought still to satisfy those who, like Dr. Black, regard suicide as a species of murder.

It is, of course, extremely revealing that Dr. Black (and others who support his views) equates homicide with suicide. To me, those two acts stand in the same sort of relation to each other as do rape and masturbation. I view homicide as the gravest crime, and suicide as the most basic human right. *Mutatis mutandis,* in my opinion, a surgical intervention, whether for real healing or for rationalized self-mutilation, is—if the client makes an uncoerced contract for it and can find a cooperating surgeon to perform it—like any other service that adults in a free society should be left free to seek or reject. However, such an intervention, regardless of its aim or outcome, is—if it is forced on a client under the threat of penal sanctions or is imposed on him in any way against his will—like any other assault on his life and liberty and should therefore be considered to be not a treatment but a grave medical crime.

First published as "Aborting Unwanted Behavior: The Controversy on Psychosurgery," *The Humanist,* July/August 1977, pp. 7-11, a response to Dr. Peter Black's essay on psychosurgery in the same issue. Reprinted with permission.

Although Dr. Black lists informed consent as one of the "conditions justifying psychosurgery," his remarks throughout the article make it clear that he does not propose to limit psychosurgical interventions to individuals who give such consent. Indeed, among the examples of "patients" potentially suitable for psychosurgery, he lists a hypothetical husband who is depressed and who, as a result, hurts his wife and others. How? Here is Dr. Black's answer: "With this [that is, a 'severe depression'] a man may lose his job, make bad decisions about his family and marriage, and even kill himself. To what extent does this involve danger to the well-being of others?" Dr. Black does not seem to want to entertain the possibility that some husbands want to hurt their wives, and vice versa, and that physicians now often call this sort of behavior "depression." The naive medicalization of morals that Dr. Black engages in—both in this connection and in treating murder and mayhem as if they were the symptoms of a sickness—requires no further comment here.

Actually, Dr. Black advocates the use of lobotomy on persons who do not consent to it. But—and this is what makes his essay and so many others like it particularly objectionable from a moral and political point of view—he does not say so. What he says, instead, is that "rarely, a claim by his [the patient's] family or by the state that he constitutes a danger to others might be accepted [as a justification for psychosurgery]." Dr. Black also asserts that most persons on whom psychosurgeons operate are not really human beings, in the political sense of that word: "In most cases the person contemplated for behavioral surgery is not a 'free' man or woman before surgery or the procedure would not be undertaken. . . . The fact that psychosurgery is done to restore rather than destroy individual autonomy sometimes is neglected by those opposed to it." The difference between this modern clinical claim, that "unfree" men and women are lobotomized to "restore their autonomy," and the medieval clerical claim, that "bewitched" men and women are burned at the stake to save their souls, is, I submit, entirely technical. Morally and politically, the relationship between those who make the claim and those who supposedly benefit from it seems to me the same in both cases.[1]

It is, of course, useless to try to clarify a concept that a person does not want to understand. A disease may disable a person, but cannot disfranchise him. If a person is struck by a car on his way to a voting booth, his ability to vote will be taken away, but his right to vote will not be. Declaring a person unfit to accept or reject a (so-called) therapeutic intervention is, par excellence, a political act. The question that Dr. Black avoids and that virtually all psychiatrists and psychosurgeons avoid, is this: Why and how does a person become converted from a free American citizen to an unfree patient on whom psychosurgery will be performed whether he likes it or not? That question, of course, leads to the questions of mental illness and responsibility, which Dr. Black does not consider and which I have considered elsewhere.[2]

To indicate my own views on psychosurgery, and to show how persistently its advocates—in this case, Dr. Black—ignore and sidestep my arguments, I quote below some of my published remarks on this subject and on the significance of consent and coercion in medical ethics.

When surgeons operate on the brain of a person with brain disease, they call what they do "neurosurgery"; when they operate on the brain of a person without brain disease, they call it "psychosurgery." It's a nice arrangement for neurosurgeons: it allows them to operate regardless of whether their patient has or has not a disease of the brain; and, because the persons without brain diseases but destined for such surgical interventions are often declared to be legally incompetent on account of "mental illness," it also allows them to operate regardless of whether their ostensible patient requests or rejects the operation.[3]

Psychosurgery changes the way a person thinks, just as plastic surgery changes the way he or she looks. The most important difference between them is that in plastic surgery the intervention is initiated by the person who seeks a change in his or her own body, whereas in psychosurgery it is initiated by a person who seeks a change in someone else's brain. Involuntary lobotomy for schizophrenia might thus be compared to, say, involuntary mastectomy for women with alluring breasts—an intervention that could be justified if those opposed to women having such breasts seized power, decreed the condition a mental disease, and defined mastectomy as the treatment for it.[4]

What justifies a therapeutic intervention—that is, an action by an individual called "physician" taken vis-à-vis the person or body of an individual called "patient"?

To the true believer in medicine, it is the disease which the alleged patient has; to the medical autocrat and to those who believe in him, it is the physician's judgment that the patient needs the treatment and that he—or his family or society—would benefit from it; to the loyal physician/employee of the Therapeutic State, and to those who believe in him, it is the decision of the government; and to the libertarian, it is the consent of the would-be patient.

Overlooking or confusing these conflicting moral and political premises and perspectives is the source of most of our so-called problems in medical ethics.[5]

Not satisfied with the controls of contract, some critics of psychiatric brutalities seek the remedy in the enemy—the state—for example, by advocating the prohibition of lobotomy. However, since they cannot advocate prohibiting a therapeutic procedure, they, too, must first rename what they want to remove: they say that lobotomy is not medicine but mutilation.

But who defines mutilation? Is abortion not mutilation? Or the ritual circumcision of a healthy infant?

Contract and consent suffice to protect those who want to be protected. Any attempt to extend protection beyond this limit makes the "reformers" indistinguishable from the therapeutic totalitarians they oppose.[6]

In short, I am wholly in favor of free trade in psychosurgery between consenting adults. Insofar as other critics of psychosurgery favor banning lobotomy (or any other psychosurgical procedure), I oppose them just as vehemently as I oppose those who favor banning abortion, heroin, pornography, or schizophrenia.[7]

I believe we could clarify our thinking about psychosurgery if we compared it to abortion. In both cases, a surgical intervention is performed on a person's body not for the purpose of curing a disease but for some other purpose: in one case, for removing an unwanted fetus; in the other, for removing unwanted feelings or behavior.

The analogy between abortion and, say, lobotomy yields some surprising results. Liberals, who are notoriously fuzzy-headed about medical matters, are apt to be for abortion but against lobotomy. I find it difficult to see, however, why one woman should have the right to hire a doctor to destroy the fetus in her womb, but that another woman, or a man, should not have the right to hire a doctor to destroy a part of her, or his, brain. Clearly, there are two separate and separable issues here, each extremely vexing, but each more easily dealt with alone than in combination with the other.

One issue is whether abortion/lobotomy is a good or bad thing. The answer to this question will depend, on the one hand, on the observer's medical and moral views on the nature of pregnancy and the ethically appropriate options for dealing with unwanted pregnancy and, on the other hand, on his medical and moral views on the nature of personal conduct and its relation to the human brain and the ethically appropriate options for dealing with unwanted behavior.

The other issue is whether abortion/lobotomy should be outlawed altogether, dispensed by medical discretion, imposed according to medical/legal criteria, or be made contractually available at the request of the person seeking the service. Although our choice among these options is likely to be informed and influenced by our views on the nature of abortion/lobotomy, it is possible to articulate an unambiguous policy concerning these procedures without debating the complex medical and moral questions that lie behind them.[8]

Humanists and libertarians—whatever they might think about the fetus as an actual or potential person—endorse the proposition that a woman should be free to seek an abortion. But they would, and should, recoil in horror from the proposition that—under certain circumstances, say where the fetus is a threat to the mother or vice versa—a pregnant woman ought to be aborted whether she likes it or not. I submit that humanists and libertarians—whatever they might think about frontal lobes and free will—ought similarly to endorse the proposition that a person should be free to seek a lobotomy. But they ought to recoil in horror from the proposition that—under certain circumstances, say where the person is dangerous to himself or others—a "psychotic patient" ought to be lobotomized whether he likes it or not.

Accordingly, in my opinion, any physician who endorses, much less advocates, the use of coerced abortion—that is, killing a mother's fetus against her will—is a menace to medicine, morals, and our most treasured personal and political liberties; and so is any physician who endorses, much less advocates, the use of coerced lobotomy—that is, killing a person's soul against his will. Since psychosurgeons in general, and Dr. Black in particular in the present article, endorse and advocate such a policy, they continue to constitute a grave threat to our personal freedom and dignity.

Notes

1. See T. S. Szasz, *The Manufacture of Madness: A Comparative Study of the Inquisition and the Mental Health Movement* (New York: Harper & Row, 1970).

2. See Szasz, *The Myth of Mental Illness: Foundations of a Theory of Personal Conduct,* revised ed. (New York: Harper & Row, 1974).

3. Szasz, *Heresies* (Garden City, N.Y.: Doubleday Anchor, 1976), p. 94.

4. Ibid., pp. 98-99.

5. Ibid., pp. 87-88.

6. Ibid, p. 134.

7. See Szasz, *Ceremonial Chemistry: The Ritual Persecution of Drugs, Addicts, and Pushers* (Garden City, N.Y.: Doubleday, 1974).

8. See Szasz, *The Theology of Medicine: The Political-Philosophical Foundations of Medical Ethics* (Baton Rouge: Louisiana State Univ. Press, 1977).

The Electroshock Dilemma

Should civil libertarians support or oppose the law banning electric-shock therapy (electric convulsive therapy, ECT), passed by the voters of Berkeley, California on November 2, 1982, and currently being challenged? The proponents of the law argue that it protects mental patients from brain damage by electroshock. The opponents argue that it prevents psychiatrists from giving, and mental patients from getting, an essential and effective treatment. I shall argue that civil libertarians should reject both of these options and refuse to be satisfied with anything less than freedom of choice of medical treatment safeguarded from state-sanctioned fraud and force.

To understand this dilemma it is necessary to understand the legal-psychiatric context in which the movement to ban electric-shock treatment in Berkeley arose. The context combines two complex elements: medical paternalism (the principle that "doctor knows best") and the ostensibly scientific claim that electrically induced grand-mal seizures are therapeutic. In its psychiatric version, paternalism is a particularly nefarious principle enabling those who wield it not only to impose their will on their victims but also to rationalize their rapine as the realization of their victims' own most deeply felt, albeit unarticulated, desires. Acts of patent violence are thus transformed into acts of putative therapeutic benevolence. Without the long, shameful history of involuntary mental hospitalization and treatment in America, and without the horrifying history of ECTs being given to persons against their will, it is unlikely that the residents of Berkeley would have had much interest in an anti-ECT proposition or that they would have approved it.

While objections to the use of ECT are as old as ECT itself, the notion of placing a proposition prohibiting it on the Berkeley ballot for the November 1982 election was the brainchild of former mental patient Theodore Chabasinski. Now forty-six, Chabasinski was diagnosed as suffering from schizophrenia when he was only six years old. The twenty electroshock treatments he received for it as a child evidently left him with a lasting passion for avenging this wrong. In 1982, Chabasinski organized a small cadre of ECT-victims and their friends into a group called the "Coalition to Stop Electroshock," which drafted "Measure T," as the proposition was called,

Reprinted, with permission, from *Inquiry*, July 1983, pp. 26-29.

and obtained the 1400 signatures necessary to place it on the ballot. With that seemingly quixotic move began a fight between a David and a Goliath—the miniscule Coalition to Stop Electroshock and the giant American Psychiatric Association (APA). The APA immediately invested $15,000 in the campaign against the measure, with a promise of "further technical and financial assistance."

The Coalition to Stop Electroshock spent about $2000 on the campaign. Despite being outspent by more than 7 to 1 (and despite the fact that all of the "authoritative opinion" fed to the public by the press opposed Measure T), the initiative passed by a large margin: 25,883 votes for the ban, 16,609 against it. Thus, on December 3, 1983, the use of ECT became illegal in Berkeley. The law, known as "Berkeley City Ordinance 5504-NS," reads as follows:

> The people of the City of Berkeley do ordain as follows: Section 1. *Title:* The title of this ordinance shall be "An Act to Protect the Human Rights of Psychiatric Patients by Prohibiting the Use of Electric Shock Treatment in Berkeley." Section 2. *Declaration of policy.* It is hereby recognized and declared that all persons within the City of Berkeley, including all persons involuntarily confined, have a fundamental right against interference with their thought processes and states of mind through the use of electric shock treatment. Section 3. *Prohibition:* The administration of electric shock treatment to any person within the City of Berkeley is hereby prohibited.

Violating the ordinance is a misdemeanor punishable by "not more than six months imprisonment, a fine of not more than $500, or both."

The passage of the anti-ECT proposition in Berkeley has not gone unchallenged. The Northern California Psychiatric Society, the American Psychiatric Association, the California Psychiatric Association, the National Association of Private Psychiatric Hospitals, and Ronald Bortman, M.D., quickly joined forces, as plaintiffs, and promptly sued the City of Berkeley for "declaratory and injunctive relief" on the ground that the ban on ECT was unconstitutional. The plaintiffs were joined by the American Medical Association and the California Medical Association with a friend-of-the-court brief. Their brief rests on two basic contentions: first, that ECT is a lawful and scientifically established psychiatric treatment, essential and effective in the management of certain mental diseases; second, that the ban on ECT deprives patients from getting, and psychiatrists from giving, this valuable treatment.

Although official psychiatry now credits ECT with miraculous healing powers, it is not difficult, even among orthodox practitioners, to find opinions condemning ECT in the harshest terms. Just as the controversy about ECT was heating up in Berkeley, a prominent Swiss psychiatrist, Paul Kielholz, disavowed its use: "We prohibited the use of electroshock years ago."

The City of Berkeley (the defendant) presented its opposing brief, stating:

> The people of Berkeley enacted a ban on electric shock treatment because they agreed . . . that its efficacy had not been proved in any scientific manner . . . that there was significant evidence of adverse long-term effects, including permanent brain damage . . . [and] that the inherently coercive nature of the psychiatric context coupled with the zeal of ECT proponents makes it very difficult for an individual to give informed consent to the procedure.

Both the brief for the defendant and for the plaintiffs share an important similarity: Each rests on the legitimacy of paternalism in medical matters, be it governmental or "scientific." Both briefs look to "guardians" to protect adult Americans from their own ill-advised choices. Both postures infantilize the citizen: one with the familiar political claim that "government knows best," the other with the equally familiar medical claim that "doctor knows best." The option of enlarging the peoples' freedom by enlarging their own choices is completely absent from these considerations. Moreover, the brief for the defendant plays into the hands of the plaintiffs' argument by sharing not only its paternalistic presumptions but also by going out of its way to reassure the court that the ban ". . . does not imply that mental disorders do not exist, or that we have no help, but that such questions come down to subjective opinion." But mental illness has nothing to do with the matter. We have a right to reject Holy Communion (or any other religious ritual) regardless of whether or not God exists; similarly, we ought to have a right to reject ECT (or any other psychiatric procedure) regardless of whether or not mental illness exists. Having these rights comes down simply to withdrawing the sanction of the state from violence, whether committed in the name of God or in the name of Mental Health. Indeed, not only is banning ECT undesirable in principle, it is unlikely to be effective as practical policy. Psychiatrists can invent brain-damaging "treatments"—such as "antipsychotic" chemicals— faster than ex-mental patients can get them banned. Thus, prohibiting the use of ECT is like chopping off the head of the legendary Hydra.

The Berkeley controversy over banning ECT combines two quite separate issues: One is the alleged therapeutic effectiveness of ECT; the other is whether a practice said to be an effective "therapy for mental illness," such as ECT, should or should not be imposed on a person against his will. Resolving the question of the effectiveness of ECT is at once impossible and easy— some maintain that ECT is an effective therapy; others that it is not, or that it is harmful, or that it is not, in any meaningful sense of the term, a "therapy" at all. The same difference of opinion prevails today about many medical practices, from blood transfusion to laetrile.

However, we must not let these differences of opinion distract us from the far more important issue at hand, namely, whether or not any so-called therapeutic measure should ever be imposed on an adult person against his declared will. In this respect, we have the following options: Either we impose the views of the proponents of a particular practice on those who object to them; or we impose the views of opponents on those who object to them; or we allow only consensual therapeutic relations. Present laws regulating the use of ECT illustrate the first option, permitting the electroshocking of individuals against their will. Present laws regulating the use of laetrile illustrate the second option, prohibiting the use of this drug by persons who want it. Present laws regulating the use of aspirin illustrate the third option, allowing anyone to use or not use it as he sees fit.

To reiterate: If the helpfulness of a practice does not justify its coerced use, and if its harmfulness does not justify its prohibition—in other words, if the decision to employ or eschew an alleged remedy remains with the consumer or patient—then the helpfulness or harmfulness of ECT becomes irrelevant to whether or not it should be banned. The electroshock contestants' claims concerning the rights of mental patients are equally misleading: The proponents of ECT want only to protect the "patient's" right to *receive* ECT; the opponents of ECT want only to protect his right to *reject* it. Neither position offers the individual the option of a fully responsible choice: to decide—with all the help anyone cares to give him, but in the end on his own—whether to receive or reject ECT.

The banning of ECT in Berkeley is an important event for two reasons. First, because it raises, in a public forum, the question of whether or not ECT constitutes a bona fide medical treatment. Second, because it condenses and symbolizes, in concrete and dramatic form, the basic moral-political problem that has so long bedeviled psychiatry, namely: Should persons in a free society be able to choose—that is, accept *or* reject—so-called psychiatric interventions? In effect, then, the controversy over ECT is a small-scale version of the larger controversy over involuntary mental interventions of all kinds (especially incarceration in so-called hospitals). Clarifying the assumptions and aspirations of the proponents and opponents of coercion in the name of mental health—a principle that undergirds the whole psychiatric profession—should help to clarify our judgments concerning the current controversy over ECT.

The difference between the proponents and opponents of involuntary psychiatric interventions is rooted in the different views they have of the world about them. Looking at psychiatry, the former see the horrors of psychotic illness, the latter the horrors of psychiatric coercion; the former focus on and fear the dire consequences of psychiatric neglect, the latter focus on and fear the dire consequences of compulsory psychiatric "treatment." This is why the proponents and opponents of involuntary psychiatric interventions do not really speak the same language. With no way of amicably resolving the conflict, this controversy has instead been settled the way all such conflicts typically are—by the party possessing more power imposing its will on its adversary. With power traditionally in the hands of the psychiatrists, psychiatric coercion has been the rule: That is why psychiatric confinement is called "hospitalization" instead of "imprisonment," why ECT is called a "treatment" instead of a "torture."

The ban on ECT in Berkeley in November 1982 is a historic event because, for the first time ever, ex-mental patients and the general non-psychiatric patient population of Berkeley took to the polls to impose their view about a particular psychiatric intervention on the medical profession and the rest of the public. No one can deny that the ban on ECT deprives the psychiatrists who want to give ECT, and the patients who want to get it, from entering into a mutually agreed-upon contract concerning this so-called psychiatric treatment. But before the ban—when ECT could be, and was, administered to individuals against their will—in effect every man, woman, and child was deprived of the right to reject this "treatment."

Where, then, does this leave us? Because the psychiatric context in which "patients" consent' to treatments, especially ECT, is saturated with coercion, and because psychiatrists passionately believe they have a right, indeed a duty, to force treatment even on competent patients, there is an obvious judicial need to protect the mental patient either from psychiatric coercion in general or from specifically dangerous procedures, such as ECT. An illustration of the APA's uncompromising opposition to the patient's right to refuse treatment, regardless of whether he is legally competent, may be found in a recent friend-of-the-court brief it has filed in a case now before the Massachusetts Supreme Judicial Court. A report in *Psychiatric News* (the APA's newspaper), January 21, 1983, titled with rare candor "APA files brief supporting forced medication," sets forth this position as follows:

> The patient's liberty interests are best served by taking medication. The concepts of "competency," "informed consent," and "substitute judgment" sound good in theory but, in fact, work against the patient's independence. Being found competent protects the civil rights of a committed patient, but it was never intended to cover medication decisions. . . . Even competent patients remain seriously mentally ill and are often unable to understand attempts at informed consent. . . . [A] patient needs to be treated quickly and effectively so he can regain liberty. . . .

Symbolically, there is a serious lesson to be learned from the fact that a group of American citizens would go so far as to prohibit a practice officially defined and established as "medical" and "therapeutic." For centuries, men, women, and children in the West were the victims of religious violence. Finally, there came a time when people revolted against the priest as a persecutor. In the United States, the result was the separation of church and state, protecting people from religious coercion and leaving them free to be helped or harmed by religion, as they saw fit. In the communist world, the result was the prohibition of religion, protecting the people not only from the cleric's coercion but from the (alleged) harmfulness of his teaching as well.

Let us not deceive ourselves. Today, the psychiatrist is empowered by the state to give ECT not only to persons who want it but, under certain circumstances, also to those who do not want it. Faced with this situation, we have three basic options: We can take away the psychiatrist's power, we can take away his ECT, or we can leave things as they are. Taking away the psychiatrist's power would be like the Founding Fathers' abolishing priestly power: Psychiatric help, like religious help, could be given to anyone who wants it, but it would no longer justify the use of force. Taking away the psychiatrist's ECT would be like the communists' abolishing religion: People would be "protected" from psychiatry and its coercive practices—albeit paternalistically, for they would be regarded as children who need the state's protection from their wicked "exploiters" and their weak selves. Leaving things as they are would be like continuing to support the Inquisition: We would continue to prattle about the "rights of mental patients," as if heretics could have rights in a theocratic society; and we would congratulate ourselves on our humanitarian laws guaranteeing the "mental patient's right to treatment," as if inquisitors had ever wanted to deprive heretics of their right to worship God.

On January 13, 1983, Alameda County Superior Court Judge Donald P. McCullum issued an injunction restraining the City of Berkeley from enforcing the law prohibiting the use of ECT. The case is now pending further adjudication in the courts. I would not venture to predict the ultimate outcome—in the courts or in the forum of public opinion—of the struggle over ECT in Berkeley. As I suggested, this controversy is but a symptom of a more general conflict in our society between the values of submitting to psychiatric authority on the one hand, and of exercising personal autonomy on the other. Banning ECT is a far cry from victory for libertarian principles over psychiatric violence. But once placed on the ballot, not banning ECT would have been a convincing victory for psychiatric violence over the elementary human right to reject unwanted "psychiatric help."

Ironically, neither sustaining the ban in the courts nor overturning it will have the slightest effect on the root problem of psychiatry—the fraud and force that permeate its practices (especially those directed toward "helping" persons said to be "seriously mentally ill"). We in the West have long ago repudiated the legitimacy of violence in the name of God. So long as we do not similarly repudiate the legitimacy of violence in the name of Mental Health, the very term "psychiatric help" will carry an impossible load of ambivalence, rendering it useless, if not obscene.

Terror by Tylenol

In the same breath in which the world learned about murder by cyanide-laced Tylenol, it also learned what sort of person did it: a madman. Such has been our progress since the Middle Ages. When unexplained tragedy struck then, people were no less able and ready to account for it: the witches did it! The Jews did it! It doesn't matter that such explanations are not true, do not explain and even impede the genuine understanding and rational solution of the problem.

The mass mind is like the child's. It cannot bear unexplained events that frighten it. Since it lacks the means for rational understanding, it "explains" by means of fantasized images and magical incantations.

Presumably, no one knows who is responsible for the Tylenol murders or why he or she has done these deeds. Nor will we know the answer to these questions until we have identified the killer or killers. But we seem unable to bear the burden of such rational uncertainty. Simultaneously with the announcement of the Tylenol murders, the media as well as the persons responsible for apprehending and convicting the culprit were informing the public that the killer was a "madman." On Oct. 2, after the sixth victim died but before the news of the seventh victim had reached the press, one news story spoke about the FBI's mounting a broad investigation to find a "crazed madman" responsible for the kilings. Mind you, they are not looking for just a plain madman, they are looking for a "crazed madman"! The Oct. 11 *Newsweek* story on the case stated matter-of-factly: "The death of seven people who took the drug triggers a nationwide alert—and a hunt for a madman." It must be nice to be so sure.

An editorial in the *New York Times* on Oct. 5, taking for granted that the Tylenol terrorist was mentally ill, intoned: "The acts of aberrant minds are hard to guard against, impossible to accept. Hurricanes are easier to cope with than psychopaths." This is simply not true. Worse, it is true only if and because we equate viciousness with mental illness and thus incapacitate ourselves both from understanding the deed and punishing the doer.

Let us recall in this connection that in his first news conference after being shot by John Hinckley, Jr., President Reagan asserted, as if it were the

First published as "Tylenol Killer: Mad—or Just Bad?" the *Washington Post* (Op-Ed), November 3, 1982, p. A-23. Reprinted with permission.

most obvious thing in the world, that Hinckley was "sick." That hint was evidently not lost on the federal prosecutor who, in concert with the defense, managed to secure a psychiatric "acquittal" for the would-be assassin. Hinckley was not permitted to talk during his trial. But there has been no stopping his self-revelations since his "acquittal." In view of the letters Hinckley has sent to *Newsweek* and others, can anyone really doubt that, the sworn lies of the psychiatrists notwithstanding, Hinckley is not mad but bad? What else must he do to prove that he is not a sick patient but a sickening punk?

But the magic of madness is a powerful lure and is useful to boot. A variation of the Hinckley scenario is unfolding already. Instead of preparing to prosectue and convict the Tylenol terrorist, the highest-ranking law-en-forcement authority of the state of Illinois is diagnosing him and thus laying the ground for his insanity defense. In an Oct. 2 news story, State Attorney General Tyrone C. Fahner is quoted as saying: "This was not the act of the McNeil people [the manufacturer], but the act of a crazed madman." But isn't it possible that the Tylenol killer is a terrorist who, instead of planting car bombs, is planting cyanide? Isn't it possible that he has (or they have) made certain demands on the government that we haven't been told about because our "betters" do not believe we could take such news?

Such reflections are evidently considered to be foolish or irrelevant. No one seems to entertain them, at least not publicly. Why, indeed, should we be uncertain, cautious and punitive, when we can be certain, decisive and thera-peutic. Never mind that madness cannot explain the events in question. There are millions of people in the world who are said to be mad. Do they poison people unknown to them with cyanide?

Finally, there remains the bitter fact that poisoning people who have harmed no one has been a favorite pastime of governments and government officials. How many people have been poisoned by our government with Agent Orange or with marijuana sprayed with paraquat? How many people were poisoned by government psychiatrists with cocktails laced with LSD and God-knows-what-else?

The Tylenol terrorist is not a clever killer, he is a "crazed madman." *Credo quia absurdum.*

The Church of America

No one denies that there's a Church of Rome or a Church of England. But practically no one admits that there's also a Church of America. How can there be? After all, the First Amendment to the Constitution is unequivocal when it declares: "Congress shall make no law respecting the establishment of religion, or prohibiting the free exercise thereof . . ."

Nevertheless, I contend that a Church of America does exist, that doctors are its high priests and apostles, that the faith it propagates is the conceit and pretense that medical science is the panacea for moral problems. It's not difficult to see how this national "religion" came into being, the First Amendment notwithstanding.

No government can be indifferent to morality—the ways in which its citizens behave. So every society—through custom, law, and religion—seeks to encourage certain values and conduct, and to discourage others. Thus, by offering freedom both *from* and *of* religion, the First Amendment promises more than any government could possibly deliver. We need look only at our Blue Laws and the prohibition of Mormon polygamy (among countless other measures) to see that the United States has been anything but neutral about religious behavior.

That lack of neutrality becomes even more apparent if we ask a naive question: Exactly *what* qualifies for the protections guaranteed by the First Amendment? Why, anything that's deemed to be a religion, of course. And there's the rub: Who does the deeming?

While each of us undoubtedly has his own ideas about what constitutes a religion, we can all pretty well agree with Webster's broad definition of religion as "a cause, principle, or system of tenets held with ardor, devotion, conscientiousness, and faith; a value held to be of supreme importance . . ." If we accept that definition, then we must also regard such diverse moral principles as individualism and collectivism, capitalism and Communism, and even nationalism and one-worldism, as either constituting religions, or resembling them in significant ways.

How we classify such systems of belief is no idle pastime. For anything that's considered a religion qualifies for the protections guaranteed by the

First published as "In the Church of America, Psychiatrists Are Priests," *Hospital Physician,* October, 1971, pp. 44-46. Reprinted with permission.

First Amendment; and anything that is not, does not. That's why the government and the "democratic majority" find it so useful to transform religious problems into psychiatric disorders—to define moral quandaries as problems of mental health.

This process of transforming the moral into the medical, the religious into the psychiatric, is clearly symbolized in the M'Naghten Rule, the criminal responsibility principle in effect in most states. Essentially, it's a legal-psychiatric formula that establishes "scientific" criteria of "criminal insanity." To see how it works, let's assume that a Mr. Jones is accused of murder, an immoral, irreligious, and illegal act. Under due process, he is entitled to a fair trial, with either punishment or acquittal as the ultimate result.

The M'Naghten Rule, however, specifies that Jones is not guilty, if "at the time of the committing of the act, the party accused was laboring under such a defect of reason, from disease of mind, as not to know the nature and quality of the act he was doing; or if he did know it, that he did not know he was doing what was wrong." Several points are worth noting:

The first is that the M'Naghten Rule was formulated in the middle of the nineteenth century, when the industrial-scientific revolution went into high gear, shifting attention and emphasis from *what for* to *how to*.

Under the twin banners of science and rationalism, M'Naghten continues to ride roughshod over moral principle. In cases of suspected insanity, it tramples the defendant's traditional protection—presumption of his innocence—into oblivion. M'Naghten makes absolutely no sense without an a priori assumption of guilt—that the defendant did, in fact, commit the crimes with which he is charged. For if he did not commit them, how could he not know that "he was doing what was wrong"?

Worst of all, the M'Naghten Rule places the judgment of what is right and wrong smack in the hands of physicians—specifically psychiatrists—another case of rationalism and science "debunking" religion; a case of the law itself driving the last nail into the coffin of Christianity. Luther obviously preached in vain that every man be his own ethicist and theologian.

Unable or unwilling to shoulder that responsibility, Everyman has cast it away. But the clinician—heir to the cleric—has been only too happy to pick it up. In exchange, of course, for the power and privileges that go with the job of telling people what is right and wrong. Examples abound:

In our schools, the state can't compel a child to say a prayer or to receive religious instruction. But it can compel him to submit to psychiatric examination, and—despite his own or his parents' moral-religious feelings—to receive sex education or drug-abuse information.

In courts and jails, neither defendants nor prisoners can be compelled to accept visits by priests, ministers, and rabbis. But they are compelled to submit to psychiatrists—with consequences far more devastating than visits by clergymen could possibly produce.

We thus accept, as perfectly obvious and reasonable, that a judge should order an alcoholic to report to a pharmacist to take Antabuse. But we consider it unthinkable that a judge should order the alcoholic to report to a priest to take Holy Communion. That's because alcoholism is defined as a disease, and Antabuse is recognized as a medical method for controlling it. But resistance to temptation—in this case, to drink to excess—may be enhanced, not only by drugs that make the person suffer when he yields to it, but also by strengthening his powers of self-control to help him not yield to it. Is there any doubt that the religious neutrality of the American system of government is wholly chimerical?

There was a time when our proclaimed religious neutrality was not so easily exposed as the impossibility it is. That was in the days when individuals structured their lives around their families, and families sustained a Judeo-Christian ethic. But the family has been replaced by the state as the primary agency of socialization, and formal religiosity had declined. Result: The image of the First Amendment has created a conceptual and moral vacuum, thus producing a craving for a moral order.

This hunger is being appeased in two ways: First, by the people themselves, with unflagging appetite for an ever-growing menu of creeds, cults, and communities. Second, by the state's fake ethical system served up under the pretense—as it obviously must be—that it's scientific, not moralistic.

We don't deny that there's a Church of Rome, and that it propagates a faith called Catholicism; or that there's a Church of England that propagates Anglicanism. But we deny that there's a Church of America—better known as the National Institute of Mental Health—and that it propagates a faith called psychiatry. It would have us believe that we can lead lives of ambition without anxiety; that we can have success without strife, sociability without conflict, reward without punishment, and pleasure without pain. All this and Heaven, too, is the promise, if only we have faith in mental health.

III

THE INSANITY DEFENSE

Some Call it Brainwashing

Like all persons accused of a dramatic crime, Patty Hearst has managed, for however brief a period, to make people pay attention to her. Although the play in which she now appears is likely to have a short run, she is its undisputed star—the victim of mind-rape. Truly, life imitates art. We have had *The Manchurian Candidate* and *A Clockwork Orange.* Now we have the Brainwashed Heiress.

Gone are the days when people asked: "Did she or didn't she?" Who cares any more what people do—legally or sexually? What people now want to know is what's in other people's brains. So they ask: "Was she or wasn't she brainwashed?" Having asked it they demand an answer with the same impatience with which a spoiled child demands an ice cream cone. And the experts on brainwashing will give them an answer as eagerly as doting parents give ice cream cones to their whining children. In fact, although people are asking for only one answer, they shall inevitably get two: yes, she was brainwashed; no, she was not.

But the question is meaningless. Asking it is an intellectual and moral copout; answering it is psychiatric prostitution; and believing the answer is self-deception.

Nietzsche was right when he said that "a criminal is frequently not equal to his deed: he makes it smaller and slanders it." Patty Hearst, the victorious SLA soldier, with gun slung snappily over her shoulder, seemed proud and self-assured. Her lawyers claim that she was then "brainwashed." Patty Hearst, the victim of kidnapping, with a decorous dress draped over her slender frame, seems shrunken and bewildered. Is this what Nietzsche had in mind when he remarked that "lawyers defending a criminal are rarely artists enough to turn the beautiful terrible mess of the criminal's deed to his advantage"?

Has there been any significant change in Patty Hearst's behavior? Before her arrest, she demeaned and denounced those who "helped" her as a child; now, she demeans and denounces those who "helped" her as a fugitive. For whatever reason, she seems to be inclined to make her life exciting at the expense of the dignity, liberty, and property of others.

The basic facts in the Hearst trial are simple and uncontested. The

Reprinted, with permission, from the *New Republic,* March 6, 1976, pp. 10-12.

defendant engaged in numerous acts which, unless legally excusable and excused, constitute serious crimes. What legal excuses mitigate or negate "criminal responsibility" for such acts? There are only a few. One is actual, physical duress. If a person forces another to commit an illegal act—say, literally at gunpoint—then the coerced actor is not legally responsible for his act. Another excuse is insanity. The illegal act, according to this claim, is not something that the defendant has done; it is something that has happened to him. The defendant is therefore no more responsible for his illegal act than a patient with myocardial insufficiency is responsible for his abnormal electrocardiogram. Patty Hearst does not claim this defense.

What excuse is left? Only what used to be called "temporary insanity," a concept that has become as unfashionable in forensic psychiatry as narrow ties have in menswear; hence, being "temporarily insane" has been refashioned into being "brainwashed." The defendant, according to this claim, was not "really" himself when he committed the illegal acts; he was "really" someone else, that is, his "brainwashed" self; hence his "unbrainwashed" self cannot be held responsible for these acts. This is Patty Hearst's defense.

The crucial question thus becomes: What is "brainwashing"? Are there, as the term implies, two kinds of brains: washed and unwashed? How do we know which is which?

Actually, it's all quite simple. Like many dramatic terms, "brainwashing" is a metaphor. A person can no more wash another's brain with coercion or conversation than he can make him bleed with a cutting remark.

If there is no such thing as brainwashing, what does this metaphor stand for? It stands for one of the most universal human experiences and events, namely for one person influencing another. However, we do not call all types of personal or psychological influences "brainwashing." We reserve this term for influences of which we disapprove.

In other words, "brainwashing" is like "perversion": as the latter term refers only to those sexual activities that one disdains, so the former refers only to those educational or psychological influences one abhors. While she was with the SLA, Patty Hearst was no doubt influenced by her captors and associates; Hearst, F. Lee Bailey, the press and nearly everyone else calls this "brainwashing." Between the time of her arrest, when she identified herself as an "urban guerrilla," and her appeareance in court as a demure and dutiful daughter, Patty Hearst was no doubt influenced by her new captors and associates: no one calls this "brainwashing."

In short, trying to ascertain whether Patty Hearst has been brainwashed by having her examined by psychiatrists is like trying to ascertain whether holy water is holy by having it examined by priests. Terms like "brainwashing" and "holy water" are invented and deployed strategically by these very "experts" for their own purposes. If we really want to understand what holy water is, we must examine priests, not water; it we really want to understand what brainwashing is, we must examine psychiatrists, not brains (or criminal defendants).

What, then, are the psychiatrists doing in the Hearst trial? They are "testifying" for whoever pays them. More than 300 years ago, an English aristocrat defined an ambassador as an honest man sent abroad to lie for his country. I would define a forensic psychiatrist as an honest doctor sent into court to lie for his masters.

We have done away with canon law and no longer look to priests to tell us about the purity or pollution of the soul. But we have substituted for it mental hygiene law and look to psychiatrists to tell us about the purity or pollution of the brain.

Mercenary Psychiatry

It is difficult to say whose behavior in the Patty Hearst trial is more distasteful—the defendant's, her lawyers', or her psychiatrists'. However, some
revelations about the antics of the alienists have at least injected an amusing
note into the repellent proceedings. These disclosures have also added a few
fresh facts to the story, a commodity in notoriously short supply in dramatic
criminal trials.

In June 1975, before Patty Hearst was apprehended, Dr. Louis J. West,
chairman of the department of psychiatry at the University of California at
Los Angeles, wrote a letter to Patty Hearst's parents telling them not to
despair "because she might be restored to health" if she was returned to them
alive; and advised them that "powerful legal and medical arguments can be
mobilized in her defense."

Such testimony-chasing by a psychiatrist is no more surprising than is
ambulance-chasing by a lawyer. Each has a sacred professional duty to
protect his client's "best interests." And what better way is there to do this
than by finding a client who doesn't even know he has any interests that need
protecting.

There is, however, an important distinction between psychiatrists and
lawyers, at least in the eyes of the courts and the public. The lawyers are
seen, correctly, as gladiators, hired to do battle for their client. The psychiatrists are seen, incorrectly, as experts, impartially testifying about the truth,
or at least about their "expert opinion" about it. It is, after all, just this fact
that defines the psychiatrist's role in the courtroom: he is neither judge, nor
prosecutor, nor defense attorney, nor ordinary witness; he is an "expert
witness." True to form, according to the newspaper reports of the trial, even
after his testimony-chasing tactics were exposed in court, West, the supposedly impartial expert, "vehemently denied that he showed bias toward the
Hearst family by writing them letters of sympathy and advice." As he did for
Patty Hearst's behavior, West had an "explanation" for his own, too: "I
wrote to them," he said, "as one parent to another." How touching. The fact
that the Hearsts are rich and powerful obviously had nothing to do with it. I
suppose one has to be an orthodox psychiatrist to believe that.

The performance of another defense psychiatrist exuded the same odor

Reprinted, with permission, from the *New Republic*, March 13, 1976, pp. 10-12.

of arrogant self-advertisement. Dr. Robert Jay Lifton, professor of psychiatry at Yale University, testified (as quoted by the *New York Times)* that Patty Hearst "came under the category that I wrote about in my book of the obviously confused about what had happened to her." In the style character-istic of the courtroom psychiatrist, he thus makes Hearst into a "case" about whose conduct he, the "brainwashing expert," knows more than does the "patient" herself. Such psychiatric self-flattery is acquired at the expense of the "patient's" self-esteem, not to mention, in this case, her father's money.

The comparison between the people "brainwashed" in Chinese captivity and Patty Hearst is, moreover, contrived, to say the least. The former lived in the most closed of societies, with no opportunity to walk away from their captors; the latter lived, during most of her alleged captivity, in the most open of open societies, with an opportunity not only to walk away from her captors, but also to make use, as she is now doing, of the resources of an influential and wealthy family.

A serious inconsistency between what Lifton told the court and what he told Steven Weed further impugns the validity, and even the veracity, of his testimony. Toward the end of his "search" for Patty, Weed remembers "telling Lifton that, given who Patty was and what had happened to her, there was really no other path she could have taken," and Lifton replied: "I think that's the definition of tragedy." Oedipus Rex and King Lear were tragic heroes. Does Lifton claim that they were not responsible for their actions? And if they were, and if Miss Hearst is a tragic heroine, then why does he claim that she is not responsible for her actions? It's only too obvious why.

To be sure, there is nothing new about the fact—perhaps I should call it the "contention"—that forensic psychiatrists sell their testimony for cash, and for other considerations. Still, it remains remarkably unappreciated how disastrous the consequences of this psychiatrization of the law have been for virtually every segment of American society, except the mental health estab-lishment. More than a hundred years ago, this corruption was denounced by the managers of the New York State Lunatic Asylum, who were moved, in their 1873 annual report to the legislature, to offer this warning:

> It may not be amiss to observe that this matter of the testimony of experts, especially in cases of alleged insanity, has gone to such an extravagance that it has really become of late years a profitable profession to be an expert witness, at the command of any party and ready for any party, for a sufficient and often exorbitant fee.

Unfortunately, when Santayana warned that "Those who cannot re-member the past are condemned to repeat it," he did not count on the psychiatrists, who, like other Orwellian totalitarians, rewrite history, so that there is nothing left to remember. Thus I am bitterly opposed to forensic psychiatry not merely because it is a fraud, but rather because it is so profoundly inimical to the loftiest moral principles of Anglo-American criminal law. Those principles, summed up by the phrase "the Rule of Law," are, simply put, to acquit the innocent and to convict and punish the guilty, giving the defendant the benefit of the doubt, and the prosecution the burden of proving guilt. This sounds simple enough, and it would be without psychiatry. Psychiatry corrupts this process by confusing the issues—especially in much publicized cases of violent crime. The fundamental issue in such a case is whether the accused did or did not commit the acts with which he or she is charged. Forensic psychiatrists—masquerading as medical doctors, which technically they are, but actually are not—cannot add one iota to the accurate and fair determination of such facts. But they can take away a great deal from this process. How? By offering strategically contrived speculations, disguised as medical determinations, about the "mental condition" and "responsibility" of the defendant.

In criminal trials such as the Hearst case, there are two types of psychiatrists: excusers and incriminators. The former, hired by the defense, are paid to offer psychiatric prevarications that tend to excuse the accused. The latter, hired by the prosecution, are paid to offer psychiatric prevarications tending to incriminate the accused. If a psychiatrist is unwilling to offer such testimony, he is not hired. To the extent West or other defense psychiatrists claim that they are not excusing, protecting, or trying to help Hearst, they are deceiving the public. Similarly, to the extent that prosecution psychiatrists maintain that they are not accusing, incriminating, or trying to harm Hearst, they are equally disingenuous.

It is instructive and ironic to recall in this connection that this is not the first time that the paths of the Hearst family and forensic psychiatry have crossed. More than 50 years ago William Randolph Hearst had offered Sigmund Freud $25,000 or anything he named to come to Chicago to "psychoanalyze" Leopold and Loeb. This offer, explains Ernest Jones in his biography of Freud, was made so that Freud could "presumably demonstrate that they [the murderers] should not be executed." To his credit, Freud, though in straitened circumstances, declined the offer.

West, on the other hand, seems to have solicited, and eagerly accepted, the opportunity to testify in the Hearst trial. Perhaps he and Dr. Lifton know something about human behavior that Freud didn't. In any case, at least they and their colleagues are presumably recouping some of the financial loss that psychiatry suffered when Freud refused an earlier Hearst offer.

Reply to Louis West

Dr. Louis West protests *(New Republic,* Correspondence, April 24) about the purity of his motives in the Hearst trial. My criticism of forensic psychiatry has, however, little to do with the motives of psychiatrists. It has to do with their acts, that is, with their using the courtroom as a forum for advancing their particular theories of human behavior, and using such theories, capriciously and meretriciously, to excuse some defendants, to incriminate others, and to ignore the rest. I object to psychiatric excuses (and incriminations) not because the "experts" who supply them are paid for them, but because such interventions subvert the rule of law. Indeed, when psychiatric opinion or testimony is sought by the court, and is supplied by ostensibly impartial psychiatrists without compensation (or for only a token fee), the result is an even more pernicious—because it is more insidious—subversion of the rule of the law than when the psychiatric intervention is obviously "bought."

Dr. West's claims that he has never "accepted a fee for testimony or consultation in a criminal trial," and that his colleagues' "professional accomplishment(s) and impeccable character" place their morals beyond the scrutiny of ordinary mortals also deserve a brief reply. In the first place, no psychiatrist ever accepts a fee for his "testimony" in a criminal trial: he is always paid for his "time." Secondly, although in the Hearst trial we received, thanks to Mr. F. Lee Bailey's inquiry about it, a full disclosure of the fee paid to Dr. Joel Fort, we have received no similar disclosure of *all* fees and expenses paid to *all* of the psychiatrists and psychologists who in any way assisted the Hearst defense. Until we do, certain important facts about the use of psychiatry in this trial will remain concealed. *Honi soit qui mal y pense.*

First published as "Psychiatry in Courtrooms," the *New Republic* (Correspondence), May 8, 1976, p. 31. Reprinted with permission.

Twice Brainwashed

On September 24, 1976, Patricia Hearst was sentenced to seven years in prison on the charges of armed robbery and use of a firearm to commit a felony. That sentence was even more severe than what the prosecution had requested. In her trial, Miss Hearst was represented by one of the most famous defense lawyers in America, and had a galaxy of psychiatric experts testifying on her behalf. If the outcome of her trial with their help was such a heavy sentence for her, what might have been its outcome without their help? I submit that she would have received a much lighter sentence; that Miss Hearst was victimized, and victimized herself, twice: first by her lowly kidnappers and by her own ill-advised decision to join them in venting her resentment against her parents and her society; and second, by her lofty psychiatrists and her ill-advised decision to join forces with them in reneging on her responsibility for her crimes.

It is clear that Miss Hearst was kidnapped and hence restrained in her freedom of action; but it is equally clear that within the range of the freedom of action that remained to her, she chose to attack her parents and her society, instead of attacking her kidnappers. As a responsible adult, she had a right to make that choice and benefit, or suffer, from its consequences.

Likewise, it is clear that Miss Hearst was arrested and hence again restrained in her freedom of action; but it is also clear that within the range of the freedom of action that remained to her, she chose to listen to the advice of the lawyers and psychiatrists her parents retained to defend her, instead of listening to herself.

The question that Miss Hearst's conviction and sentencing now raises is this: Did she fare so badly at the hands of the law because, as Mrs. Randolph Hearst put it, "She never had a break at all, not in the press or in the courts"? Or rather, as I believe, because she allowed herself to be victimized by psychiatrists?

To be sure, the possibility that Miss Hearst is a victim of a sort of reverse discrimination against the rich cannot be ruled out. But even to the extent that she is such a victim, the defense tactic chosen for her, and accepted by her, contributed heavily to that outcome.

Poets and playwrights have always understood that the rich and the

Reprinted, with permission, from the *New Republic,* October 23, 1976, pp. 6-8.

famous invite the envy of the gods and of those who create such envious gods. Miss Hearst's fame and her family's fortune were, therefore, liabilities for her defense right from the outset. In view of that fact, and in view of the evidence the prosecution possessed to convict her, it would have been reasonable for her and for those defending her (and it is not just perfect hindsight that makes me say this) not to attract any unnecessary attention to the Hearst family's wealth and power. That would have meant avoiding a highly dramatic and dramatically expensive defense. It would have also been reasonable for Miss Hearst to have acknowledged her guilt, as that would have obviated the impression, which psychiatric testimony invariably creates, that she was trying to get away with something for which an ordinary person would be severely punished. In other words, it should have been obvious to all concerned that introducing high-powered and high-priced psychiatrists into the Hearst trial might not only serve to solidify the popular prejudice that Patty Hearst was the pampered daughter of super-wealthy parents, but that it might do something even more damaging, namely, create the impression that she was trying to cop a plea by means of a contrived psychiatric defense.

Actually, everything I assume and assert above seems to have been entertained by Miss Hearst. According to the *New York Times* (April 12, 1976), "Immediately after Patricia Hearst was arrested last September on armed bank robbery charges, she was ready to negotiate for leniency in return for a guilty plea." Why, then, didn't she plead guilty? Because "Instead, lawyers and psychiatrists began to talk with her. From those talks emerged a defense plan based on a story that pictured her as a brainwashed victim of a revolutionary conspiracy."

Psychiatrists are experts in making up stories, at their patients' expense. In the mental hospital, those stories are called "psychodynamics" and "psychopathology." In the courtroom, they are called "brainwashing" and "diminished responsibility."

As we know, the story fabricated for Miss Hearst by the doctors was exposed for the deception it was. At whose expense? Not the psychiatrists. They got their picture in *Time,* and were paid for their efforts. The hoax of brainwashing has hurt only Patricia Hearst. That, it seems to me, is unjust.

The psychiatric advice Miss Hearst received, and which turned out to be so bad for her, raises an interesting question about the responsibility not only of Miss Hearst for following it, or of Mr. Bailey for implementing it, but also of the psychiatrists for offering it. Were the psychiatrists who advised Miss Hearst to plead "brainwashing" guilty of medical malpractice? If a physician advises a patient to follow a course of action, whether diagnostic or therapeutic, and if he does not advise the patient of both the potentially beneficial and harmful consequences that may accrue to him or her from following that advice, he is guilty of malpractice, having diagnosed or treated his patient without the patient's informed consent.

There is massive evidence to support the view that psychiatric testimony in the courtroom can be a kiss of death for the defendant on whose behalf it is ostensibly employed. Was Patricia Hearst adequately apprised of the risks she was taking when she was advised to abandon her decision to plead guilty and plea bargain and accept instead the decision of the doctors to deceive the court with a psychiatric "story"? If she was not, perhaps she has a case against the psychiatrists who were so eager to save her from a punishment she herself admitted she deserved.

The Psychiatrist as Accomplice

Since World War II psychiatry has had an exceedingly good press, especially in the United States. A combination of physician and priest, the psychiatrist, it seemed, could do no wrong. He dealt with the most "difficult" patients and even if his methods were sometimes "heroic," his aim was always, we were told, "therapeutic."

In the last few years, especially when looking at Russian psychiatry, the press has discarded its rose-colored glasses. The fact that, in the United States, psychiatrists not only do the same things their colleagues in the Soviet Union do, but, in addition, systematically act to exonerate individuals who have killed other innocent individuals, seems so far to have escaped the attention of civil libertarians and journalists.

There are countless ways in which psychiatry may be "abused." With respect to incarceration, psychiatry may be abused in two ways: by inculpating the innocent and by exculpating the guilty. For example, when a "mentally healthy" dissident is diagnosed as schizophrenic and committed to a mental hospital in Russia, we have an instance of the psychiatric inculpation of an innocent person as permanently insane. Such acts are now condemned by Western intellectuals and journalists as the psychiatric abuses of a totalitarian government. When, on the other hand, a so-called mad killer is diagnosed as suffering from some form of mental illness and is acquitted by reason of insanity in America, we have an instance of the psychiatric exculpation of a person as temporarily insane. Such acts are now praised by Western intellectuals and journalists as the scientific applications of humane psychiatry. In my opinion these two sets of acts are symmetrical: In the one, the psychiatrist acts as an accessory to what—morally speaking— is a crime by the state; in the other, he acts as an accessory to what—morally speaking—is a crime by an individual. Moreover, since killing an innocent person is a graver offense than imprisoning him, the American psychiatrist who helps to acquit a killer as not guilty by reason of insanity should be regarded as having committed a graver "psychiatric abuse" than his Russian colleague who helps to imprison an innocent person as a schizophrenic.

The death of Randolph Evans and the subsequent trial of his killer illustrate a typically American psychiatric abuse. Its professional acceptance

---

Reprinted, with permission, from *Inquiry,* April 3, 1978, pp. 4-5.

and popular approval illustrate that Americans love their own "abuses" of psychiatry (which, of course, they regard as its "proper uses") at least as much as the Russians love theirs.

Randolph Evans was a black youth who lived in Brooklyn. On Thanksgiving Day in 1976, when he was 15 years old, he was shot and killed by a white policeman named Robert H. Torsney. Officer Torsney was charged with murder while on duty. He pleaded insanity. On December 1, 1977, an all-white jury acquitted Torsney as not guilty by reason of insanity. To my knowledge, no reporter, no politician, no civil libertarian, domestic or foreign, has denounced the Torsney verdict as another instance of the American abuse of psychiatry.

Why was Evans killed? Why was Torsney acquitted? The shooting took place shortly before midnight, when Officer Torsney and his partner answered a radio report of an armed man in an East New York housing development where young Evans lived with his family. As the policemen left the building, Torsney was approached by the boy and five others. According to the *New York Times,* "Young Evans paused to speak to Officer Torsney, who pulled his gun from his holster and shot the boy in the head. He died several hours later."

Although Torsney claimed that he acted in self-defense, his legal defense was that "he was insane because of an epileptic psychomotor seizure suffered at the time of the crime." The 32-year-old policeman had no record of any previous epileptic attacks. Until the homicide, according to police personnel files, Torsney "had never fired his gun, had an unblemished record, and had no signs of emotional handicap." On the witness stand, the policeman testified that he had shot Evans "after he saw the boy reach into his waistband for what appeared to be a gun." No gun was found and none was seen by witnesses.

To maintain a defense of insanity, the accused needs a psychiatrist to support the claimed defense by means of expert testimony. Torsney had such a psychiatrist in the person of Dr. Daniel Schwartz, chief of forensic psychiatry at Kings County Medical Center (who had earlier testified that David Berkowitz, otherwise known as the Son of Sam, was schizophrenic and was psychiatrically unfit to stand trial). Dr. Schwartz lent his prestige and persuasive powers to the task of convincing the jury to acquit Torsney. Not only did he claim that Torsney suffered from psychomotor epilepsy, but also that the policeman had had an attack at the moment of the shooting, that the shooting was the result of the epilepsy, and that Torsney "acted automatically and suffered from organically caused amnesia."

It is, of course, the task of the prosecution to demolish such psychiatric claims. In this case, however, the prosecution called on a psychiatrist who believes that virtually everyone is mentally ill. Dr. Herbert Spiegel, clinical professor of psychiatry at the Columbia University College of Physicians and Surgeons and a well-known "hypnotist," testified that the policeman "suffered from hysterical dissociation, an emotional rather than an organic disorder that is not categorizable as legal insanity."

The judge gave the jury a choice among five possible verdicts: second-degree murder, first-degree manslaughter mitigated by extreme emotional disturbance, second-degree manslaughter, not guilty by reason of insanity, or self-defense. The jury brought in a verdict of not guilty by reason of insanity.

Torsney has been ordered confined for observation for 60 days in a facility of the State Mental Hygiene Department to determine whether he is a "danger to himself or to the community." According to the *New York Times,* because Torsney's "insanity had a specific organic cause," he may retire from the police force on a full medical disability pension.

The facts speak for themselves. Randolph Evans, a 15-year-old black, is killed by a white policeman before numerous witnesses. The killing was unprovoked, a fact tacitly acknowledged by the defendant's own insanity plea (which implies that, but for his alleged insanity, he would be guilty of the killing). A white psychiatrist testifies for the defense that Robert Torsney was "legally" insane at the time of the offense; another white psychiatrist testifies for the prosecution that Torsney was "illegally" insane. Finally, a white jury acquits Torsney, leaving the unprovoked killing of an innocent person unpunished. I hold my fellow psychiatrists largely responsible for this stubborn and willful destruction of law and justice.

Such, at least, is the message I draw from these facts. When I say that "the facts speak for themselves," I speak, of course, metaphorically. Facts don't speak, only persons do. What, then, do other psychiatrists hear when listening to these facts? Remarking on this same case, as well as on several other recent cases of "trying the mad"—such as that of the Michigan woman, also acquitted as not guilty by reason of insanity, who killed her husband by pouring gasoline on him while he was sleeping and then setting him on fire— Alan A. Stone, professor of law and psychiatry at Harvard University, comes to a totally different conclusion. "Reading about these developments," he writes in the *New York Times,* "the public seems to get angry at psychiatry and psychiatrists. Yet the current situation is the work of judges, lawyers, and legislators; psychiatrists play a minor if inept role."

Although partly true, such a judgment exonerates psychiatrists of a responsibility that is, in my opinion, wholly theirs—that is, the responsibility for supporting the insanity defense. Let us again recall in this connection the accusations now so fashionably leveled against Russian psychiatrists for "abusing their profession." Dr. Stone has not, to my knowledge, defended these Soviet psychiatrists by claiming that they "play a minor if inept role" in incarcerating dissidents in madhouses. Why not? Surely, because of the differences between Soviet and American societies, such an excuse would be more valid for Russian psychiatrists than for American psychiatrists. Why, then, should we accept Stone's plea of ineptness on behalf of his colleagues, the true nature of whose deeds is becoming increasingly difficult to disguise?

I submit that the courtroom psychiatrist who seeks to exonerate a killer of responsibility for his act is, from a moral point of view, an accomplice to the act of taking an innocent life. Psychiatrists choose whether to testify in court or not, just as people choose whether to kill or not. Psychiatrists who aid and abet the insanity defense are no more inept than their accomplices are insane. Instead of calling such acts inept or insane, we ought to call them wicked and immoral. Not until we do so will our homes and streets be safe from criminals, and our laws and courts from psychiatrists.

The Torsney Scandal

Despite intense Western scrutiny of Russian psychiatric "abuses," critics of Soviet psychiatry have been unable to turn up a single case in which Russian psychiatrists have "hospitalized" and "treated" someone who, in the hospitalizing psychiatrist's own opinion, was not mentally ill and did not need psychiatric treatment. However, precisely such a case exists now in the United States.

The case is that of Robert H. Torsney, a white policeman in New York, who on Thanksgiving Day in 1976 shot and killed a 15-year-old black youth in Brooklyn. After being acquitted of the manslaughter charge on a plea of insanity, Torsney was committed, as required by law, to the custody of the New York State Department of Mental Hygiene. According to the legal-psychiatric fiction that was henceforth to govern his fate, he was confined in order to be observed, examined, and if necessary treated—not in order to be punished. He was, after all, "not guilty" of any crime. In due course, again as required by law, the Department of Mental Hygiene reported back to the committing court about the "patient's" status. The report, based on observing Torsney for about a year, was that he was not mentally ill, was not a danger to himself or others, and should therefore be released forthwith. Justice Leonard Yoswein, the New York State Supreme Court judge in Brooklyn who had to rule on the case, held nine days of hearings, during which eighteen psychiatrists testified. All the expert witnesses agreed that "Officer Torsney was not psychotic and was not a danger to himself or others." In the decision he handed down, Judge Yoswein noted that "evidence also indicates that the patient was not suffering from mental illness during the entire period that the patient has been in the custody of Mental Hygiene . . . Mr. Torsney was not insane at any time during his committal." Accordingly, Judge Yoswein ordered Torsney released.

Predictably, this judicial decision led to an outcry in the black community in Brooklyn. It also led to what the *New York Times* characterized as a "rare appeal by the District Attorney's office of the lower court's finding in an insanity-defense case." Predictably, the appeal was successful. On February 6, 1979, the Appellate Division of the State Supreme Court reversed

---

First published as "'Mental Illness and Police Brutality," *Libertarian Review*, April 1979, pp. 32-33. Reprinted with permission.

Justice Yoswein's ruling. In a unanimous, 20-page decision, the five-judge panel ordered that Torsney's commitment be continued. "We may not shirk our responsibility to the community by prematurely releasing Mr. Torsney while he continues to suffer from a dangerous personality disorder," the panel said. The appeals court also justified continuing Torsney's psychiatric confinement and "treatment" by noting that "he might face continued stress from a departmental hearing, possible suits, financial stress, and threats."

In an editorial remark on these goings-on, the *New York Times* (February 11) laconically observed that "Freedom [is] fleeting for Officer Torsney." In the same issue of the *Times,* in a story about Pakistan's recent turn to Islamic laws, we learned that in the case of two Pakistanis sentenced to have their hands chopped off, the sentence could not be carried out because the "military courts have been unable to find a surgeon willing to perform the operation." It is surely worth noting that American courts never encounter any difficulty having their sentences carried out by psychiatric executioners— as the case of Robert Torsney dramatically illustrates.

Consider the brutal facts—and the psychiatric fictions—in this case. After observing and examining Torsney for more than a year, psychiatrists in the New York State Department of Mental Hygiene—at all levels, from those directly in charge of the case to those in the highest ranks of the bureaucracy—have declared that Torsney is not mentally ill, is not dangerous to himself or others, requires no psychiatric treatment, and should therefore be released from psychiatric "hospitalization." In this ostensibly medical judgment, the psychiatric experts have been overruled by a group of laymen, called judges. Despite the Mental Hygiene Department's own determination that Torsney is not mentally ill and should be released, the courts—and the Department—have evidently had no trouble finding psychiatrists to imprison and "treat" Torsney. In my opinion, these facts make this a more obvious and more convincingly demonstrated case of psychiatric abuse than any of those reported from the Soviet Union.

Of course, Torsney should never have been acquitted as insane. No one should be. The "psychomotor epilepsy" allegedly causing him to kill his victim was pure psychiatric fiction. No neurologist testified in the case. Actually, neurologists do not believe that epilepsy (real or pretended) causes crime. Only psychiatrists believe that. And even psychiatrists believe it only when it suits their purpose. When, at the Appeals Court hearing, Alfred B. Annenberg, the attorney representing the New York State Mental Hygiene Department, was chided by the justices for insisting that Torsney was sane despite having been acquitted as insanse, Annenberg, probably quite unwittingly, tore the mask off the official face of institutional psychiatry. "Your Honor," he reminded the court, "the Department of Mental Hygiene bears no responsibility for what happened at the trial—miscarriage of justice or whatever. . . . No one could find one violent act in this man's life except for two seconds killing Randolph Evans." Unrelenting in their quest for a diagnosis of insanity, the judges badgered Annenberg, asserting that Torsney "suffered from a rare form of epilepsy." Evidently losing his cool, Annenberg shot back that, had he been at the trial, "I would have had four experts to testify there's no such thing."

Of course, Torsney should not have been, and should not continue to be, imprisoned in a mental hospital. No one should be. The game Torsney, the psychiatrists, the lawyers, and the courts have played lays bare the evil inherent in psychiatric justice—namely, the principle that two wrongs make a right. The insanity acquittal was—and always is—a grave wrong. Imprisonment in the insane asylum was—and always is—another grave wrong. These two wrongs add up to a practical right. A crime has been explained, excused, and avenged. Who could ask for more?

Pathetically, Department of Mental Hygiene psychiatrists—trying, for a change, to be honest—claim to be unable to "find" any mental illness in a "killer" like Torsney. Piously, State Supreme Appeals Court judges—trying, as usual, to cater to the public passions which they think is justice—remind them of their duty to find it. Voltaire is reputed to have said that if there were no God, we would have to invent Him. Obviously, if there is no mental illness, we must invent it. *Le plus ça change, le plus c'est la même chose.*

How Dan White
Got Away with Murder

There is no question that a travesty of justice occurred in the trial of Dan White. How could the killer of San Francisco Mayor George Moscone and Supervisor Harvey Milk—who fired nine bullets into his victims and shot each one twice in the back of the head, execution-style—not be found guilty of murder?

The answer is: Easily.

Anything is possible in human affairs if one has the power to redefine basic concepts—to say that day is night, that two plus two make five—and get away with it. In the trial of Dan White, the defense, aided and abetted by the prosecution, had the power to hand the case over to the psychiatrists, and the psychiatrists had the power to redefine a political crime as an ordinary crime, and an ordinary crime as a psychiatric problem. How did psychiatry gain such power? By having seized it, long ago; and by society not resisting—indeed welcoming—that seizure of power.

To understand the White affair, we must understand some things about the recent history of American psychiatry. During World War II, American psychiatry became very useful to the military authorities by offering an ostensibly medical mechanism for disposing of useless or unwanted military personnel. That mechanism was the so-called NP (for neuropsychiatric) discharge. Approximately half of those separated by "medical" discharges from the military services received NP discharges. At the time, this was considered to be a great medical-humanitarian achievement. It is still so considered. The psychiatrist most responsible for it, William Menninger, was hailed as a great physician and a benefactor of the nation. Why? Because he, and the countless psychiatrists who participated in that gigantic con game, offered to obscure, and thus to de-ethicize and depoliticize, one of the most obvious and painful moral problems that then faced the nation—namely, the obligation to serve in the armed forces, with the grave risks to life and limb attendant on that obligation. That wartime psychiatrization of fear, self-protection, cowardice,

First published as "J'accuse: How Dan White Got Away with Murder, and How American Psychiatry Helped Him Do It," *Inquiry*, August 6 & 20, 1979, pp. 17-21. Reprinted with permission.

pacifism, wisdom—call it what you may—laid the foundation on which American psychiatrists and the other enemies of freedom and dignity have been building their castles ever since.

At the end of the war, American psychiatry lost no time demonstrating its usefulness to the country at peace. Ezra Pound, one of the greatest poets of his time, was indicted for treason—a charge he vehemently denied. Whether he was innocent or guilty of that crime, psychiatry spared the nation the need to undergo the political soul-searching that his trial would have generated. Prosecution and "defense" conspired to declare Pound mentally unfit to stand trial, condemning him instead, without a trial, to serve a thirteen-year sentence in St. Elizabeths Hospital, the nation's model psychiatric dungeon in Washington, D.C. Pound's jailer was hailed as a great psychiatrist, the benefactor of Pound as well as the nation.

Neither the mass stigmatization of American servicemen as mad, nor the psychiatric diversion of the Pound case from the criminal to the mental-health system, was considered to be an abuse of psychiatry. The American public has been led to believe that only in Russia do psychiatrists abuse psychiatry; that in the West, psychiatrists use psychiatry only to do good. But what is the nature of that good? With its service to the nation richly rewarded, postwar psychiatry proudly declared its lofty aims. "The belated objectives of practically all effective psychotherapy," declared Brock Chisholm in 1946, "are the reinterpretation and eventual eradication of the concept of right and wrong. If the race is to be freed from its crippling burden of good and evil, it must be psychiatrists who take the original responsibility." The physician who uttered this much-neglected self-revelation of the moral and political mandate of psychiatry was the former director general of medical services in the Canadian army, the head of the World Federation of Mental Health, and the director of the World Health Organization. Thirty-three years later, the men and women who sat on the jury in San Francisco in the case of Dan White proved themselves to be apt pupils of the psychiatric perverters of our system of justice.

In the postwar years, psychiatrists continued their crusade against homosexuals, whom they called, among other things, "inverts" and "perverts," and whose incarceration as "sex offenders" they enthusiastically supported. "If it is considered the will of the majority," declared one of the then leading American psychiatrists, "that large numbers of sex offenders . . . be indefinitely deprived of their liberty and supported at the expense of the state, I readily yield to that judgment." That opinion was uttered in 1951 by Manfred Guttmacher, in whose honor the American Psychiatric Association offers an annual award "for outstanding contribution to the literature of forensic psychiatry"—in other words, for the most valuable contribution to the psychiatric subversion of the rule of law.

In 1974, the American Psychiatric Association (under pressure from gay liberationists) dropped homosexuality from the official roster of mental diseases, while still maintaining that the conversion of homosexuals to hetero-sexuality is a bona fide treatment. Thus it would be a serious mistake to believe that these long-standing enemies of homosexuals have really changed their minds about one of their most dearly hated scapegoats. For example, Karl Menninger, the undisputed dean of postwar American psychiatry, has never retracted the following views, which he set forth in 1963. After deni-grating homosexuals by classifying their "condition" as a species of "Second Order of Dyscontrol and Dysorganization," Menninger asserts: "We do not, like some, condone it [homosexuality]. We regard it as a symptom with all the functions of other symptoms—aggression, indulgence, self-punishment, and the effort to forestall something worse." While Menninger thus stigma-tizes and slanders homosexuals, he tries, in every way possible, to relieve real criminals of responsibility. His crowning achievement in this enterprise is epitomized in the title of one of his most celebrated books: *The Crime of Punishment.* According to Menninger, the punishment even of persons guilty of the most heinous crimes, is, quite literally, a crime—whereas their crime is not a crime. Lest anyone think that Menninger is championing liberty for lawbreakers, let me hasten to add that he is not championing liberty for anyone; instead, he seeks to lump the "criminal" together with the rest of humanity—everyone being a fit subject for indefinite psychiatric incarceration at the whim of the psychiatrist. In his magnum opus, *The Vital Balance,* Menninger declares "that all people have mental illness of different degrees at different times, and that sometimes some are much worse, or better."

This brings us, historically as well as logically, to the present psychiatric-legal situation in California: in particular, to the concept of "diminished mental capacity" as a defense in criminal law.

Modern medicine has revealed that the capacities of various organs to perform their functions may be impaired or abolished by disease. The liver, for example, may have a diminished capacity to metabolize certain nutrients and to secrete bile—the result of which may be jaundice and death. Similarly, the kidneys many have a diminished capacity to secrete metabolites and excrete urine—the result of which may be uremia and death. And so on, with the capacities of the lung, the heart, and other organs.

Psychiatry has always been living off a succession of medical metaphors. Its whole idea of mental illness, as I have shown elsewhere, is one colossal metaphor. In postwar America, psychiatry was hungry for fresh concepts to live off. Thus, the psychiatrists borrowed from medicine the idea of the "diminished capacity" of an organ and applied it, literally, to "criminal responsibility." The authority widely acknowledged to be most responsible for popularizing the doctrine of "diminished capacity" is Bernard Diamond, a professor of psychiatry and law at the University of California at Berkeley. With this mendacity through metaphor, Diamond helped to lay the ground for decisions such as the jury reached in the White case. Let us keep in mind, however, that Diamond's opinions are hardly novel, following, as they do, upon decades of psychiatric attacks on criminal responsibility as a moral concept.

Diamond writes: "[S]cientific evidence proves that there is no such thing as free will. . . . Each [criminal] case should be judged on its own clinical merits." Diamond thus takes it for granted that every defendant is a "patient" whose "case" has "clinical merits."

All human behavior—each "act of will"—is, moreover, nothing but a physiological process: "Each act of will, each choice, presumably made on a random basis, turns out to be as rigidly determined as any other physiological process of the human body."

Diamond writes as if the metaphor of diminished responsibility were an established "fact": "We thus arrive at a legal spectrum of an infinitely graduated scale of responsibility which corresponds, or could be made to correspond closely, to the psychological reality of human beings as understood by twentieth century medical psychology."

Of course, no one can see, smell, taste, or measure "criminal responsibility," normal or diminished. This makes it different from the diminished capacities of the liver, the lungs, the kidneys, and other organs, all of which are readily measurable. Nor is this a matter of technological sophistication. Criminal responsibility will *never* be measurable—because it just isn't that sort of thing. That it is not is something psychiatrists know perfectly well, which supports the impression that they are not fond of telling the truth. In the very article in which he touts the concept of diminished capacity, in the *Stanford Law Review* of December 1961, Diamond writes: "I concede that this whole business of lack of mental capacity to premeditate, to have malice or to entertain intent, is a kind of sophistry [that is, a kind of lie] which must not be allowed to remain an end in itself. Right now we must utilize these legal technicalities to permit psychiatrists to gain entrance into the trial court."

Why didn't the prosecutor read these lines to the White jury? And why didn't he read Diamond's further psychiatric-imperialistic declarations published in the same article? "The next step after *Gorshen* [a 1957 trial at which Diamond testified] is to expand the principle of limited or diminished responsibility of the mentally-ill offender to include all definitions of crime. . . . The ultimate step will be the extension of the treatment principle to all prisoners—sane, insane, fully responsible, and partially responsible."

Here it is, in black and white. Diamond is not the least interested in justice—and like Menninger he says so. What he is interested in is treatment—that is, in medicalizing law, crime, and punishment.

Against this backdrop we can better reconsider the killing of George Moscone and Harvey Milk and the psychiatric exoneration of the man who killed them. Most of the facts of this case have been well-publicized and are familiar, especially to those who have paid attention to this astonishing judicial-psychiatric spectacle. It is a spectacle for which we do not have a proper vocabulary. We have a rich lexicon to describe unjust punishments meted out to innocent victims—judicial lynching by a kangaroo court being a succinct and picturesque way of describing that sort of legal crime. Revealingly, we have no comparable words to describe the inverse aberration of justice, such as occurred in the White affair. "Getting away with muder" is the closest we can come to it. This is not inaccurate, but is inadequate since it neglects to suggest how the judicial crime in question was perpetrated.

Keep in mind that according to the experts—one more of whom I shall quote in a moment—there is no such thing as a political assassination in America. In America, only "mental patients" kill political figures.

—The mayor of one of America's great cities is killed by five shots, two of them fired into his head at close range after he is gunned down with three previous shots. The mayor is a "liberal" protector of the rights of sexual minorities. The assassin is a "conservative" foe of "social deviants." The killing is not a political crime, asserts prosecutor Thomas Norman.

—The most prominent self-declared homosexual politician in America is killed by four shots, two of them fired into his head as he lies fatally wounded. The killer is the mayor's assassin, who reloaded his gun after the first killing. That's not a political crime either, says Norman.

What else do you expect? In an America poisoned by psychiatry, any political embarrassment or crime can be psychiatrized. James Forrestal, former secretary of the navy and the first U.S. secretary of defense, begins to act erratically and is imprisoned by psychiatrists in a suite on the top floor of the National Naval Medical Center, from which he allegedly jumps to his death. Ezra Pound is, as I have noted, incarcerated in a madhouse for thirteen years. Major General Edwin Walker, implicated in an integration riot, is imprisoned in a federal insane asylum in an effort to deprive him of his right to stand trial.

John Kennedy is assassinated. The explanation? A lone psychotic named Lee Harvey Oswald shot him. Oswald, in turn, was shot by another lone psychotic, called Jack Ruby. If you don't believe that, you are paranoid.

Robert Kennedy is assassinated. The explanation? Another lone psychotic, this time a Palestinian-American called Sirhan Sirhan, shot him. Sirhan did it, the psychiatrists claimed, because he fell off a horse when he was a child. If you don't believe that, you are paranoid.

You are paranoid because American psychiatry has established that in our "sick society" what seem to be political assassinations are, in reality, not political acts at all. As Edwin Weinstein, a professor at Mount Sinai Medical School, wrote in 1976 in one of the most prestigious American psychiatric journals: "Assassinations of heads of state of foreign countries have usually been carried out by organized political groups seeking to overthrow the government or change its policies. In the United States, on the other hand, Presidential assassinations have been the work of mentally deranged individuals."

How many more cases or authorities must one cite to prove that not only Russian psychiatry, but American psychiatry also, is a political weapon?

To return to the most recent case of a psychiatrically depoliticized political assassination—that of the assassination of George Moscone and Harvey Milk—consider the following:

—The killer of Moscone and Milk had been informed that his political hopes had been destroyed by Moscone's refusal to reappoint him supervisor, a refusal in which Milk was thought to have had a hand. The next morning the killer came to City Hall with a well-hidden gun and ten extra bullets; gained entrance to the building through a window, thus avoiding the metal-detectors at the door; shot Moscone five times; reloaded his gun; then shot Milk four times. To the psychiatrists all this proved diminished capacity to premeditate.

—One psychiatrist insisted that the killer was a "good man"; this also proved that he had diminished capacity.

—White sat at home consuming Cokes, Twinkies, and other "junk food" before the killings, said another psychiatrist—additional evidence that he had diminished capacity.

—The defense and the prosecution collaborated in deliberately depoliticizing the assassinations. After the trial, defense attorney Stephen Scherr told the San Francisco Examiner that "the defense was wary of having gays serve on the jury. He said the attorneys feared that a gay might believe that the slaying of Milk, San Francisco's first openly homosexual supervisor, was a political assassination committed to block gay power. Scherr said such a belief would be contrary to the facts in the case. . . ." This is like excluding black jurors from the trial of the accused assassin of Martin Luther King (the alleged assassin was, of course, never tried)—on the grounds that they might mistakenly believe that the killing had something to do with the fact that King was black.

When patients do not want to face unpleasant facts, psychiatrists love to tell them that they are practicing "denial" and "repression." That may be true—although we must remember that patients have a right to deny or repress any fact they please. But witnesses in criminal trials are sworn to tell the truth. Journalists saw the truth—and they saw it withheld, evaded, and obscured by the psychiatrists (and the prosecution).

Charles McCabe, San Francisco Chronicle columnist, wrote:

[Quoting free-lance writer Mike Weiss:] "The San Francisco image-mongers—the politicians and the flacks—don't talk out loud about the seething frustrations and angers aroused by this confrontation [between straights and gays]. But, out in the neighborhoods, everybody knows San Francisco has a sexual integration crisis." . . . White [McCabe continues] had all the old-fashioned prejudices and bigotries. He hated blacks and "queers" and made no secret of it. . . . The man [Moscone] who double-crossed him had offended his manhood. Moreover, the mayor was the most powerful friend the homosexuals had in this city. . . .

Herb Caen, another *Chronicle* columnist, was equally candid:

"What's wrong with San Francisco?" was being asked again yesterday . . . one can kill, twice, complete with coup de grace, and get away with it. The grateful defendant was a staunch defender of law and order . . . a religious man who went straight to church after he killed. . . . This is a city of undercurrents, not all of them well hidden. Many police made an open secret of their support for Dan White and their dislike (understatement) of homosexuals. . . .

If these journalists are telling the truth, what did the psychiatrists tell us and the jury? A "higher" version of the truth—or strategic untruths? Since "psychiatric expert testimony" is, legally speaking, *opinion,* it can never be perjured. This fact points to the role of the single prosecution psychiatrist in the White case. This physician was foolish enough actually to examine Dan White on the day of the killings. He testified that he found White to be sane, competent, and responsible for his actions. The jury, no doubt, concluded that he was an inept doctor who couldn't find the "diminished capacity" so easily detected by four other doctors and a clinical psychologist.

The very act of examining White was stupid and totally inconsistent with mounting a strong case for the prosecution. The fact that the DA had White examined must have proved to the jury—and rightly so—that there was something a psychiatrist *could* discover by examining him that would be relevant for establishing White's "capacity" to commit first-degree murder. Therein, precisely, lies the utter hoax of "diminished capacity." In my opinion, the prosecution should have led the jury to infer malice and premeditation from the facts of the case—just as a jury is supposed to infer malpractice when a surgeon leaves a sponge in the patient's stomach.

White's defense thus rested on two separate pillars: psychiatry and the plea of "diminished capacity" was one; a subtle but persistent appeal to the jury's antihomosexual prejudices was another. This latter aspect of the defense strategy has seemingly been overlooked by most previous commentators on the trial.

"Good people—fine people with fine backgrounds—simply don't kill people in cold blood," was defense attorney Douglas Schmidt's premise in interpreting, to jury and press alike, what "really" happened to Dan White. "Seeing Mrs. White," wrote a reporter for the *San Francisco Chronicle,* "it was impossible for the jury not to believe that White came from a decent, hard-working background that they, the jury members, shared and admired. Repeatedly, Schmidt used the word 'background'. . . ."

"Background" was, indeed, the code word. For what? Primarily for "straight" (as against gay)—and secondarily, for white, Christian, policeman (as against black, Jewish, "deviant"). But if Schmidt's bigoted premise—

which the prosecution never challenged and hence the jury readily accepted—is allowed to stand, then no heterosexual, married, policeman jogger will ever be convicted of first-degree murder in America again.

Thus with great skill Schmidt successfully replaced the reality of Dan White, the moral actor on the stage of life, with the abstractions of White's "diminished capacity" and his "background"—and then instructed the jury to focus on those fictions and ignore the facts.

As soon as the trial was over, one of the defense psychiatrists gave an interview in which he flatly contradicted his own testimony. As a witness for the defense, Martin Blinder, a San Francisco psychiatrist, "told the jury [according to *Newsweek,* June 4] that White's compulsive diet of candy bars, cupcakes and Cokes was evidence of a deep depression—and a source of excessive sugar that had aggravated a chemical imbalance in his brain." Two weeks later, Blinder—who says he has been "involved in thousands of cases"—told a *San Francisco Chronicle* reporter: "Judges and juries should determine issues of guilt and innocence, sanity and insanity . . . psychiatrists are often pushed into making that decision for them. . . . There is a tendency for psychiatrists to find mental illness in every instance of emotional stress. I personally resist this."

But who is "pushing" Blinder or any other psychiatrist to testify in a criminal trial? No one! In each and every case, a psychiatrist who testifes in court is a hired gun. He does what he does for money or fame or because he believes in it, or as Bernard Diamond implied, to gain eventual control of the entire judicial system. Assuredly, he does not do it because anyone forces him to—just as no one forces him to go to court to commit innocent people to mental hospitals, which hired psychiatric guns also love to do.

After the war, the German people could not claim that they did not realize what the Nazis were planning for the Jews. Hitler had warned them of his intentions clearly enough—in *Mein Kampf* and the voluminous anti-Semitic literature that accompanied the National Socialists' rise to power. After they awaken from their psychiatric stupor, the American people will not be able to claim that they did not realize what the psychiatrists were planning for all of us. The psychiatrists have warned them of their intentions clearly enough—in books with such telling titles as *The Crime of Punishment* and the voluminous anti-responsibility and pro-commitment literature that accompanied these pseudomedical prevaricators' rise to power.

When psychiatric testimony is used as it has been in the White trial, where are the so-called critics of psychiatry—those who timidly chastise the sensational foreign or marginal domestic abuses of the profession, and thus make headlines for themselves as humanitarians? Do they speak out against gross psychiatric abuses, such as have occurred in the White case and in other cases of political assassination? The fact is they never do.

Mrs. Rosalynn Carter is so tireless a promoter of this fake religion that she seems to be veritably thrice-born: as a human being, a Baptist, and a votary of psychiatry. One could reasonably expect that a person so lavish in her praise of the "good" that psychiatry has done would feel duty-bound to speak out when psychiatrists make a mockery of justice. But she has not.

Where were our conservative and neoconservative journalists and thinkers, who so lament the decline of the sense of personal responsibility in our "permissive" society? Where, when all is said and done, were the ever-ready crusaders for human rights and justice throughout the world? Did they protest the injustice of the White verdict? No, they did not.

In the struggle against the psychiatric perversion of responsibility and justice, I propose that we make Voltaire's famous battle cry—*Écrasez l'infâme!* ("Crush the infamous thing!")—our own. The infamous thing that Voltaire sought to crush was the political power of the Roman Catholic church. The infamous thing that we ought to crush is the political power of the Church of Psychiatry.

Or, to take another famous example from French history, of another crusade for justice—at the end of the last century, French society was wracked by the trial and conviction of Captain Albert Dreyfus. What the Dreyfus affair was for the French at that time, the Dan White affair ought to become for us now. In the Dreyfus case, the judicial system was used to convict a demonstrably innocent man. In the White case, the judicial system was used to exonerate a demonstrably guilty one.

Dreyfus, the Jew, was the victim. White, the policeman, is the victimizer. Dreyfus became the symbol of what happens to an innocent individual when anti-Semitic hatred in the community, unacknowledged but powerful, is allowed to masquerade as justice. White should become a symbol of what happens to a guilty individual when antihomosexual hatred, unacknowledged but powerful, is allowed to masquerade as justice.

Who allowed—who, indeed, engineered—these carefully orchestrated miscarriages of justice? In the Dreyfus case, it was the French military and the power it then wielded in the French courts. In the White case, it is American psychiatry and the power it now wields in the American courts. As Emile Zola then accused the French generals of having perverted the legal order in *l'affaire Dreyfus,* so I accuse organized American psychiatry of perverting the legal order in the White affair.

I maintain that American psychiatry is White's accomplice in crime. While White pulled the trigger of the gun that killed Moscone and Milk, American psychiatry pulled the wool over the eyes of the lawmakers and journalists and the public—leading to the courtroom scenario of psychiatrists fabricating fantasies and having their fantasies legitimized by the courts as "expert medical testimony."

On Mondays, Wednesdays, and Fridays, the psychiatric prevaricators thus go to court to exonerate the guilty: That is called "psychiatric defense." On Tuesdays, Thursdays, and Saturdays, the same prevaricators go to court to incriminate the innocent: That is called "civil commitment." The lawmakers, the judges, and the attorneys (for both sides) all shamelessly use these fakes—which is why each of them is as reluctant to expose and demolish the psychiatric defense of the guilty as he is to expose and demolish the psychiatric incrimination of the innocent.

Long before Dreyfus's days, the homosexual was already one of psychiatry's favorite scapegoats. Amerian psychiatry's true feeling about homosexuals showed in all its ugliness once more in the trial of Dan White. Let us hope that the White affair will arouse the sense of justice in the gay community in America and in the hearts of all who sympathize with such victimization; and that the result will be the long-overdue expulsion of the psychiatric liars from the courtroom—whether they come to pervert justice by imprisoning the innocent or by exculpating the guilty.

Reagan's "Diagnosing" Hinckley

With the dramatic unfolding of events after the attempted assassination of President Reagan, even his bitterest critics were forced to concede that his behavior under fire was courageous and inspiring. Veritably, Reagan seemed to possess all of the virtues of the Western hero he had portrayed so often and so well on the screen. Unfortunately, on April 22, in the first interview he gave the press after the shooting, he fell off his horse and didn't even seem to know it. Quite unwittingly, Reagan offered some comments about John W. Hinckley, Jr. that were, in my opinion, unfounded and misguided and that have gravely prejudiced his trial.

What President Reagan said was this: "I hope, indeed I pray, that he can find an answer to his problem. He seems to be a very disturbed young man. He comes from a fine family. They must be devastated by this. And I hope he'll get well, too."

I believe that these remarks are important enough to justify my taking them one sentence at a time.

"I hope, indeed I pray, that he can find an answer to his problem." In the old Westerns, if memory doesn't deceive me, the good men first hanged the bad men and only then did they pray for their souls. Elsewhere in the same interview Reagan also said that he prays daily for Brady's recovery. As I do not pray, I grant that my views on prayer may be impious and "incorrect." Nevertheless, I believe that the dignity of prayer is cheapened when it is bestowed as indiscriminately as this. Is there anyone for whom Reagan would not pray? Would he pray for Brezhnev's health? For Stalin's soul? If not, then why for Hinckley? Surely, Solzhenitsyn is no less pious than Reagan, but I do not recall Solzhenitsyn's ever mentioning that he prays for communist murderers. Perhaps capitalist would-be murderers who fail to kill anyone and succeed only in lobotomizing a press secretary are more deserving.

One more comment on this brief but psychiatrically significant sentence needs to be added here. President Reagan's statement implies that Hinckley has a "problem" and is looking to "find an answer" to it. But I think Reagan

---

First published as "Reagan Should Let Jurors Judge Hinckley," *Washington Post* (Op-Ed), May 6, 1981, p. A-19. Reprinted with permission.

(and the conventional psychiatric mind-set he so naively displays) may have got this backwards. Hinckley had a *problem* before the assassination attempt. The criminal act was his *solution* to it. Now other people, especially poor Jim Brady and his family, have got a problem. I, for one, find the compassion for Hinckley premature. Like the men Reagan used to impersonate, I believe that Hinckley deserves punishment first, compassion and forgiveness later, if ever.

"He [Hinckley] seems to be a very disturbed young man." Anyone with any respect for language—and without such respect there can be neither truth nor justice—must realize that while this may be a piece of received psychiatric truth, it is a big lie nevertheless. Hinckley is not disturbed, he is disturbing. He is not sick, he is sickening.

"He [Hinckley] comes from a fine family." How does Reagan know this? All we were told so far is that Hinckley comes from a wealthy family.

There is one more thing we know, and I cannot emphasize its importance enough: namely, that Hinckley has not been allowed to speak for himself. In effect, he has been muzzled, he has been silenced, while everyone, including the president of the United States, is busy explaining that he is "disturbed." For all we know, Hinckley may now feel quite undisturbed.

"They [Hinckley's family] must be devastated by this." That is likely and is probably one of the reasons for Hinckley's dastardly deed. But this is a speculation. And so is the possibility that the Hinckley family might have preferred George Bush for president. But that is heresy. We treasure our received psychiatric truths about mentally-ill assassins precisely in order to banish such thoughts from our collective consciousness. In America, political motives for the murder of the high and mighty exist only in the half-forgotten pages of Shakespeare's tragedies.

"And I hope he'll get well, too." By thus acknowledging that Hinckley is ill, Reagan here implicitly supports an insanity defense for him. Should Hinckley plead insanity, his lawyers would be able to appeal to the "expert testimony" of the president of the United States to support the contention that Hinckley is innocent because he was insane when he wounded Reagan instead of killing him.

President Reagan made a mistake in answering any questions about Hinckley at all. Respect for the law should have made him say, quite simply, that Hinckley's fate—and in particular the question of whether he is disturbed or depraved—will be for the jury to determine. The fact is that the distinction between disturbance and depravity—between madness and badness, between mental illness and criminality, call it what you will—is not a specialized or technical judgment doctors can make because they possess a medical degree; or psychiatrists can make because they possess training in diagnosing and treating mental illness; or the president of the United States can make because he occupies a lofty office. That distinction is a *moral judgment,* which is why a jury, and no one else, is supposed to make it. If we forget that, we might as well forget about America.

The Case of John Hinckley

John W. Hinckley, Jr., the man accused of shooting President Reagan, is now being "studied" by psychiatrists. According to press reports, his "tests" may take up to three months to complete. President Reagan was shot, hospitalized, tested, treated, and released, all in less than two weeks. Thus, the mere length of time seemingly necessary for "examining" Hinckley lends weight to the impression—implied, asserted, or simply taken for granted by mental health experts and others—that Hinckley is indeed sick.

Hinckley's parents, who may perhaps be forgiven for tilting the truth, spoke with what seemed to me arrogance when they said: "We simply ask that you realize John is a sick boy . . ." But John Hinckley's alleged sickness (presumably "mental") is not like cancer, that a person may have and not "realize" (or not want to "realize") that he has. Hinckley's parents also asked that we join them "in prayers for our son John . . ." Since I do not pray, I must decline the invitation. But I must add that I find the idea of people praying for a person who tries to assassinate the president distasteful, to say the least.

But then we live in an age in which right and wrong, guilt and innocence, are hopelessly confused, especially by psychiatrists. For example, *Time* magazine quotes a Harvard psychiatrist, Thomas Gutheil, referring to Hinckley as a "victim" of a disease—"erotomania"—manifested by "obsession with celebrity."

Crime is a disease. Punishment is a crime. The criminal is a victim. And America, poverty, and, of course, mental illness are the "causes" of everything that interferes with unremitting human happiness. Consider these typical comments about Hinckley.

William Buckley (who should know better) writes: "John Hinckley, like the killer of Allard Lowenstein, is for all intents and purposes as inexplicable as Mount St. Helens, and probably as uncontrollable." Not so. John Hinckley is a person, a moral agent. Mount St. Helens is a part of the earth's crust, a mountain. Hinckley is easily controllable: that, indeed, is what he had obviously asked for, back in Nashville and perhaps earlier.

Anthony Lewis compares Hinckley to other presidential assassins (in-

---

Reprinted, with permission, from the *Spectator* (London), July 11, 1981, pp. 9-10.

cluding those who killed Lincoln, McKinley and Kennedy), considers them all obviously insane, and concludes—comfortably and no doubt comfortingly—that the "attempt on President Reagan was in the historic mold of derangement." Jane Brody assures us that "nearly all [presidential assassins] were mentally unstable," and supports this by explaining that "psychiatrists have emphasised the schizophrenic personalities of American assassins."

Carl Rowan counsels sympathy for the parents, taking it for granted that the would-be killer is sick since he "has been a drug abuser [and] . . . has been under the care of a psychiatrist." *Newsweek* speaks of Hinckley's "lunatic mission" and of a public unsafe "from the fantasies of madmen." Alas, if that were all we had to fear.

Since several prominent commentators have casually coupled the assassination of President McKinley and the attempted assassination of President Reagan, I thought it would be interesting to see whether McKinley's assassin had been examined by psychiatrists, and, if so, what they had found. Believing that, if we want to, we can learn from history, I herewith offer a brief account of the encounter between the man who killed McKinley and the experts who examined him.

Leon F. Czolgosz shot President William McKinley in Buffalo, on 6 September, 1901. He was tried on 23 and 24 September, the entire proceedings occupying only eight and a half hours. Found guilty by the jury, Czolgosz was sentenced to death on 26 September and was electrocuted at Auburn prison (about 20 miles west of Syracuse) on 29 October. The time that elapsed between the murder and the execution was less than eight weeks.

In January 1902, the *American Journal of Insanity* (the official organ of what is now the American Psychiatric Association) published a lengthy report of the case by the principal defense psychiatrist in it. Entitled "The Trial, Execution, Autopsy, and Mental Status of Leon F. Czolgosz, Alias Fred Neiman, the Assassin of President McKinley," the report was written by Carlos F. Macdonald, M.D., Professor of Mental Diseases and Medical Jurisprudence at the Bellevue Hospital Medical College, and included "A Report of the Post-Mortem Examination" by Edward Anthony Spitzka of the College of Physicians and Surgeons. All subsequent quotations are from this article.

"There are many persons," wrote Macdonald, "who are disposed to hold that the enormity of such a crime is in itself sufficient evidence to warrant the opinion of the existence of insanity, merely because it seems to them inconsistent with the principles of rational conduct . . ." Denying that this is so, he instead urged upon his readers the view that "medical science [now] holds that the whole question of responsibility should rest upon the presence or absence of mental disease and not upon a knowledge of right and wrong as regards the nature and consequences of the act in question . . ."

In keeping with this belief, Czolgosz was closely studied by five psychiatrists, three appointed by the prosecution, two by the defense. Like many defendants charged with the murder of a political figure, Czolgosz did not want to be examined by psychiatrists. This did not prevent them from finding Czolgosz to be mentally healthy. He also objected to being represented by court-appointed counsel and wanted to plead guilty. He was, of course, forced to plead not guilty and received a defense that consisted, according to Macdonald, "mainly of an apology [by the chief defense counsel, a former judge] for appearing as counsel for the defendant and a touching eulogy of his distinguished victim . . ." The jury brought in a verdict of guilty in less than half an hour.

On the morning of 29 October, 1901, the superintendent of State Prisons assembled with several prominent New York state officials, among them Macdonald and Spitzka, to witness Czolgosz's execution. During the preparations for the electrocution, Czolgosz "addressed himself to the witnesses in a clear and distinct voice in the following significant language: 'I killed the President because he was an enemy of the good people—the good working people. I am not sorry for my crime. I am sorry I could not see my father.' The Warden then signaled the electrician to close the switch, sending the first charge of current through Czolgosz's body. A few moments later Macdonald —the principal defense psychiatrist!—ordered the electrician to make a second contact 'as a precautionary measure.'"

The experts who have spoken out on the Hinckley case and who have compared him with Czolgosz have all asserted or implied, as if it were an obvious "fact," that Czolgosz was mentally ill. Carlos Macdonald thought otherwise. He ended his report with this conclusion: "The writer having reviewed the case in all its aspects, with due regard to the bearing and significance of every fact and circumstance relative thereto that was accessible to him, records his opinion unqualifiedly that Leon F. Czolgosz on September 6, 1901, when he assassinated President McKinley, was in all respects a sane man—both legally and medically—and fully responsible for his act."

The grisly scenario of proving Czolgosz sane was still not over. Less than an hour after Czolgosz was led into the death chamber, his body lay on the autopsy table. The post-mortem examination was performed by Spitzka under Macdonald's supervision. After reporting that the autopsy findings were negative and apologizing for not finding any evidence of "insanity" Spitzka concluded: "Why not rejoice at the occasional discovery of a—I will not say normal—but nearly normal anatomical subject, instead of resorting to miscitation to deprive us of so rare a consolation?"

And therein lies the final irony of the psychiatric study of the Czolgoszs, Oswalds, and Hinckleys—ante-mortem and post-mortem, with or without "examining" the subject: that regardless of whether the "diagnosis" is sanity or insanity, it is a lie.

On Hinckley's
''Innocence By Insanity''

Since the Hinckley trial, the insanity defense has been discussed ad nauseam. However, the most important things about this particular instance of it have generally been ignored or denied.

The widely held idea that John Hinckley, Jr. "got away with (attempted) murder" is inconsistent with the fact that he was willing, indeed eager, to take responsibility for his criminal acts. Hinckley did not want to plead insanity. In a letter to *Newsweek* (Sept. 20, 1982), he wrote: "In return for four concurrent life sentences and a parole possibility in 15 years, I would have pleaded guilty. . . . I was not allowed to plead guilty, without any sort of plea bargain."

Thus, the idea that Hinckley "got away" with something by being adjudged insane is not only untrue, but is the very opposite of the truth: Given that at the time of his trial, John Hinckley, Jr. was competent to stand trial (had he not been mentally and legally competent, he would not have been *allowed* to stand trial), and that he nevertheless was not permitted to choose his own defense tactic (the insanity plea was, in effect, *imposed* on him), one could reasonably argue that Hinckley was denied his Fifth Amendment right to a fair trial.

Why, then, did Hinckley plead insanity? My guess is that he was misled into doing so, partly by believing the plea would fail and partly by believing that if it succeeded he would, sooner or later, be released from captivity. (I venture to predict that the only way the authorities charged with determining Hinckley's fate will let him leave St. Elizabeths Hospital is in a pine box.)

The role played by the defendant's parents—JoAnn and John Hinckley, Sr.—in their son's insanity defense and the ongoing publicity about it has been almost totally ignored. It was, in fact, Hinckley's parents' idea and wish that their son plead insanity. In an interview with Barbara Walters on ABC's "20/20" (April 28, 1983), John Hinckley, Sr. acknowledged that his son "wanted to plead guilty." In the interview JoAnn and John Hinckley, Sr. make it very clear that they want to present their son to the public as "ill," not "evil."

First published as "A Look at John Hinckley's Parents," *Washington Times* (Op-Ed), May 12, 1983, C-1. Reprinted with permission.

In this connection, it is important to note, also, that while Dr. John Hopper was, and still is, consistently referred to as John Hinckley, Jr.'s psychiatrist, he was nothing of the sort. Hopper was JoAnn and John Hinckley, Sr.'s psychiatrist: They paid Hopper to help rid them of their unwanted son. John Hinckley, Jr. did not want Hopper or psychiatry. He wanted his parents and their home; he also wanted the money his father held in trust for him and would not give him . . . and he wanted Jodie Foster. The parents' efforts to have their son defined as insane also were supported by the prosecution, which arguably failed to prosecute: It selected a psychiatrically gullible jury; it supported the defense contention that Hinckley was "mentally ill"; and it never introduced the evidence that Hinckley had acknowledged his guilt by wanting to plead guilty.

Let us not deceive ourselves about mental illness and the insanity defense: Much as we may try to disguise desires as diseases and dispositions as diagnoses, in the long run the only people we fool are ourselves. The insanity defense has nothing to do with disease but has everything to do with disposition. We see this clearly enough when the Russians dispose of "dissidents" by imposing insanity pleas and acquittals on them.

The fact is that a lot of people wanted to dispose of John Hinckley, Jr. as insane. President Reagan himself implied as much when he called Hinckley "sick" in his first press conference after the assassination attempt. More important, Hinckley's parents wanted such a disposition: Despite their protestations to the contrary, they bought the lawyers and psychiatrists needed to mount an insanity defense for their son and they seduced or coerced him into pleading insanity.

If all the world is a stage, we have, in the last two years, watched a play featuring not only John Hinckley, Jr. but his parents and their hirelings as well. The plot, scripted by JoAnn and John Hinckley, Sr., is the decriminalization of John Hinckley, Jr.—that is, his systematic transformation from attention-seeking malcontent trying to kill an American president to "schizophrenic patient" not knowing what he is doing and therefore not responsible for his actions.

Let us ask: *Cui bono?* Who has profited from this recasting of John Hinckley, Jr. from bad to mad? Perhaps John Hinckley, Jr., but that remains to be seen. Assuredly, JoAnn and John Hinckley, Sr. Their apologetics in the *Readers' Digest* (March 1983), and their recent performance on ABC television make it clear, through their own deliberate self-revelations, that they are the primary beneficiaries of John Hinckley, Jr.'s insanity acquittal. The successful insanity defense they mounted and the subsequent publicity campaign they have orchestrated have established them as loving parents and their son as a "victim of schizophrenia." Moreover, they can rest safely with the knowledge that their troubled and trouble-making son is securely out of the way—his embarrassing infantilism, his failure to live up to his parents' expectations, his dastardly deeds all neatly obscured by an outpouring of psychiatric rhetoric.

Alas, Hinckley *père et mère* succeeded precisely where Lord Macbeth failed—namely, in procuring medical (and legal) legitimization for redefining familial evil as individual illness.

Writing People Off as Crazy

For the past century and more, the insanity defense—now in the public eye again in connection with the case of John Hinckley—has been debated ad nauseam. These debates have been fruitless because they focus on the abstract concepts of insanity and responsibility and because they treat the insanity defense in isolation. In the context of the insanity defense, the abstract notions of insanity and responsibility effectively distract attention from the obvious social-psychological function of this so-called defense, a function I will describe presently. In addition, by treating the insanity defense in isolation we fail to consider its relations to other social strategies of claiming and disclaiming, accepting and rejecting an actor's responsibility for his act.

To illustrate both points, consider the case of modern political terrorism. Typically, we are here confronted with murders committed by stealth so that the killers are unknown and are likely to remain so. As a rule, the terrorists do not want to be captured but do want to get credit for their deed. They accomplish this by anonymous messages delivered to the media in which they *claim* responsibility for their act. The result is that news accounts of bombings and shootings carried out by terrorists are now usually followed by the stock phrase that "such-and-such a group or organization has claimed responsibility" for them. This public acknowledgment of the terrorists' responsibility for their deeds implies respect for them as human beings and recognition of the legitimacy (at least in their own eyes) of their aims and of the violent tactics with which they seek to attain them.

All this stands in sharp contrast to the instant, almost reflexive response of the press to crimes of violence carried out by individuals deemed to be insane. The media immediately label an Oswald or a Hinckley crazy, thus implying that because of their insanity, such persons are not responsible for their violent acts. This view satisfies a collective urge—to which the media cater—to deny that such persons are fully human and that their "abnormal" acts do not differ fundamentally from those of "normal" persons.

"A normal person does not kill the president" is what the normal person tells himself. At the same time, this hypothetical normal person does not doubt for a minute that an Irish, Italian, or Palestinian terrorist who kills many persons is quite normal. This drama of recognizing or rejecting the

---

Reprinted, with permission, from the *Washington Post* (Op-Ed), April 16, 1982, p. A-29.

meaning of certain violent acts, and of dignifying or disdaining certain violent actors is now performed through the images and vocabularies of politics and psychiatry. Political actors are recognized as sane and their deeds are dignified as responsible acts, whereas psychiatric actors are rejected as insane and their deeds are demeaned as non-responsible acts.

The labeling of Soviet citizens who defy the Communist system illustrates this theme. In America, such persons are viewed as responsible—engaging in political protest—and are hailed as heroic "activists" and "dissidents." In Russia, the same persons are viewed as irresponsible—engaging in the psychotic slander of the state—and are diagnosed as schizophrenics requiring psychiatric confinement and treatment.

It would be fair to say, then, that the insanity defense, despite its name, has nothing to do with insanity; nor, despite the legal emphasis put on it, does it have anything to do with criminal responsibility. What it does have to do with is whether or not we want to take a particular person charged with a crime seriously. If we do not want to take him seriously, we will support his "acquittal" as insane and will, in general, be favorably disposed toward the retention of this legal-psychiatric mechanism. On the other hand, if we want to take a particular defendant seriously, we will support his conviction for the crime he has committed. And if we want to take everyone seriously, then we will support the abolition of the insanity defense.

IV
PSYCHIATRY AND POLITICS

The Martyrdom Of Ezra Pound

It has been your habit for long to do away with good writers,
You either drive them mad, or else blink at their suicides,
Or else you condone their drugs, and talk of insanity and genius,
But I will not go mad to please you.

So wrote Ezra Pound in 1914. What Pound failed to understand is that if we
want to consider a person insane, we need not "drive" him mad; we can
simply "declare" him mad. Like Pound, many people do not grasp the
double meaning of the concept of madness, and, like Pound, they often pay
dearly for their ignorance. The word "mad" may refer to a person's existential
condition: For example, a man may *go* mad because of unbearable dis-
appointment and grief. It may also refer to a stigmatized social role into
which a person may be cast: For example, a man may be *called* mad because
his conduct disturbs those about him. When, in 1914, Pound resolved not to
go mad to please the "enemies" of art in America, he did not anticipate that,
thirty-one years later, his "friends" would call him mad. But this is precisely
what they did. How they did it may be learned from this book, written by
Pound's lawyer.

Julien Cornell's *The Trial of Ezra Pound* (John Day, 1966), which he
calls "A Documented Account of the Treason Case by the Defendant's
Lawyer," is falsely titled and falsely subtitled. It is not the story of Ezra
Pound's "trial," but rather of his nontrial. It is not a "documented account,"
but rather a collection of documents strung together with a few transitional
explanations. Finally, it is not, in an important sense, written by the
"defendant's lawyer" (although, to be sure, Mr. Cornell was recognized by
the court as Pound's counsel), but rather by an attorney who, by adopting a
tactic which made his position as counsel for the defense indistinguishable
from that of the prosecution, chose not to help his client stand trial.

Ezra Pound had long resided in Rapallo, Italy. When, in May 1945, Allied troops reached the north of Italy, Pound sought out the American

First published as "There Was No Defense," a review of *The Trial of Ezra Pound*, by Julien
Cornell, *New York Times Book Review*, November 13, 1966, pp. 4, 34; the present longer
version is reprinted, with permission, from the *Rutgers Law Review*, 21 (Winter 1967), pp.
367-374.

authorities and requested permission to return to the United States. He believed that he would be allowed to do so, in order to give President Truman the benefit of his intimate knowledge of conditions not only in Italy but also in Japan. Instead, to his surprise, he was placed in solitary confinement in a military prison at Pisa. In November 1945, he was flown back to Washington, and was charged with treason.

Pound, however, was never tried. Instead, the court, the prosecution, and the defense, together with their respective psychiatrists, unanimously agreed that he was mentally unfit to stand trial. In this way, his right to trial, guaranteed by the Sixth Amendment to the Constitution—a right which Pound was eager to exercise—was denied him, and he was "imprisoned" (the term is Cornell's) for more than twelve years at St. Elizabeths Hospital in Washington, D.C. Franz von Papen, a leading figure in the Nazi regime, was allowed to stand trial at Nuremberg and was acquitted. Justice? Perhaps not moral justice, but a fine case, indeed, of psychiatric justice.

When Pound first realized that he was accused of making treasonous broadcasts during the war, he wanted to conduct his own defense. He was prevented, however, not only from pleading his own case, but from standing trial altogether, by his friends, his wife, and his lawer. I do not doubt that their intentions were good; I doubt, however, that their judgment was. Pound, too, had misgivings about this.

Mr. Cornell was asked to defend Pound by James Laughlin, who was Cornell's friend and Pound's publisher. When he tentatively accepted, Laughlin wrote to Arthur Moore, a member of a firm of London solicitors for Mrs. Pound, recommending Cornell. A letter from Moore to Laughlin, written in October 1945, provides the first of many insights into the basic rift between what Pound thought was best for him and what his friends thought was best for him. "I am however rather troubled," wrote Moore, "with the thought that whatever his friends may think or wish to do for him, he will much prefer to conduct his defense in his own manner, and by such means as may seem expedient to him."

In the same month, in reply to Moore's advice not to address the court when he came to trial, Pound wrote: "I am not sure that your advice is given in full knowledge of certain essential facts of my case. For example, I was not sending axis propaganda, but my own. . . . I want very much to know the source or reason for your opinion that I should not address the Court. Is it due to your not knowing what I actually said on the air? . . . The investigator for the American Department of Justice expressed himself as convinced that I was telling him the absolute truth months ago, and has since with great care collected far more proof to that effect than I or any private lawyer could have got at." Is this the writing of a man incapable of standing trial? "My instinct all along," Pound continued, "has been to leave the whole matter to the U.S. Department of Justice, the good faith of whose agent I have had no reason to doubt." Is this the writing of a person afflicted with paranoia, as Pound was said to have been? In addition, Pound suggested that Roger Baldwin of the American Civil Liberties Union be contacted as someone who might help him in his defense.

A month after this thoroughly lucid letter was written, Pound was declared insane and incapable of standing trial.

It is unclear whether Pound really wished to be represented by Mr. Cornell, or whether—as it appears—he simply went along with the recommendations of his friends and wife. After Cornell first met Pound, he described him, in a letter to Laughlin, in November 1945, as a "poor devil" whose mind was "wobbly," but whose talk was "entirely rational." "I discussed with him the possibility of pleading insanity as a defense," Cornell writes, "and he had no objection." But this was not what Mr. Cornell did: Instead, he petitioned the court that Pound was unfit to stand trial. (Pleading insanity and pleading unfitness to stand trial are two quite different legal-psychiatric gambits and have vastly different practical implications for the defendant.) Moreover, Cornell's claim that Pound agreed to the insanity defense is flatly contradicted by Thurman Arnold, who was instrumental in securing Pound's release. "He [Pound] could not be tried and acquitted on the ground of insanity," writes Arnold in his book *Fair Fights and Foul,* "because he refused to make that defense. . . ."

One wonders if Mr. Cornell then understood, or now understands, the practical consequences of various legal-psychiatric maneuvers. In the above-mentioned letter, he explained that "the trial of such an issue [i.e., of insanity as a defense] is almost always a farce, since learned medicos who testify for each side squarely contradict each other. . . ." (I infer from this that Mr. Cornell was well aware that it is possible to secure almost any kind of psychiatric expert testimony, a fact which will assume special significance later on.)

By the end of November 1945, "Pound's trial was not my immediate concern," writes Cornell. "The man was too ill for that. He was in dire need of medical care." It is not clear on what medical authority Mr. Cornell bases this opinion. Pound was examined by Army psychiatrists in Italy before being flown back to the United States and was declared sane; as physicians, they would, presumably, have been able to diagnose Pound's medical condition as well as Mr. Cornell. Moreover, Cornell's evaluation of Pound's health is flatly contradicted by the four physicians who examined Pound a short time later; they declared Pound to be "in generally good physical condition." Mr. Cornell's emphasis on how very "sick" Pound was thus appears to be a rhetorical device to justify sparing him the burden, or taking from him the right—which depends on our point of view—of standing trial.

Having decided to declare Pound unfit for trial, Mr. Cornell instructed his psychiatrist to discover the necessary infirmities. "In examining Mr. Pound," wrote Cornell to Dr. Wendell Muncie, "I wish you to bear in mind that there is another question involved in addition to his sanity, namely, the question whether even if he is sane, he is sufficiently well to stand the ordeal of a lengthy trial. This would require several weeks of conferences with his attorneys in preparation for trial, and probably two weeks at least of proceedings in court. I have some reasons to fear that even if he were sufficiently sane to understand the proceedings, the ordeal of the trial might bring on a relapse."

Pound, we must remember, was eager to stand trial. He wanted to address the court. There is good reason to believe that he would have loved the role he would have had to play in the proceedings. If so, standing trial for Pound would have been no more of an "ordeal" than it is an ordeal for Mr. Johnson to be president. Whether a particular human situation is a painful ordeal or an exhilarating experience for a person cannot be decided by someone else.

It is also necessary to recall that Pound survived five months imprisonment in Italy, in what Mr. Cornell calls a "concentration camp." Compared to this, two weeks in a courtroom in Washington, D.C., should have seemed like a vacation. Lastly, if Pound needed medical attention, why could he have not received it in the District of Columbia prison where he was confined prior to the psychiatric intervention? After all, he was a famous poet awaiting trial in Truman's Washington—not an unknown kulak banished to Stalin's Siberia.

Pound was examined by four psychiatrists; one was retained by the defense, three by the prosecution. In December 1945, they unanimously declared Pound "insane and mentally unfit for trial." It would be an error to conclude that this unanimity meant that theirs was indeed a valid—truly "scientific"—finding. Actually, the agreement among the four psychiatrists was deliberately sought and carefully contrived. "In Overholser's [Superintendent of St. Elizabeths Hospital] opinion," writes Cornell, "a dispute between doctors was unworthy of the profession, degrading to the doctors involved, and a hindrance to the judicial process." There is no mention here of the "patient" to whom physicians, at least according to the Hippocratic Oath, are supposed to owe their primary loyalty. Was it not degrading to Pound to be characterized as insane—unanimously, no less—so that ever since he has usually been referred to as "paranoid"? Moreover, this ostensibly unanimous psychiatric expert opinion did not even reflect the full truth, as known to Cornell and Overholser. Before Pound's sanity hearing, the two men had a private meeting, in which, according to Cornell, the following transpired: "Dr. Overholser asked me to wait a moment, as he wanted to talk to me. When I was ushered into his private office he told me abruptly that he wished to disclose something to me which he had not told Matlack [attorney for the Justice Department] and was not going to tell him. This was a great surprise to me, as Overholser was the government's 'star witness' who would not ordinarily volunteer any information to the defense attorney, much less information which he had not disclosed to the prosecution. . . . He told me that he remained firm in his opinion that Pound was mentally unfit to stand trial, but, he said, many of the young doctors on his staff disagreed."

Dr. Overholser, a medical expert for the prosecution in a criminal case, was thus suppressing information from the legal representatives who retained him and who paid for his services. Indeed, he did more than just suppress the divergent opinions of the other physicians at St. Elizabeths Hospital about Pound's mental condition; he falsely implied that they were in agreement with him. Testifying at Pound's sanity hearing, in reply to the question: "Has he [Pound] been under constant observation?" Overholser answered: "Yes, he has been under constant observation. I spent a long time on consultation with him and other doctors last Thursday and I have before me the report made by the other physicians at the hospital, and I have no reason to change my opinion." Actually, the psychiatric reports which Dr. Overholser withheld would have declared Pound sane and fit to stand trial.

This admission from Overholser is additional proof that Cornell knew he could as easily obtain psychiatric expert opinion to the effect that Pound was sane as he could that Pound was insane. If he chose the latter course in preference to the former, it could only have been because he believed that this would best serve his client's interests. But was Cornell's judgment sound?

Apart from using insanity as a tactical device, it appears that Cornell wanted to believe that Pound was *really* crazy. He mentions with dismay that Albert Deutsch, a newspaperman and the author of several outstanding books on psychiatric subjects, "wrote at length in the newspapers [about the Pound case] in an unfriendly vein." To consider Pound sane is, in this view, to take "an unfriendly" view of him. Deutsch suggested that the prosecution "adopt the line of argument that Pound's insanity was no different from the insanity of other war criminals and traitors"—a reasonable suggestion if ever there was one. The prosecution, however, was quite happy to go along with Cornell's strategy, which promised a sure way of locking Pound up for a good long time in St. Elizabeths Hospital. Could this have been because of the possibility, if not probability, that Pound could not have been convicted of treason, because his broadcasts were, in fact, not treasonous?

Still more doubts about the validity of the dismal pronouncements about Pound's mind arise when we note some of Cornell's observations and comments about it. Barely a month after Pound was declared mentally unfit to stand trial, Cornell wrote to Mrs. Pound: "You need not be alarmed about the report on your husband's mental condition. . . . I believe that his condition is just about normal. . . . Those who have known him for some time, such as James Laughlin, tell me that he is very much his old self. . . ." But if Mr. Cornell believed this to be true, was it not his duty—not only to his client, but to his profession—to petition the court to proceed with Pound's trial without delay?

In the same letter, Mr. Cornell asserted that "the mental aberrations which the doctors have found are not anything new or unusual . . . In fact I think it may be fairly said that any man of his genius would be regarded by a psychiatrist as abnormal." If this were true, no "genius" could ever be tried in an American court. Moreover, Cornell's last comment is a slur on the psychiatric profession, for it applies only to those psychiatrists—and they are probably in the minority—who do not understand, or who deny, the tactical uses of psychiatric diagnoses in courts of law.

Not only did the law treat Mr. Pound shabbily, but so did many individuals associated with his nontrial. In addition to his responsibility for incriminating Pound as insane, Mr. Cornell published a book about his case in which he included several letters which Pound wrote him. Permission for printing these letters was obtained from Mrs. Dorothy Pound, "as Committee for Ezra Pound, incompetent. . . ." Are we to believe that Pound was incompetent not only to stand trial, but *totally,* to do anything? If not, why did Cornell fail to obtain permission for the use of these letters from Pound himself? This omission is further evidence—if more were needed—of how the actions ostensibly intended to protect Pound's mental health actually served to destroy his status as a human being. Eight years after his release from psychiatric confinement, Pound's letters were published without his permission, but with the permission of his wife, thus according Ezra Pound continuing recognition as a childlike madman with no rights to his person or property, and according to Dorothy Pound continuing recognition as a motherlike guardian, the rightful owner of the person and property of her insane child-husband.

The moral insults showered on Pound were almost limitless. His lawyer did not respect his dignity and privacy and helped to deny him his right to trial. His judge and his psychiatrist did not consider him innocent until proved guilty. In dismissing the charges against Pound in 1958, Judge Bolitha J. Laws wrote that "there is a strong probability that the commission of the crime charged was the result of insanity. . . ." Dr. Overholser concurred, finding "a strong probability that the commission of the crime charged was the result of insanity. . . ." These may seem like well-intentioned statements, further exonerating Pound from guilt. Perhaps that's how they were intended. But that is not what they mean!

If we declare Jones "not guilty by reason of insanity" of the murder of Smith, we *imply* that we believe two things to be true: one, that Smith is dead; and two, that Jones killed him. Our statement about Jones' "innocence"—by reason of insanity—is thus, simultaneously, a declaration of our belief, first, that Jones did commit the crime with which he had been charged, and, second, that he has a valid excuse for doing what we believe he did (and what he often admits to having done). Suppose, however, that Jones is accused of murdering Smith, but denies the act. By saying that Jones "committed the crime he is charged with probably because of insanity"—as Judge Laws and Dr. Overholser said Pound did—we judge Jones to have taken Smith's life. Herein lies the moral and legal core of the Pound case, and generally of the denial of the right to trial by declaring the defendant mentally unfit to be tried. Pound insisted that he committed no treasonous act. The only facts not contested are that Pound made several broadcasts during the war over the Rome radio. The text of two of these is included in this book. Mr. Cornell flatly asserts that they are not treasonous. I agree. The reader can judge for himself. But if these broadcasts were indeed not treasonous, and if Pound had a sound defense and a fair trial, then he might very well have been acquitted. As it happened, he was not tried, but was imprisoned nevertheless. Moreover, although he may not have committed the crimes with which he was charged, he could not—and cannot ever—prove his innocence.

All this was accomplished by means of a sanity hearing in which Pound had no adversaries—only "friends." Three of the psychiatrists who testified were chosen and paid by the prosecution; they also happened to be full-time career employees of the United States Government. One was a private psychiatrist chosen by the defense and presumably paid by Mr. Cornell. Yet, ironically (or by mistake?), all four psychiatrists are listed in the transcript of the sanity hearing as appearing "on behalf of the defendant."

The upshot was that every one testified "for" Pound, and no one "against" him. His "sentence": more than twelve years at St. Elizabeths Hospital as an involuntary mental patient, and a lifetime—or perhaps even an historical—dehumanization as an "incurable paranoid." In April 1958, in a sworn statement, Dr. Overholser asserted that Pound has been "suffering from a paranoid state . . . which is permanent and incurable . . . and which renders him permanently and incurably insane." Camus realized—but Pound, unfortunately, did not—that "the executioners of today, as everyone knows, are humanists."

Ezra Pound was sixty years old when he was placed, against his will, in Dr. Overholser's "care." Throughout all his adult years, he was a self-reliant and creative individual, responsible for himself and his family, and notably helpful to aspiring artists and writers, among them James Joyce and T. S. Eliot. (In a letter to Ford Madox Ford in 1932, Joyce wrote: "It is nearly twenty years since he [Pound] first began his vigorous campaign on my behalf and it is probable that but for him I should still be the unknown drudge that he discovered.") To be sure, Pound had ideas that might have been wrong, and made utterances that might have been unwise. Who hasn't? But what did he do—beside being intransigently critical of certain aspects of American life—to deserve the vicious character assassination and the long imprisonment without trial meted out to him by his country which, in his own way, he loved deeply?

Although he might not be a Socrates, Pound's stature as a martyr—partly because of his own undisputable gifts, and partly because of the reaction of his countrymen which he managed to provoke—seems firmly established. Those responsible for Pound's post-war fate—our legal system, our psychiatry, and especially the persons instrumental in depriving him of the opportunity to clear his name in court—have placed a black mark on the pages of contemporary American history. We cannot erase this black mark. The best we can do is to expiate it by mending our ways. If, from the martyrdom of Ezra Pound, we have learned our lesson about the inhumanity of modern legal psychiatry, then, in a larger sense, Pound will not have suffered in vain.

The Hazards of Zeal

Woodrow Wilson's personality and presidency have always been and still are a delicate subject. Inevitably, any critical biography of an American president, whether the author so intends or not, is considered an exposé of his secret weaknesses. This effect is greatly heightened when, as in *Thomas Woodrow Wilson: A Psychological Study,* by Sigmund Freud and William C. Bullitt (Houghton), the subject is a great and "martyred" president, and one of the biographers, a great but still controversial psychiatrist. This book, then, is sure to make the fur fly.

Because of the criticisms already leveled against it on the grounds that it impugns Wilson's greatness by demeaning him as mentally deranged, I shall first address myself to the psychiatric aspects of the work. Freud, it must be noted, foresaw this criticism. "We must attack the misconception," he writes in the Introduction, "that we have written this book with a secret purpose to prove that Wilson was a pathological character, an abnormal man, in order to undermine in this roundabout way esteem for his achievements. No! That is not our intention. For belief in a stiff frame of normality and a sharp line of demarcation between normal and abnormal in the psychic life has been abandoned by our science." This claim of Freud's bears the same relation to the realities of psychiatry as Wilson's claims about the Treaty of Versailles bore to the realities of politics. The fact is that millions of persons all over the world have been defamed and imprisoned by having been declared "mentally ill"; but Freud never even alludes to any of this. Similarly, in a speech on September 24, 1919, Wilson characterized the Treaty of Versailles as "the most remarkable document . . . in human history," and asserted that the Great Powers "did not claim a single piece of territory"; the facts were blatantly otherwise.

Freud's disclaimer, that he was not trying to prove that Wilson was a "pathological character," is contradicted by what he and Bullitt actually say about Wilson. For example, they cite Wilson's false characterization of the Treaty of Versailles and conclude that Wilson was "not consciously lying," but was "very close to psychosis." The authors thus use psychiatric diagnostic

---

Review of *Thomas Woodrow Wilson: A Psychological Study,* by Sigmund Freud and William C. Bullitt, reprinted, with permission, from the *National Review,* March 21, 1967, pp. 307-10.

terms, as do others, to explain behavior which they dislike or disapprove of, and thereby stigmatize the person whom they label. Herein lies one of the valuable lessons contained in this volume. If the reader believes that mental illness is a disease like any other, then he must be ready to accept the possibility that the experts capable of diagnosing such diseases may find them not only in unimportant people, but also in national leaders. Moreover, if psychiatric diagnoses demean great men, they also demean little men. How, then, do we reconcile crying "Foul!" when Wilson is diagnosed mentally sick, with practicing the same kind of name-calling with great fervor on our less important citizens?

As psychiatric analysis, this book thus exemplifies what has become commonplace in our day: the substitution of the language of medicine for the language of morals, and the consequent condemnation of individuals as "sick" rather than as "bad." This perspective on human affairs suffers from a fundamental misunderstanding of the differences between physical science and (so-called) social science. In physical science, we desire knowledge of an object in order to control it better; by understanding electricity, we can produce light, heat, and send messages. If social science is merely an extension, to man and society, of the aims and methods of physical science, then it follows that we will wish to have a greater understanding of people, the better to control them. But the control of man by his fellow man is supposed to be a problem for ethics, law, and politics—not for "science." Moreover, although it is true that we must know physics to control electrons, it is not true that we must know psychology to control men: to control man, we need power, not knowledge, and the desire and will to use that power.

Despite these defects, this is a valuable book. To be sure, it is a personalistic, rather than a historical, analysis of Wilson and his presidency; but that is what the authors intended it to be. It is possible to separate, to some extent, the portrait of Wilson here presented from the authors' "psychoanalysis" of his character; the former may stand even if the latter does not. The following quotations illustrate the sort of picture which Freud and Bullitt paint of Wilson. In his mature years, they say, Wilson was "an ugly, unhealthy 'intense,' Presbyterian, who had little interest in women and none in food, wine, music, art or sport, but enormous interest in speaking, in himself, in his career and in God." At Princeton, when reminded of a promise he had made, Wilson retorted: "We must not lay too great stress on 'commitments.'" In Paris, he was said to be the man who "talks like Jesus Christ and acts like Lloyd George."

The picture of Wilson which thus emerges is consistent with that painted by others, notably by Thomas Bailey, a distinguished professor of American history at Stanford University, who characterizes him as follows: "He called for 'peace without victory' early in 1917 (he ultimately settled for victory without peace). After trying 'armed neutrality' (it was essentially unarmed unneutrality), he asked for a war to make the world 'safe for democracy' (it ended with the world made unsafe for democracy) and for 'a war to end war' (there were twenty or so wars being waged after the big one jarred to a halt). At Paris he fought desperately for his Fourteen Points, including 'open covenants for peace, openly arrived at' (he met secretly with the Big Four). . . ."

Undeniably, Wilson managed to entangle the United States in a war purely on economic conflicts between two groups of European powers, "right" and "wrong" being as evenly divided between the combatants as they have ever been in war; and he managed to superintend a peace treaty unwittingly guaranteed to breed discontents and wars the likes of which mankind had never seen. Bullitt, on the other hand, resigned in 1919 (when he was only 28 years old) from his position as attaché to the American Peace Commission, because, as he wrote to the President, "our government has consented now to deliver the suffering peoples of the world to new oppressions, subjections and dismemberments—a new century of war. And I can convince myself no longer that effective labor for 'a new world order' is possible as a servant of this Government . . . [The] duty of the Government of the United States to its own people and to mankind is to refuse to sign or ratify this unjust treaty, to refuse to guarantee its settlements by entering the League of Nations, to refuse to entangle the United States further by the understanding with France." Still, Wilson, not Bullitt, is honored as a great American and a great "peacemaker"; and Wilson, not Bullitt, was awarded the Nobel Prize for Peace.

Herein lies one of the crucial differences between science and politics. We revere Giordano Bruno, not those who burned him at the stake. We remember Ignaz Semmelweis, not those who persecuted him and committed him to an insane asylum. But we do not similarly honor men, like Bullitt, who had courageously warned about and sagely predicted the consequences of Wilson's "therapeutic" politics—and who were proved right by future events as fully as any scientist predicting the motion of planets could hope to be. In human affairs we thus continue to focus on motives rather than consequences, and to honor lofty aims rather than decent deeds.

Freud, we may recall here, taught psychiatrists about the risks lurking in excessive therapeutic zeal. In this book Freud and Bullitt show us the dangers lurking in the reforming zeal of the politician and statesman. If proof were needed that Samuel Johnson was right when he exclaimed, "Hell is paved with good intentions," this book would amply supply it.

Although written more than thirty years ago, this study of Wilson is astonishingly timely today. One of the reasons for this is that Wilson was the first important meliorist liberal in modern American politics. His failure and tragedy were not just the failure and tragedy of a particular individual—as Freud and Bullitt make it appear—but also the failure and tragedy of evangelical liberalism as a psychological perspective and political ideology. As Kenneth Minogue has so brilliantly shown, one of the hazards the liberal faces is that while he "is concerned with vague general ends, it is in fact the means which are crucial in society—for the simple reason that the ends are never reached. Especially where the end is vague and utopian, the politician will be particularly liable to misunderstand the actual implications of his work. How many visionaries have unwittingly prepared a Hell on earth because their gaze was stubbornly fixed on Heaven? And when Hell comes—well, there is always some *ad hoc* theory of sinister interests or Judas-like betrayal to extricate the theorist from his disaster. What his illusions have prevented him from understanding are the forces he in fact served; and good intentions are quite beside the point. Stupidity is a moral as well as an intellectual defect."

Wilson was the quintessence of the ascetic, self-sacrificing, salvationist liberal who denies his own desires and needs and claims to represent the interests and welfare not of his own person or nation, but of all mankind. Historians sympathetic to Wilson view his inability to impose this vision on others as a "tragedy." But should we not rather rejoice that men who seek to deceive others, even with the best of intentions, in the end only deceive themselves? So long as that remains true, there is hope for mankind.

Patriotic Poisoners

Continuing revelations about medical crimes by American physicians indistinguishable from those of the Nazi "doctors of infamy" hanged at Nuremberg raise troubling questions, not only about the precise nature of the deeds in question, but also about these physicians' legal and moral accountability for their acts. Whereas, decades after their deeds, the perpetrators of Nazi atrocities are hounded for their crimes and brought to justice, the perpetrators of analogous American medical atrocities reap nothing but rewards for their pioneering "research" in psychopharmacology.

Surely it is no accident that the major medical crimes in Nazi Germany were committed by psychiatrists. It is conservatively estimated that German psychiatrists murdered at least 30,000 German (non-Jewish) mental patients. I submit it is similarly no accident that most of the physicians so far identified as having participated in what the American press calls the CIA-sponsored "drug tests" have been psychiatrists.[1]

The Rockefeller Commission's report on CIA activities within the United States, released in June, 1975, lifted the lid, albeit ever so slightly, from what may yet prove to be a veritable Pandora's box of psychiatric atrocities. Buried in that report—occupying less than three pages and naming no names—is a section on "The Testing of Behavior-Influencing Drugs on Unsuspecting Subjects Within the United States."[2] After an initial paragraph attributing the rationale of the program to the supposed use of psychochemicals by the Soviets, the report goes on to say: "The drug program was a part of a much larger CIA program to study possible means for controlling human behavior. Other studies explored the effects of radiation, electric-shock, psychology, psychiatry, sociology, and harassment substances."[3] The bracketing of the "mental health" disciplines with "harassment substances" is surely revealing of the uses to which these supposed sciences are often put.

The report contains very little actual information about the clandestine CIA drug program because, the Commission explains, "unfortunately, only limited records of the testing conducted in these drug programs are now available. All the records concerning the program were ordered destroyed in 1973, including a total of 152 separate files."[4]

The Commission does state, however, that "commencing in 1955 under

---

Reprinted, with permission, from the *Humanist,* November/December, 1976, pp. 5-7.

an informal arrangement with the Federal Bureau of Drug Abuse Control, tests were begun on unsuspecting subjects in normal social situations." And it reports one fatality. The victim was "an employee of the Department of the Army [who] was administered LSD without his knowledge while attending a meeting with CIA personnel working on the drug project [who] developed serious side effects and was sent to New York with a CIA escort for psychiatric treatment. Several days later, he jumped from a tenth-floor window in his room and died as a result." This last sentence is significantly footnoted as follows: "There are indications in the few remaining Agency records that this individual may have had a history of emotional instability."[5] In other words, the Commission is not satisfied with passing over in silence the fact that the CIA agents in charge of protecting the drugged victim's mental health placed him in a tenth-floor room, but it goes out of its way to defame the victim as mentally ill, implying that he killed himself not because he was poisoned but because he was psychotic.

The Rockefeller Commission's report was soon followed by a series of revelations about medical crimes whose details still continue to trickle in: the anonymous suicide mentioned in the report was identified as Frank Olson; and another victim, not mentioned in the report, was identified as Harold Blauer.

In 1953, Dr. Frank Olson was a forty-three-year-old biochemist employed at the Army's Fort Detrick, Maryland, germ-warfare laboratories. That fall, the CIA suddenly switched his role—by slipping LSD into his after-dinner Cointreau—from researcher into guinea pig. After downing his spiked liqueur, Olson became upset and depressed. His colleagues concluded that he was mentally ill and needed psychiatric attention. Two of them, Vincent Ruwet and Robert Lashbrook, took Olson under their wing and flew him to New York to see Dr. Harold A. Abramson, a former psychiatric consultant for the Army. Abramson diagnosed Olson's problems as "delusions and severe psychosis" and recommended that Olson enter a mental hospital. On November 28, 1953, while seemingly contemplating admitting himself to a mental hospital, Olson escaped from his "protectors" by jumping to his death from a tenth-story hotel room.[6]

The second fatality directly attributable to the secret CIA psychochemical program occurred on January 9, 1953, when Harold Blauer was killed at the New York Psychiatric Institute. In the fall of 1952, Mr. Blauer, a former Army colonel and a professional tennis player, was divorced by his wife. He became depressed, sought psychiatric help, and in December, 1952, voluntarily entered the New York Psychiatric Institute. He had been scheduled to be released from the hospital the day after the fatal injection. According to the *New York Times,* "Documents explaining the experiment with Mr. Blauer indicate that he protested the injections and Miss Barrett [his daughter] says she believes he was forced to take the drug."[7] An internal Army report made public on August 3, 1976, confirmed Miss Barrett's suspicions. It quotes a

Department of Justice memo as saying that "neither the patient nor his family were advised of the proposed therapy [*sic*] or gave permission."[8] Blauer died on January 8, 1953, less than two and a half hours after being injected with a "mescaline derivative."[9]

In addition to these two known fatalities, thousands of persons, Americans and foreigners, were drugged with hallucinogenic and related substances in "research programs" sponsored by the Army, the Navy, and the Air Force. The Department of Defense claims to have discontinued these programs in 1967. The Air Force has admitted that it continued them until 1972. The scope and the cost of these programs may be gleaned from press reports published during the past year.

For example, on September 9, 1975, the *Times* reported that "the Army disclosed today that it had surreptitiously given LSD to soldiers in cocktails in much the same way the Central Intelligence Agency did in an experiment that led to the death of one of its subjects."[10] Gradually, the categories from which subjects were selected for drugging by the CIA were expanded. On April 27, 1976, the *Times* reported: "For nine years, beginning in 1954, employees of the Central Intelligence Agency randomly picked up unsuspecting patrons in bars in the United States and slipped LSD into their food and drink."[11] The next day we learned that "Army officers gave LSD to unsuspecting American soldiers, Europeans, and Asians in the late 1950s and early 1960s."[12] This information was based on a report by the Inspector General of the Army after an eight-month investigation of the service's more than twenty years of experimentation on humans with drugs. "In its more than 250-page report, the Inspector General's office said it had found numerous irregularities and violations of policies and regulations."[13] This particular program alone was said to have cost 110 million dollars.

An earlier report in the *Times* (September 10, 1975) gave us this glimpse of the money psychiatrists made from the poisoning business: "Less than a year after a patient died in an Army-sponsored experiment with an hallucinogenic drug at the New York State Psychiatric Institute, the Army gave the Institute another contract for nearly $143,000 to continue experimenting on humans for four more years."[14]

All this raises an obvious question: Who were the physicians responsible for these medical crimes? Who were the doctors who participated in, and profited from, these ostensibly patriotic and professional "research programs"? The Rockefeller Report named not a single one. It must remain a matter of conjecture whether this is because one of the "principal investigators" in one of the largest of these projects was the Commissioner of Mental Hygiene of New York State under Governor Rockefeller.

When in August, 1975, the Army released some of the details of its LSD program, it identified Dr. Paul Hoch as one of the "principal investigators" of this project.[15] Dr. Hoch, a refugee from Nazi Germany, was one of the most influential and respected psychiatrists in the United States. From 1952 until his death in 1964, he was the Commissioner of Mental Hygiene of the State of New York. Before his appointment to that important position, he was Principal Research Scientist at the New York State Psychiatric Institute and clinical professor of psychiatry at the Columbia University College of Physicians and Surgeons.

Another physician identified as responsible for these druggings is Dr. Sidney Malitz, who at the time of the Blauer-Olson experiments was doing "drug research" as a captain in the Army assigned to Walter Reed Hospital in Washington, D.C.[16] Dr. Malitz is now an accredited psychoanalyst, the acting director of the New York State Psychiatric Institute, and vice-chairman of the Department of Psychiatry at the Columbia University College of Physicians and Surgeons. Among his publications is a paper titled "The Role of Mescaline and D-Lysergic Acid in Psychiatric Treatment."

In August, 1976, another "principal investigator," and the only one still alive who was associated with the project in which Blauer was killed, was named.[17] He is Dr. James P. Cattell, who was then a senior research psychiatrist at the New York State Psychiatric Institute. In 1959, Dr. Cattell co-authored a paper with Dr. Hoch on "pseudoneurotic schizophrenia." The patients at the Institute were, I assume, in no position to counter with a paper on "pseudotherapeutic poisoning."

A few other physicians directing "drug-testing" programs in other states and at other institutions have also been named. One of them is Dr. Amadeo Marrazzi, presently the chairman of the Division of Neuropharmacology at the University of Missouri Institute of Psychiatry.[18] In November, 1975, Dr. Marrazzi was accused at a Senate subcommittee hearing of having "devastated" a young psychiatric patient with LSD in an Air-Force-funded experiment in 1965. His accuser, Mrs. Mary Ray, then a psychometrist at the University of Minnesota Hospital, said that "the patient, an eighteen-year-old girl being treated for a 'personality disorder,' definitely did not want to be part of the experiment. I saw her and they were taking her in, and she said she won't go, and they said, 'Yes, you will!'. . . When [Mrs. Ray] next saw the patient, about an hour or two later, 'she was totally disintegrated; she was absolutely psychotic.'"[19]

All of the above-named physicians participated in these programs of their own free will; and all were, or are, psychiatrists. Indeed, they all were, or are, highly respected and prominent members of the American Psychiatric Association. The pundits of that organization have steadfastly maintained for these past twenty years that a person who takes LSD because he wants to is a "drug abuser," is "mentally ill," and is a fit subject for coerced psychiatric treatment; and that a person who sells LSD to a willing buyer is a fit subject for some of the harshest punishments permitted under our system of criminal law.[20] At the same time, the officials of this organization have not only failed to object to these grave abuses of the physician's role, but have implicitly condoned them. On August 11, 1975, confronted with the sorts of revelations

I have reviewed here, Dr. Judd Marmor, then the president of the American Psychiatric Association, offered this comment: "One might argue as to whether [the Army] has obtained informed consent, but if you tell the subject everything you might well invalidate the experiment."[21]

But the German doctors who killed unsuspecting persons did not practice euthanasia; they murdered people. Similarly, the American doctors who drugged unsuspecting persons did not perform "experiments"; they poisoned people. The facts are clear enough: prominent American psychiatrists are implicated in the most serious and systematic violations, not only of medical ethics, but also of the criminal law, that have ever been brought to light in the United States. The question is: What are we going to do about it?

Notes

1. J. B. Treaster, "Report on Army's Drug Tests Tells of Efforts at Concealment," *New York Times,* Aug. 3, 1976, pp. 1 and 21; and Treaster, "Army Discloses Man Died in Drug Test It Sponsored," *New York Times,* Aug. 13, 1975, pp. 1 and 13.

2. Commission on CIA Activities Within the United States, *Report to the President, June 1975* (Washington, D.C.: U.S. Govt. Printing Office, 1975), pp. 226-28.

3. Ibid., p. 226.

4. Ibid.

5. Ibid., p. 227.

6. See S. M. Hersch, "Family Plans to Sue CIA Over Suicide in Drug Test," *New York Times,* July 10, 1975, pp. 1 and 18; J. B. Treaster, "Detective Said Scientist Had 'Severe Psychosis,'" *New York Times,* July 11, 1975, p. 34; and "The Casualty," *Newsweek,* July 21, 1975, pp. 17-19.

7. Quoted in J. B. Treaster, "Efforts at Concealment."

8. Ibid.

9. See also Treaster, "$8.5 Million Sought from Army in 1953 Drug Death," *New York Times,* Sept. 4, 1975, p. 22; and "Drug Death Data Omits Army Link," *New York Times,* Aug. 14, 1975, p. 37.

10. Treaster, "Army Tricked GIs into Drug Testing," *New York Times,* Sept. 9, 1975, p. 1.

11. Treaster, "Report Says CIA Agents Picked up Bar Patrons for LSD Experiments," *New York Times,* April 27, 1976, p. 25.

12. "GIs, Foreigners Used in LSD Tests," *New York Times,* Apr. 28, 1976, p. 9.

13. Ibid.

14. Treaster "Drug Death Brought No Halt to Tests," *New York Times,* Sept. 10, 1975, p. 12.

15. See Treaster, "Army Discloses Man Died."

16. See Treaster, "Drug Death Brought No Halt to Tests."

17. See Treaster, "Efforts at Concealment."

18. See Treaster, "LSD Researcher Is Under Inquiry," *New York Times,* Aug. 3, 1975, p. 23.

19. "Latest LSD Charge: Forcible Air Force Experiments," *Medical World News,* Nov. 3, 1975, p. 22.

20. See, generally, T. S. Szasz, *Ceremonial Chemistry: The Ritual Persecution of Drugs, Addicts, and Pushers* (Garden City, N.Y.: Doubleday, 1974).

21. Quoted in Treaster, "Mind-Drug Tests a Federal Project for Almost 25 Years," *New York Times,* Aug. 11, 1975, p. 42.

The Method in
Martha's Madness

"If it hadn't been for Martha [Mitchell]," said former President Richard M. Nixon to David Frost in their final videotaped conversation, "there'd have been no Watergate . . ." If there would have been no Watergate without Martha Mitchell, then she must have been a very powerful person indeed.

Wherein did her power lie? It lay in a web woven of the following facts and of what she made of them. Certain crimes had been committed in high places. Because of her close familial and personal ties to the lawbreakers, she suspected that the persons she ostensibly loved the most were in fact criminals. Finally, out of her own need for notoriety, her hatred toward her husband, or whatever other motives may have been buried in her bosom, she proceeded to malign the malefactors in a manner bound to be damaging not only to them but to herself as well. In short, Martha Mitchell's situation was in some ways like Hamlet's.

The Prince smelled "something rotten in the state of Denmark." He was right in his suspicions and was declared demented for them by precisely those persons who knew that he was right. The Princess of the Potomac smelled something rotten in Washington. She was right in her suspicions and she, too, was pronounced paranoid for them by those who knew that she was right.

Through the Ghost, Shakespeare reveals Hamlet's awareness of his father's "foul and most unnatural murder," and his own resolve to "revenge" it. Hamlet's mother and uncle, his father's murderers, declare Hamlet to be mad and deputize Rosencrantz and Guildenstern to therapize him.

Through Nixon, Frost reveals John Mitchell's foul and most unnatural mad-doctoring of Martha and her reaction to that deed. "You see," Nixon tells Frost, "John's problem was not Watergate. It was Martha. . . . In 1968, during the campaign, John had to send Martha away for about five or six weeks."

When Nixon asked Mitchell to come to Washington as his attorney general, Mitchell was reluctant to accept because of his wife. "You know, she's not really up to it, emotionally," Mitchell told Nixon. Like Gertrude,

Written in September 1977. Not previously published.

the Queen of Denmark, Nixon, the president of the United States, thereupon proposes a psychotherapeutic program: "I said, 'Look,' now being an amateur psychiatrist—we all are, aren't we? I said, 'If you move her to Washington, she may be better.' So he brought her to Washington. She was much better for a while."

What made Martha Mitchell seem "better" was, perhaps, her newly acquired access to the press. Nixon's description of this phase of Martha's behavior is extremely revealing: "Then the midnight calls came, and so forth, and so on. And then came the campaign. And then it began to go up and up and up. I mean the tempo of her calls and she busted her hand through a window out in, here in California, and all the rest. And she said that she was going to blow the whistle on everybody . . ."

Martha Mitchell made it clear to all who were willing to look and listen that she was out to get her husband and whomever else she could in high places. Nixon was concerned—he says about Martha, but it seems impossible that he could not have been concerned for Mitchell and himself as well—and asked his friend Bebe Rebozo to talk to Mitchell about Martha. This is Nixon's recollection of the incident: "And he [Rebozo] said, 'John,'—and they'd had a couple of drinks, and John was talking a little freely to him—and he said, 'John, why don't you put her away like you did in '68?' Bebe said, 'Tears came into John's eyes and he says, 'Well, because I love her.'"

Alas, we have learned much about the nature of science since Shakespeare but have forgotten even more about human nature. Nixon quotes Martha as telling him: "Mr. President, I just want you to know that there are only three men in the world I love: I love John; I love Bebe; and I love you." Then Nixon adds: "The next night she was on the phone at midnight raisin' hell about everything."

What should concern us here is not what Martha Mitchell did, but how it was generally interpreted. Her behavior was viewed—by her husband, by Nixon, by the press—as symptomatic of an "underlying mental illness" that she "had." Nixon's own concluding comments to Frost are important in this connection: "I've talked too long about it, but just let me summarize it by saying: I'm convinced that if it hadn't been for Martha, and God rest her soul, because she, in her heart, was a good person. She just had a mental and emotional problem that nobody knew about."

I disagree. A person is what he or she does. By that standard Martha Mitchell was—at least during her final years when she was a public persona—not a good person. But neither was she a madwoman. Paraphrasing Hamlet, she might herself have said, "I am but mad north-north-west. When the wind is southerly I know a coverup from a coverlet." As Polonius said about Hamlet's behavior, "Though [it] be madness, there is method in it," so we ought to acknowledge that there was method in Martha's "madness" also.

That consideration brings me to the point of these remarks. The legal and political aspects of Watergate have been exposed and the guilty parties have been punished. But what about the psychiatric aspects of Watergate? The Nixon–Frost tapes provide irrefutable evidence of the "political abuse of psychiatry" in the United States (as such practices are called when they occur in the Soviet Union). The fact that John Mitchell chose not to commit his wife in 1972—the act to which Nixon now attributes his fall from power— establishes, beyond the shadow of a doubt, that her commitment in 1968 was not "medically necessary" (whatever that fatuous phrase may mean); that, in short, it was an instance of the use of involuntary mental hospitalization for the suppression of a political troublemaker—a psychiatric intervention which, when it is practiced in Russia, the American press condemns with great enthusiasm.

On the Incarceration
of Martha Mitchell

On September 1, the general assembly of the World Psychiatric Association, meeting in Honolulu, approved, by a vote of 122 to 66, a resolution introduced by the American Psychiatric Association opposing "the misuse of psychiatric skills, knowledge, and facilities for the suppression of dissent wherever it occurs." On September 4, in the published version of the transcript of the final videotaped conversation between former President Richard M. Nixon and David Frost, Mr. Nixon was quoted as saying: "In 1968, during the campaign, John [Mitchell] had to send Martha away for about five or six weeks." Mr. Nixon also alluded to a conversation between Bebe Rebozo and John Mitchell, Mr. Rebozo saying: "John, why don't you put her [Martha] away like you did in '68?"

If this story is true, I submit that Martha Mitchell's psychiatric incarceration constitutes the latest in a long series of "the misuse[s] of psychiatric skills, knowledge, and facilities" in the United States. Some of the previous victims of such misuse are: Ezra Pound, Secretary of Defense James Forrestal, Gen. Edwin Walker and Senator Barry Goldwater. (Unlike the others, who were involuntarily hospitalized, Senator Goldwater was only involuntarily diagnosed.)

For decades, and especially in recent years, the *Times* has rendered the American people an incalculable service by exposing financial and political crimes in high places. I hope it will now render similar service by exposing psychiatric crimes in high places—by investigating and publishing the precise circumstances under which Martha Mitchell was "put away," and by identifying the psychiatric institution in which she was imprisoned and the psychiatrists who imprisoned her.

Reprinted, with permission, from the Letters column of the *New York Times*, September 25, 1977, p. E-14.

Jim Jones as Jesus

Although neither psychiatrists nor laymen can satisfactorily define sanity, they all "know" that if a person claims to be Jesus, then he is mad—insane, psychotic, schizophrenic, whatever. But crazy, for sure. Similarly although no one can clearly define the criteria for commitment to an insane asylum, everyone "knows" that if a person announces that he is going to kill himself, then he ought to be locked up—to protect him from himself, to cure his psychosis or schizophrenia, or whatever. Ernest Hemingway, for example, was locked up and given electric-shock treatments against his will for precisely such reasons.

For several years before the carnage in Guyana, the Reverend Jim Jones repeatedly claimed that he was Jesus. He also repeatedly threatened to kill himself—and to take his followers with him in a mass suicide—if people didn't do as he told them. Many knew that Jim Jones made such a claim about himself and uttered such a threat against others. Many who knew this were intelligent and influential persons, some of them physicians and lawyers. But not one of them said that Jones was mad or suggested that he ought to be committed to a mental hospital.

Why didn't anyone "discover" that Jones was "mentally ill" before he died, especially since that "diagnosis" seems now so obvious to everyone? Because he had powerful political friends? That cannot explain it. Secretary of Defense James Forrestal had much more powerful political friends and sought only his own death, whereas the Rev. Jones sought the death of his family and followers as well. Nevertheless, Forrestal was captured, confined, and psychiatrically destroyed, but Jones was not.

Did Jim Jones escape psychiatric diagnosis and detention because he had made a good impression on people? That cannot explain it either. Marilyn Monroe made a much better impression, but was made to suffer the indignity of involuntary mental hospitalization nevertheless.

The answer, I think, is simple. The American people—and, most importantly, journalists and judges and politicians—have opened their eyes and ears and are beginning to look at and listen to madmen as well as mad-doctors. When Jones declared that he *was* Jesus, people interpreted this to mean that he wanted to be *like* him, that he wanted to be admired *like* he is,

Reprinted, with permission, from the *Libertarian Review*, January 1979, pp. 34-35.

and so forth. This view of madness is both a cause and a consequence of a dramatic shift in the public perception of madness and the public policy toward it (each affecting the other).

Until recently, when madmen asserted certain (possibly) metaphorical claims, their assertions were invariably interpreted literally. If the "patient" said he was Jesus, then everyone insisted that that is what he meant; ergo, he was crazy. It was of no avail if the "patient" subsequently explained, in word and deed, that what he *really* meant was that he wanted love, fame, respect, and all the other spiritual "goods" that many crave but few obtain. He was crazy, and that was that.

Now the tables are turned. Jones said he was Jesus. We don't know, we cannot possibly know, whether he meant that claim literally or figuratively (or both). But everyone—the public, journalists, politicians—acted as if Jones were asserting a metaphorical claim; ergo, he was not crazy. The more Jones escalated his claims, the more "charismatic" (confident)—and the less "crazy" (deluded)—he appeared. Indeed, even in his penultimate performance, one could not distinguish the literal from the metaphorical, the real from the fake, from what Jones said. The truth about Jones became known only after the bodies were counted. Then, the chorus called him crazy.

"Why," asks Patrick J. Buchanan uncomprehendingly, "wasn't the Secret Service alerted to keep Mrs. Carter miles away from a certifiable madman like the Rev. Jim Jones?" What Buchanan does not understand, perhaps does not want to understand, is that whether a person is considered mad depends not on what he does but on how we interpret what he does. For a number of reasons (among which the changing attitude toward madness is probably only one), Jones's self-definition as Jesus was regarded as a symbol of his "humanitarianism"—rather than as a symptom of his megalomania; similarly, his rituals of mass suicide were viewed as the thunderings of an angry prophet—rather than as the blackmailings of a blood-thirsty terrorist.

President and Mrs. Carter say that they are "born-again" Christians. We interpret that claim metaphorically—and either approve it or ignore it. But what if we gave that message a literal reading? We might then expect each of them to produce two birth certificates to substantiate their claim or to die twice before we bury them. Clearly, if we gave such a claim a literal interpretation (and had the power to implement it), then the claim of having been born more than once would be called a delusion symptomatic of a psychosis. The Carters' claim that they are born-again Christians is not likely to be so (mis)interpreted. But the analogous claims of countless other persons have been (mis)interpreted in just such a way. Some years ago, after one of my public lectures in which I made this point, a colleague came up to me and told me this story. As a supervising psychiatrist in a state mental hospital, he was asked to review a recent admission. The patient was a middle-aged woman who had complained of intense anxiety. In the admission record she was described as "delusional" and was diagnosed "psychotic." When the patient said nothing to the consultant that he considered "delusional," he turned to the admitting psychiatrist, who was a recent immigrant from Eastern Europe, for an explanation. "She kept saying she had butterflies in her stomach," replied the doctor, who might have been a poet in his native tongue but was deaf to the music of a metaphoric butterfly fluttering in an English-speaking stomach.

"All the world's a stage," observed Shakespeare. He was right. Poetry, politics, and psychiatry all come down to language—to the ancient truth which we forget at our own peril: namely, that it is by controlling words that we control men.

The Freedom Abusers

Since the death of the Reverend Jim Jones, the diagnosis of paranoia has been falling on his memory like snowflakes in a winter storm in Syracuse. I suggest that we take another look at some of the facts reported about this Marxist-Christian minister before the sordid truths about his behavior and that of his followers are completely buried beneath a blanket of psychiatric speculations and diagnoses.

Virtually everyone who knew Jones—among them some prominent and presumably perceptive and intelligent men and women—regarded him as perfectly healthy mentally. For instance, during the 1976 Carter presidential campaign, Rosalynn Carter and Jim Jones dined together in San Francisco. Mrs. Carter, who is, as we know, one of America's foremost experts on mental health, found no sign of mental illness in Jones—on the contrary: In March 1977, she wrote him a letter praising his proposal to give medical aid to Cuba, and after the election she invited him to attend the inauguration, which he did.

That Jones was accepted as at least "normal" in California liberal political circles has by now become notorious. That he was still widely regarded as both mentally healthy and morally admirable during the weeks and days immediately preceding the massacre is evident from the fact that a gala, $25-a-plate dinner benefit for the Peoples Temple was planned in San Francisco for December 2, 1978. Called "A Struggle Against Oppression," the affair was to feature Dick Gregory and the Temple's two lawyers, Mark Lane and Charles Garry, as speakers. It was endorsed by 75 prominent city leaders and politicians. It was cancelled after the massacre.

Actually, in view of Jones's impressive record of good "psychothera-peutic" works, the enthusiasm of evangelistic mental healthers for him should come as no surprise. Jones "cured drug addicts." He "rehabilitated" aimless Americans and put them on the road to a communitarian salvation. He was, officially at least, even against suicide—when it was a course chosen on one's own. On Memorial Day in 1977 (only 18 months before the Jonestown massacre), Jones led a delegation of Peoples Temple members on a march onto the Golden Gate Bridge in San Francisco, demanding that the city build a suicide barrier on the bridge.

Reprinted, with permission, from *Inquiry,* February 5, 1979, pp. 4-6.

In addition to these testimonials to Jones's good mental health and commendable character, we also have the word of Jones's personal physician that the minister was both psychiatrically normal and morally admirable. Dr. Carlton Goodlett, identified as a "prominent black doctor" in San Francisco who had also attended Jones in Guyana, told the *New York Times:* "I was convinced that Jones was involved in a brilliant experiment in Guyana that actually put people in better shape down there than they had been in San Francisco." Even after the massacre Dr. Goodlett offered this psychiatric opinion—not about Jones, but about his disenchanted followers: "The deserters from the church had come to me, but they were just a neurotic fringe."

To say that Jim Jones was widely regarded as mentally healthy is indeed an understatement: He was regarded as a brilliant healer of minds, a great "therapist." Many of his followers were former drug users. Two survived the massacre. One of them, Tim Carter, told the *Times* he had been "heavily involved in drugs in California" and was cured by Jones. Tim's father, Francis Carter (both of whose sons were "on drugs"), praised Jones's treatment of drug abuse to a *Times* reporter: After joining the Temple "they gave up drugs, became rehabilitated, and got better." Odel Rhodes, another survivor, "had been a heroin addict from the Detroit ghetto. [W]ith the help of Jim Jones's power he had beat heroin, he said. He felt he needed his mentor to keep him straight."

After the butchery in Guyana, Jones's followers and friends were eager to dismiss him as "paranoid." Steven Jones lost no time diagnosing his father as psychotic, an opinion he kept carefully to himself until "dad" was dead. Why did Steven Jones think his father was mad? Because he destroyed the concentration camp that young Jones evidently loved dearly. "He has destroyed everything I've worked for," said Steven Jones.

One of Jones's lawyers, Charles Garry, characterized the commune as "a beautiful jewel. There is no racism, no sexism, no ageism, no elitism [sic], no hunger." After the massacre, Garry declared: "I am convinced this guy was stark raving mad." If Garry believed this before November 18, 1978, he violated his professional responsibilities as a lawyer and his moral responsibilities as a human being; and if he concluded it only because Jones finally carried out his oft-repeated threat of mass murder and suicide, then Garry is asserting a platitude in declaring his safely-deceased client "mad."

Mark Lane, Jones's other lawyer and a renowned expert on conspiracy and paranoia, described his former client to the *Times* as "a paranoid murderer who, after four weeks of drug injections, gave the orders that resulted last weekend in the deaths of Representative Leo J. Ryan. . . ." The great conspiracy-hunter thus sought to exonerate Jones by attributing the mass murder and suicide not only to "paranoia" but also to "drugs." But the fact is that Lane accepted Jones as a client and continued to represent him, up to the very moment of the debacle.

I cite all this as presumptive evidence that, before the final moment, those closest to Jones did not believe that he was psychotic. Their subsequent conclusion that Jones was paranoid is intellectually empty and patently self-serving. (Today everyone who reads newspapers and watches television has been taught that mass murderers are mad.) While Jones was alive his friends and followers did not regard him as paranoid, quite simply because they liked what he was doing. For the bottom line is a moral judgment: Jones's supporters think that he was a good man who suddenly became mad; I think he was an evil man—and not just on the day of the massacre.

Whether or not Jones had been "crazy" long before the massacre, depends on the meaning one wishes to attach to that word. However, it is now clear that for a long time Jones's behavior had been sordid and evil. It is also clear that when his followers were faced with certain facts, they deliberately looked the other way. Consider the following reports of Jones's behavior during the period when his followers and those "outside" regarded Jones as not merely "normal" but "superior":

—Jones insisted that everyone call him "dad" or "father." When there was a disagreement in the commune, the members would tranquilize one another and themselves by repeating the incantation, "Dad knows best. Just do as dad tells you."

—Jones had a wife, several mistresses, and "had sex" with many of the women and several of the men in the commune. "He told their husbands [according to Tim Carter, an aide] that he only did it to help the women."

—Jones claimed that he was Jesus and could cure cancer.

—According to Jerry Parks, another cult member, "Everyone had to admit that they were homosexual, even the women. He was the only heterosexual."

—Several times before the final butchery, Jones conducted rehearsals of the communal carnage.

—Members of the commune had to turn their possessions over to Jones, had to work like slaves, were starved and were kept from sleeping, and could not leave the commune.

Despite these unsavory facts (and many others not catalogued here), I cannot recall, in the thousands of words I read about the Jonestown affair, a single commentator—journalist, politician, psychiatrist, anyone—characterizing the Reverend Jim Jones as an evil man. Mad, insane, crazy, paranoid, and variations on that theme—that is the consensus. James Reston's judgment of Jones was sadly typical. After quoting the opinion of "one of the most prominent members of the Carter Administration," according to whom the Jonestown massacre was a symptom of "mass lunacy in an age of emptiness," Reston delivered the craven diagnosis that liberal intellectuals, when faced with evil, instinctively issue. The Reverend Jones, declared Reston, was an "obviously demented man."

The most imaginative diagnosis was offered, not surprisingly, by a psychiatrist. Explained Dr. Thomas Ungerleider, professor of psychiatry at the University of California at Los Angeles: "I believe it was the jungle. The members got no feedback from the outside world. They did not read *Time* magazine or watch the news at night. . . ." Dr. Alvin Poussaint, professor of psychiatry at Harvard and one of the leading black psychiatrists in America, offered this shameful and revealing diagnosis: "We cannot in good conscience fault the mission of the rank-and-file because of the acute psychosis of their leader. . . . The humanitarian experiment itself was not a failure, the Reverend Jones was."

I think we can do better than that. The evidence—despite Reston and the anonymous high Carter administration official—suggests that Jones was depraved, not "demented," and that what his congregation displayed was mass cruelty and cowardliness, not "mass lunacy." I believe that plain English words such as "evil," "depraved," "cruel," and "cowardly" furnish a better description of what happened at Jonestown than does the lexicon of lunacy in which those despicable and pathetic deeds have been couched.

This instant metamorphosis of Jones from prophet to psychotic now conceals—as did previously the deliberate denial of the significance of his everyday behavior by those who knew him—the self-evident evil that animated this bestial tyrant long before his supposed "degeneration into paranoia." That is the phrase used by *Time* magazine, where Jones is described as an "Indiana-born humanitarian who degenerated into egomania and paranoia." *Newsweek* confirms the diagnosis: Jones's "mind," we are informed, "deteriorated into paranoia."

I object. It is fundamentally false and distorting to view every gesture to help the poor—regardless of motives, methods, and consequences—as "humanitarian." What tyrant has not claimed to be motivated by a desire to help the helpless? We know only too well that to those hungry for power, the prospect of "helping" life's victims presents a great temptation; one that complements the temptation that the prospect of oblivion through alcohol or drugs presents to those hungry for a simple solution to life's problems. That is why these two types of persons are drawn to each other so powerfully, and why each regards the competent, self-reliant person as his enemy. So much for Jones's "humanitarianism."

As for Jones's "paranoia," we accept the proverbial wisdom that one man's meat is another man's poison. Similarly, we should accept that one man's prophet is another man's paranoid. It is simply not true that Jones "degenerated into paranoia." Jones was the same person on November 18, 1978 (the date of the mass murder and suicide), that he was the day before, the month before, the year before. Jones did not suddenly change. What did change suddenly was the opinion certain people entertained and expressed about him.

What we need, then, is not so much an explanation of what happened in Jonestown, which is clear enough, but rather an explanation of the explanations of the carnage that the purveyors of conventional wisdom have offered us. Briefly put, such a metaexplanation might state that paranoia in a dead and dishonored "cult" leader is caused by the sudden realization of his followers and others that they have been duped, which instantly transforms them from sycophants (and sympathizers) into psychodiagnosticians.

Much could be, and should be, made of the carnage at Jonestown. What I want to make out of it here is, briefly, this: Access to drugs entails what is now smugly called "drug abuse." How, indeed, could it be otherwise? Why, then, the shocked surprise that access to freedom entails "freedom abuse"? Assuredly the abuse of freedom—like the abuse of alcohol, drugs, food, or any other good that nature or human ingenuity provides us—is a small price to pay for the boundless benefits of freedom. That the abuse of freedom entails risks to innocent persons is one of the tragic facts of life. The children murdered at Jonestown are a somber reminder of the awesome power parents have over their children—a power that, as Jonestown and other communal experiments have shown, the collectivization of the family can only amplify.

The ultimate ugly and undeniable facts are that of the 909 bodies at Jonestown, 260 were those of children, butchered by the peaceloving, "humanitarian" followers of the Reverend Jones; and that, like their leader, these butchers hated the open society and "fled" their homeland to settle in a socialist country. The men and women of Jonestown rejected liberty. It is as if they had turned Patrick Henry's maxim, "Give me liberty or give me death!" on its head, and had sworn allegiance to the maxim, "Give me death rather than liberty!"

As for Congressman Ryan and his party, they paid a heavy price for their naiveté and miscalculation, but, after being warned repeatedly about Jonestown and after being emphatically disinvited by the inhabitants, their attempt to "liberate" would-be defectors without adequate arms was as ill-advised as would be an attempt to scale the Alps without proper shoes or clothing. When Congressman Ryan insisted on staging his inspecton-invasion to foist on them the liberty they loathed, the Jonestown patriots proved that they had the courage of their convictions. The point is not merely that actions speak louder than words, which is obvious enough; it is rather that in the base rhetoric of butchers—regardless of whether they come garbed as priests, politicians, or physicians—"love" means "hate" and "I will take care of you" means "I will kill you."

The Psychiatric Presidency

Since the end of the second World War, mental health and mental illness in the United States have become progressively politicized. As a result, neither the Democratic nor the Republican Party nor any president could oppose the struggle against mental illness, for fear of appearing to oppose mental health itself. In the past 30 years, increased spending on mental health has been a more bipartisan policy than increased spending on defense, education, or welfare. Still, despite all the political and psychiatric hoopla, the actual personal support of politicians for mental health has always seemed half-hearted at best. It was like kissing babies for the photographers—something that had to be done to get oneself elected, not something one enjoyed, much less believed in.

With the election of Jimmy Carter, all this has changed. Here, for the first time in American history, a president, indeed a whole presidential family, really believed in mental health—just as they really believed in Jesus and being born twice. The upshot is a veritable "psychiatric presidency"—a fitting ornament for our Therapeutic State.

The Carters' interest in mental health antedates their entering national politics. When Carter was governor of Georgia, both he and Mrs. Carter emphasized their commitment to that cause. Between 1971 and 1975, during Carter's governorship, the number of community mental-health centers in Georgia rose from one to 18, admissions to state mental hospitals increased from 9,645 to 17,824, the number of full-time state mental-hospital employees rose from 6,467 to 8,247, and the annual state mental-hospital expenditures rose from $56,705,000 to $95,177,000. Not a bad record as madness-manufacturing goes.

During the 1976 presidential campaign, Carter ran, in part, on a mental health platform. A *New York Times* reporter described Mrs. Carter's participation in the campaign in this way: "Her schedule is carefully planned around certain campaign themes. If there is a mental hospital in the city, she tours it, talking of the need for more such facilities. . . ." Addressing a meeting of the American Association for Social Psychiatry during the campaign, psychiatrist Dr. Peter Bourne, then the director of the Washington Carter for President Campaign (and later forced to resign as presidential

Reprinted, with permission, from *Inquiry,* September 18, 1978, pp. 4-6.

assistant for health issues), promised: "I think in Governor Carter and his wife, the psychiatric and mental health fields would have a very good friend, or two very good friends, in the White House." This is true enough. But that the Carter presidency is good for the American Psychiatric Association is much more obvious than that it is good for America.

After he was elected president, Carter fulfilled at least one of his campaign promises: he appointed a presidential Commission on Mental Health with his wife as its honorary chairperson. In May 1978, after having spent an undisclosed amount of the taxpayers' money in the course of its investigations, the commission issued its much-heralded report, titled *Mental Health in America: 1978*. The report consists of an expository volume of 94 pages plus three heavy tomes of appendixes. It is unlikely that many Americans outside the mental health bureaucracy (or even inside it) will ever see this document, much less read it.

Besides the sort or psychiatric propaganda one might expect from a presidential commission on mental health, the most interesting thing about the report is its advocacy of systematic racial and linguistic discrimination in psychiatry—partly, it seems, as an expression of a trendy pseudopopulism, and partly, it is quite clear, in an effort to strengthen the legitimacy of controlling racially and linguistically handicapped persons by means of coercive psychiatry. I list below some of the statements in it which I so interpret:

According to the 1975 Special Census, the population of America includes 22 million Black Americans. . . . Like everyone else, minorities feel more comfortable and secure when care is provided by practitioners who come from similar backgrounds. Yet fewer than 2 percent of all psychiatrists in America are Black.

Language and cultural barriers have prevented some minorities from receiving appropriate care. . . . Many patients needing treatment will not seek care if providers are not sensitive to their culture or are unable to speak their language. To meet the particular needs of minority populations, the Commission recommends that: Mental health service programs should . . . provide culturally relevant services and staff them with bilingual, bicultural personnel.

At the commitment hearing, the rules of evidence should apply, and the respondent should have the right to wear his or her own clothing, to present evidence, and cross-examine witnesses. The petitioner [*sic*] should also be represented by counsel fluent in the petitioner's [*sic*] primary language. [By "petitioner" is presumably meant "respondent."]

State laws establishing rights of mentally handicapped persons should be printed in the natural or dominant language of the persons to whom they apply. . . . A copy of the rights should be given to each patient and should be read or explained in an easily understandable way and in the person's natural or "dominant" language.

The proposition that white (or yellow) psychiatrists cannot treat black (or Hispanic) patients is here advanced as a self-evident truth, supported only by the assertion that all "minorities" prefer to be treated by psychiatric "practitioners who come from a similar background." Presumably, then, so do majorities—an idea full of momentous implications for American psychiatry, a heavily Jewish profession in a predominantly Christian country. When Carl Jung dared to suggest that individuals from different cultural and racial backgrounds possess different psychologies, he was promptly branded a Nazi anti-Semite by Jewish psychiatrists. Of course, Jung was never so stupid as to suggest that membership in a particular ethnic group automatically guarantees compassion for or understanding of the problems peculiar to members of that group. He was merely emphasizing the cultural reality of human behavior. Not so the report of the President's Commisson: It urges the adoption of an explicitly racist policy with respect to psychiatric services—namely, that each racial or linguistic group be served by practitioners recruited from among its own members. Implementing such a quota system would, of course, affect Jewish-American psychiatry much the same way as National Socialism affected Jewish-German psychiatry.

The Commission's views on language are also startling. It has always been the case in America that persons who spoke no English or who spoke it very poorly were more likely to be incarcerated as mental patients than those who did speak it. If one wished to protect innocent persons ignorant of English from being deprived of their liberty by psychiatrists, the obvious way to do so would be to abolish involuntary mental hospitalization. But the psychobureaucrats responsible for the report do not want to protect non-English speakers from psychiatric oppression; they want to legitimize their oppression by extending to them the legal formalism of being read their paper "rights" in their own language.

Moreover, the report treats the inability of some persons to understand or speak English as an immutable fact. It is not the would-be client's fault that he has not mastered English. It is the fault of American society that it has not provided services in the client's own language. Nowhere does the Commission even allude to the possibility that, in the United States, failure to master the English language may be bad for one's "mental health." Accordingly, the "particular needs of minority populations" do not include learning English, but include providing them with "bilingual and bicultural" experts. But if the patients cannot or do not want to learn English, why should they be treated by bilingual psychiatrists? The recommendation is not only politically repugnant, it is also illogical. Why couldn't such persons be treated by psychiatrists fluent in the patient's dominant language alone? Moreover, in view of the ethnic and linguistic diversity that exists in America, the report's recommendation is pure humbug.

That an American president and his administration should mindlessly support mental health is, of course, hardly novel. What is novel, as I have noted, is the Carter family's own involvement in mental health. Thus, Rosalynn Carter's pet project is mental health. Her devotion to this cause has led her to endorse the "finding" that 50 million of her countrymen are "in need of" mental health services and to display special solicitude for black Americans who are mad and whose need for mental health care she considers especially neglected. Her conviction that so many black Americans are psychiatrically "underserved" should, perhaps, be seen in the context of her criteria for mental health, exemplified by her remark quoted in the French magazine *Jeune Afrique* (March 25, 1977): "I do not think that Amin Dada is crazy. He is a very intelligent man."

Ruth Carter Stapleton, the President's sister, is a famous spiritual healer. She attributes her therapeutic powers, about which she is not unduly modest, to her special relationship to God. "God speaks to my thoughts," she explained to a reporter for *New York* magazine. "That's how He talks to me. Sometimes I don't know whether I'm thinking it or He is thinking it. But often I know it couldn't be me. . . . I have found that Jesus loves a rapist, an exhibitionist, a drug addict, a communist."

The Carters' passion for mental health is particularly significant in view of the fact that psychiatrists have a similar passion for diagnosing prominent political figures as mentally ill. Indeed, while Mr. and Mrs. Carter are pushing psychiatric services on the American people, leading American psychohistorians are proclaiming the Carter family to be sorely in need of such services.

The fall 1977 issue of *The Journal of Psychohistory,* labeled "Special Jimmy Carter Issue," is devoted to a "psychohistorical analysis" of the President and his family. True to the psychohistorical form of psychoassassination, Lloyd deMause, the editor of the *Journal,* disclaims any intention to harm Mr. Carter; indeed he claims that he wants to help him. Should Mrs. Carter read this, I hope she will begin to understand how hapless Americans might feel about the psychiatric "help" she proposes to unleash on them. Writes deMause, director of the Institute of Psychohistory, publisher of the Psychohistory Press, a member of the training faculty of the New York Center of Psychoanalytic Training, and chairman of the International Psychohistorical Association: "One final word on the Carter project before I begin the presentation of my evidence. The demands of group-fantasy in America today are such that the majority of the press, including reviewers, will probably refer to these essays as an 'attack' on Jimmy Carter. Nothing could be further from the truth. Indeed, quite the opposite. I even suspect that Carter would both enjoy and profit from these studies. In point of fact, we all voted for him. . . ."

The first contributor to the special "Jimmy Carter Issue" is Paul Elovitz, a contributing editor to the *Journal.* Elovitz's "diagnostic formulation" of the President is, deMause's self-congratulatory remarks notwithstanding, hardly likely to please him. "In psychoanalytic terminology," declares Elovitz,

"Jimmy Carter can be considered a narcissistic personality with obsessive compulsive defenses. His narcissism is reflected in his need to gain praise to compensate for his own sense of inadequacy, stemming from insufficient emotional nurturance during early childhood."

The person responsible for that "insufficient emotional nurturance" is, of course, Jimmy Carter's mother, usually identified, Southern-style, as "Miss Lillian." In view of the Carters' concern for mental health, their unconcern for Miss Lillian's mental ill-health (as defined by the authorities they respect) is rather surprising. Let me hasten to emphasize that I offer this "diagnosis" not as a personal judgment but rather as a logical inference from pronouncements made by Miss Lillian and by psychiatric experts. In 1975, the American Orthopsychiatric Association's Committee on Minority Group Children declared that "Racism is the number one public health problem," adding for good measure that "Racism is probably the only contagious mental disease."

According to the evidence presented by James Wooten (author of *Dasher: The Roots and the Rising of Jimmy Carter),* Miss Lillian shows signs of suffering from just such a mental disease. "A week before her son was elected President," writes Wooten, "an erratic black preacher from a nearby city tried to worship in the Plains Baptist Church. He was ejected, rather forcefully, though not bodily. The door was literally shut in his face. It was instant news around the country—big news. It might have cost her son the White House. Several weeks later, after he had won, she remembered the incident at the church. 'Somebody,' she snarled, 'should have shot that nigger before he came on the lawn.'" The effect on "mental health" of the hypocrisy implied in the gulf between Miss Lillian's "nigger" and the capitalized "Blacks" in the presidential commission's report requires no further comment.

According to David Beisel, another contributing editor of the *Journal,* Jimmy Carter has dealt with his feelings of "maternal loss and maternal distancing" by internalizing maternal functions: "Without a mother he has become his own mother and performs domestic duties himself. Pridefully, Rosalynn proclaimed that 'Jimmy really likes to cook. . . .'" If poor Rosalynn only knew what psychiatrists can infer from the sinister symptoms of masculine domesticity which her husband displays. Our President has been known not only to cook but also to sew on buttons and wash his shirts. Better not let Anita Bryant hear about this! But why bother with psychopathological innuendos when the psychohistorical evidence clearly proves that the whole Carter clan is just plain crazy. That is the conclusion of Henry Ebel, associate editor of the *Journal:*

> The suspicion that the President may be nuts cannot—in view of his entirely projective function [*sic*]—be dissociated from the growing suspicion, by "average" Americans in "average" American families, that *they* may be nuts. . . . At the unconscious level, in other words, the Carter family, with its bizarre admixture of rednecks, faith-healers, convicts, and puritanical obsessive-compul-

sives, is perceived as being just as distorted and "crazy" as the families of "average" American voters: a Munster clan or Addams family that has somehow wandered off the TV screen and into the White House. The concern with "mental health," which for the Carters themselves may be a quasi-therapeutic involvement in other people's problems, is politically necessary to counterbalance this image. . . .

With that piece of psychoanalytic psychohistory, we come full circle: from the report of the President's Commission on Mental Health, to the demonstration of the presidential family's mental ill-health, and back to the Carters' own meddling in other people's private lives. The measure of that meddling is best reflected in its cost to the taxpayer. "In the late 1950s," observes the Commission, "the direct cost of mental illness was estimated to be $1.7 billion a year. By 1976 the direct cost of providing mental health services was about $17 billion . . ." The cost is steadily rising and the commission is recommending further sizable increases.

The President and his economists never tire of scolding us about our inability to afford imported petroleum, but they are remarkably silent about our ability to afford domestic psychiatry. Sooner or later we shall have to confront our value preferences. Perhaps the time is near when we shall have to choose between a system of "mental health care" so repugnant that it has to be financed through tax monies and imposed on the populace by means of force and fraud—and food and shelter and energy, that is, "essentials" for which individuals are quite willing to pay themselves. What President and Mrs. Carter are telling the American people is that mental health is more important than the "essentials." That is why mental health should be paid for by the government with tax monies—whereas food, shelter, and energy should be paid for by individuals with what the tax collector leaves them.

Psychodrama in
the White House

President Carter is greatly devoted to Mrs. Carter, who, in turn, is greatly devoted to psychiatry. Hence, it is not surprising that the Carter presidency has come to be characterized, first, by the replacement of a president by a marital presidential team, and second, by an imitation of the language and style of the mental health professions. Thus, the United States is now headed not by a male chief executive who is the leader of his party and the president of his country, but by a marital pair of faith healers who lust to replace politics with a religious psychodrama.

In a psychodrama, so-called mental patients are invited to enact their major life problems. The ostensible purpose of the enterprise is to help them confront and master their problems. Its only result, however, is that the performers' weaknesses are exposed. That, it seems, is what President and Mrs. Carter are doing to each other and themselves. It is to this phenomenon—which has not received the attention it deserves—to which I propose to devote my following remarks.

What does a faith healer—a term I use to mean charlatan or quack—typically do? He assumes a posture of boundless compassion and wisdom and so equipped pronounces the gravest diagnoses upon his clients. Then, he promises to cure them, provided that they place their complete trust in him. Carter's diagnosis of our condition could hardly be more gloomy; "I think it's inevitable," he told some of his guests at Camp David,

> that it's going to get worse in '80 than it was in '79, and it will get worse in '81 than in '80. The only trend is downward. . . . I think it's inevitable that there will be a lower standard of living . . . I think there's going to have to be reorientation of what people value in their own lives. I believe there has to be a more equitable sharing of what we have.

Ignoring for the moment Carter's remark about the need to "share what we have"—a precept he is obviously more fond of preaching than practicing—let me try to develop his image of our country. It is an image that fits comfortably into, and issues logically from, Jimmy and Rosalynn Carter's

---

Reprinted, with permission, from the *Libertarian Review,* December 1979, pp. 24-31.

dual infatuations with redemptive religion and rehabilitative mental health.

In this Carterian view, America is, quite simply, a sinful and sick addict: Americans are greedy for gasoline and other goodies they don't need, shouldn't have, and would be better off without. In his Baptist bull of July 15th, Carter admonished his recalcitrant addict-subjects in these words:

> I'm asking you, for your good and the nation's security, to take no unnecessary trips, to use car pools or public transportation whenever you can, to park your car one extra day per week, to obey the speed limit, and to set your thermostat to save fuel. Every act of energy conservation like this is more than just common sense. I tell you it is an act of patriotism.

President Carter here addresses us in a voice such as might have been used (but never was used) by General MacArthur addressing his vanquished Japanese charges. Indeed, while Carter is waging a metaphorical war of moral equivalents against OPEC, he is waging a real war of "therapeutic" emasculation against his own people: he is demeaning us for what we value, he is attacking us for how we behave, he is depriving us of our comforts and pleasures—all the while that he and his entourage are living more lavishly than the most profligate of private citizens, on money extracted by the Internal Revenue Service from us no-good gasoline addicts. Jimmy Carter's politics is thus the epitome of what Bernard Crick called anti-politics: "Only anti-political régimes," he wrote in his *In Defense of Politics* in 1972, "are forever preparing the individual to sacrifice his freedom of action for the collectivity, or trying to persuade him that freedom is not the positive experience of diversity, but is the euphoria that comes from making the right choice in good company. Yet people who are reborn are seldom reborn free [p. 192]."

As might be expected, some of our statist political commentators loved President Carter's castigating his fellow Americans for their addiction to oil. "Some complain that he [Carter] was 'too evangelical,'" wrote Carl Rowan.

> A leader speaking to sinners always preaches. And we have long been the energy sinners of the world. We have virtually "stolen" the petroleum of other poor nations for years and have become the gasoline junkies of the world.

Just when did we become the "gasoline junkies of the world?" Six months ago? After the Six-Day Arab-Israeli War? When Henry Ford built the Model T? As we all know, until very recently the oil industry in concert with the American government "pushed" gas—that is, they "pushed" it just as any seller pushes his product. Too, until recently, the oil-producing countries were happy to sell us a product that cost them next to nothing and whose availability seemed unlimited. Furthermore, the American government is still "pushing" oil by preventing market forces from dictating the price of petroleum in America and instead keeping that price at levels still well less than one-half of what it is in other industrial nations.

It is worth noting, in this connection, that there is a three-year backlog of orders for Mercedes automobiles, that there is no speed limit on German superhighways, and that there is no shortage of gasoline in Germany—although the Germans must, of course, import every drop of oil they use.

Mrs. Carter shares her husband's image of Americans as greedy material-ist addicts who ought to do with less and worship Jimmy. For all we know, she may even have developed this image herself and infected her husband with it. On a tour in July selling the President, she told reporters: "What I would like the people of this country to do is every time they turn out a light, every time they ride a bicycle or car pool, to think about Jimmy and that they are doing this for the country."

I submit that President and Mrs. Carter treat us, the American people, as if we were sinful addicts, given over to unpatriotic dissipations, not because that is the way we are, but because that is the way they want to see us. Theirs is the pat, time-honored priestly-psychiatric posture: I am virtuous—you are wicked; I am sane—you are insane; I know how to cure what ails you, and I'll fix you, whether you like it or not.

Politicians used to promise us two chickens in every pot. The Carters tell us we are eating too much chicken, that eating less of it is good for us—and patriotic to boot. But the facts are all the other way. There is no "shortage" of oil. That is to say, there is no more of a shortage of oil than there is of anything else in the world that people desire and the supply of which is limited. Nor are we addicted to oil—any more than are the people of all industrially advanced and politically free societies—with whom most people in the rest of the world would like to change places. Finally, we are not—and let us make no mistake about this—going to be better off by emasculating ourselves, economically, politically, or psychologically. The idea that it is sinful and wrong for one person to have more than another goes back to ancient history. The Greeks feared and sought to placate their jealous gods. The Christians elevated self-abnegation and poverty—at least in prin-ciple—to a virtue, giving Marx and Freud powerful ammunition in their efforts to replace Christianity with their own brands of anti-individualistic gnosticism. The Carters have managed to combine the worst—the most self-destructive and undignified—elements of these three creeds into a single vision, if one can call deliberately self-induced blindness vision.

The Carters' vision is one of unrelieved bleakness for America. "After listening to the American people," Carter declared in July, "I have been reminded again that all the legislatures in the world can't fix what's wrong with America." Note that Carter always knew that America was sick unto death, and was merely reminded of this once more. How does Carter know this? The same way Susan Sontag knows that "the white race is the cancer of human history."

Actually, the Carters gloat over the moral corruption of America, which, they seem to think, presents a background against which their own moral rectitude can shine forth with dazzling luminosity. Thus, on August 6, with Carter's performance as president generally rated as falling, he let the American people know of his efforts to Christianize a heathen head of state: "While teaching an adult Bible class at the First Baptist Church of Washington, Carter said yesterday that the 'roots of the weakness of the Christian church, one of them anyway, is the reluctance to assume the responsibility placed on our shoulder.'" He was referring, of course, to his responsibilities as a Baptist, not as a president: "Noting that a Christian should try to win new followers [reported the UPI news dispatch], the President said he made such an effort during his trip to South Korea in late June." President Carter, we learn, "tried to convert President Park Chung Hee to Christianity and the South Korean leader was 'very interested'—but matters now rest in 'God's hands.'" One wonders which god, or whose god, will decide this matter. After all, let us not forget that even the officially atheist Mr. Brezhnev "has" a deity, for he warned Carter that God would not forgive us if the Senate did not ratify SALT II.

Apropos of President Carter's attempts to religionize politics, what was curiously much less publicized than his efforts to convert President Park was his inviting not one, not two, not three—but five—theologians to his Camp David domestic summit. The sociologist Robert Bellah shared the evening with them and described the experience as follows: "Carter feels at home with the religiously sincere; he opened and closed with a prayer. It was actually very moving; we felt like we'd been at a religious experience." It is an altogether deliciously ironic situation: A child cannot now say a prayer in school, but abroad, on a tax-supported diplomatic mission, the President can try to convert another head of state to Christianity; while at home, at a tax-supported gathering organized to prop up his sagging authority, the President can open and close the meeting with a prayer.

Thus, we are confronted with a president who talks incessantly about making sacrifices, but is unwilling himself to make the sacrifice of, say, restricting his Christianizing efforts to non-official occasions. But, then, why should *he* sacrifice? He is not a sinner. We are. This explains why both President and Mrs. Carter feel so strongly that it is we who should make sacrifices and more sacrifices—and who should be grateful to those who so abuse us. The Carterian remedy—a veritable witch's brew of religion, socialism, and mental health—is, indeed, a fitting potion to be dispensed by faith healers.

Like all such remedies, it is, of course, for patients only. Bertrand Russell did not only preach about sharing. He believed that a man should live from what he earns and give away his inheritance. Ludwig Wittgenstein, the great Austrian linguist-philosopher, gave away an even larger patrimony. But what have the Carters and their cronies shared with the poor? What sacrifices have Peter Bourne and Bert Lance made for the country?

Patrick Caddell, the Carter's personal pollster, we learn from *Time* magazine (August 6, 1979), relaxes by "whipping around town in his gold-covered Mercedes." Let the peasants relax by riding around in car pools.

Rosalynn Carter as Big Nurse

If Jimmy Carter is the doctor, determined to wean his addict-patient off everything that makes his life worth living, then Rosalynn Carter must be his nurse-assistant. Sally Quinn, writing in the *Washington Post,* has actually suggested that Mrs. Carter is "playing nurse." As Quinn sees it, however, it is Jimmy Carter who is the patient, and we are the worried relatives whose anxiety she tries to soothe:

> She is the nurse. He is the patient. She has come to the waiting room to reassure the concerned relatives. They are not listening to what she is saying. They are listening to how she is saying it. . . . She tells them everything that can be done is being done. She tells them the patient is fine. But he needs their encouragement and support.

While Quinn's interpretation is not without merit, the facts fit the scenario I am suggesting better. Rosalynn Carter is the nurse, all right—but she is the Big Nurse, she is Nurse Ratched of *One Flew Over the Cuckoo's Nest* fame. Jimmy Carter is the emasculated doctor whose formal powers she wields. And we, the American people, are the patient-enemy, whom she/they are determined to bring to heel. With the best "therapeutic" intentions and methods, of course.

"I bring," said Mrs. Carter in Pine Bluff, Arkansas, in July, "greetings from Jimmy. I left him at home and Amy is away at camp so he's going to be very lonesome. But he said to tell you hello. I want you to know he's healthy and we're having a wonderful time at the White House. . . . He's healthy. He's happy. He's confident; and he's optimistic about the future of the country."

Quinn quotes this passage as typical of the sort of thing Rosalynn Carter says when she is standing in for the President. It illustrates, she says, "the nurse-patient image [which] arises time and again as she continues to defend her husband; to promote him in a way one would not expect a President to need."

Quinn's remark is consistent with my suggestion that while Mrs. Carter seemingly enhances her husband's image, actually she diminishes it. Since it is unlikely that she would publicly announce feeling ashamed of Mr. Carter, her protestations of "I am proud of Jimmy" strike a false note.

Increasingly, commentators are noting that although the American people elected Jimmy Carter as president, they have got Rosalynn Carter as co-president—at least. In Dallas, in July, she was called "the President's secret weapon" (an interesting metaphor), and a minister there led prayers for "those who lead this great nation, Jimmy Carter and Rosalynn Carter." In one of her speeches on her Texas tour, Mrs. Carter slipped into speaking as if she were indeed president. After touring a "camp for emotionally and physically disadvantaged children," she told an assembled group that "I have a bill now before Congress" to implement improved mental health care. Speaking in Dallas on the same tour, she modestly remarked, apropos of the Camp David domestic summit: "I sat in on the meetings; I listened with him, and we, uh, he made the decisions."

In a story that verged on being adulatory, *Time* magazine (August 6) reported on Mrs. Carter's July tour of the country in praise of the President. Under the title of "Selling True Grit—and by God She's Good at It," *Time* illustrated Mrs. Carter's effectiveness as a popular politician by citing a Los Angeles bystander who witnessed her performance and remarked admiringly: "Now why couldn't *she* be the President?"

In an unofficial sense, Mrs. Carter is, indeed, the president. She views herself, at the very least, as co-president. Her own remarks about her role are revealing. "The President of the United States [not Jimmy] cares what I think," she has told reporters. "I have influence. I know it." About her present situation, she has remarked: "I find myself in the eye of history." Since she has also claimed having "always been more political" than her husband, it would have been more truthful if she had taken more responsibility for her actions and said that she had thrust herself into the eye of history. Surely, there is nothing passive about her advice that the White House band stop playing "Hail to the Chief"—a suggestion ostensibly made to "de-imperialize" the presidency. She succeeded. "The White House discovered," commented Harry Kelly (in the *Chicago Tribune,* August 2), "that without pomp, the President was just another guy with a shoe shine." In the meanwhile, Mrs. Carter has done everything possible to insure that she is not perceived as just another woman with a rich husband.

The impresssion that Mrs. Carter is using not only her position as the president's wife but also her much-touted concern for mental health to satisfy her own cravings for power and publicity is supported by everything that has happened, or not happened, with respect to mental health during the Carter administration. Instead of a survey of official psychiatric "achievements" or statistics, I shall cite some events that, I believe, illustrate Rosalynn Carter's real stand on mental health.

Mrs. Carter, let us keep in mind, has not been unduly modest in her role as the promoter of psychiatry. She has served as honorary chairperson of the President's Commission on Mental Health. She has received numerous honors from psychiatric groups, such as the American Psychiatric Association—and for psychiatric causes, for example, from the National Council of Negro Women. She was an ardent supporter of Dr. Peter Bourne. Furthermore, as she herself has stated, *she* now has a bill before Congress—"to implement improved mental health care" (whatever that means).

Rosalynn Carter often speaks on mental health. On May 7, 1979, she addressed the World Health Organization in Geneva. On that occasion, she was, as usual, full of compassion for the psychiatrically downtrodden. "The reality of mental health care in America," she said to the guardians of mental health in, among other places, the Soviet Union, "is that in too many cases those without power or influence suffer from severe discrimination in the delivery of services." Note here Mrs. Carter's emphasis on discrimination against mental patients, a subject to which I shall return in a moment.

On May 16, only nine days after speaking in Geneva, Mrs. Carter addressed the American Psychiatric Association in Chicago. That speech—full of psychiatric platitudes praising the mental health lobby—nevertheless also contained some notable passages. She spoke of her devotion to building "a more caring society," of her "sense of compassion for those who are vulnerable," and of her determination to eradicate the stigma of mental illness. "Until we change this aura of ignorance and prejudice, our efforts to improve care will be in vain," she concluded.

But words, as an old saying has it, are cheap. They are especially cheap if they are unsupported or contradicted by the speaker's actions. Such is the case with Mrs. Carter's platitudinizings about psychiatry. As it happened, very soon after her ringing speeches against psychiatric stigmatization, delivered in Geneva and Chicago, she had a chance to show whether she meant what she said.

In June, according to press reports, two foreigners, one from England and the other from Germany, holding valid U.S. visas, were denied entry because as homosexuals they were automatically classified as "psychopathic personalities." Here, in summary, is one of these episodes, as reported by the Associated Press:

> Customs officials asked Karl Kinder if he was homosexual when they found a copy of a gay magazine in his suitcase, when he arrived in Minneapolis from his home in West Germany. Kinder, 32, said he replied: "No, I'm bisexual." As a result, U.S. Immigration and Naturalization Service inspectors denied Kinder entrance into the United States and he was forced to fly back to West Germany. . . . The incident was the second time in two weeks that a foreigner was denied entrance to the United States for reasons of sexual preference. . . . "I don't believe it," Kinder said as he held his passport open to show the large "CANCELLED" which covered the page. "They say this country is free and everything. I feel like a criminal, but I've done nothing wrong. . . . In Germany gay is legal since 1969."

Human rights, as we know all too well, are won by confronting actual, real injustices—not by protesting about abstract "discriminations." They are won by refusing to recant one's religious or scientific views, by publicly denouncing the scapegoating of a Dreyfus—or of a homosexual. Has Mrs. Carter spoken out against the U.S. Immigration code's psychiatric standards, which enshrine the very discrimination that she claims to be opposing? No, she never has. To my knowledge, she has never spoken out about *any actual case* of psychiatric violation of human freedom and dignity. Indeed, how could she? She supports the organizations responsible for these discriminations.

As I noted earlier, Mrs. Carter brags shamelessly about having a bill of her own before Congress "to implement mental health care"—a remark all too revealing of her personal vanity rather than of her concern for individuals accused of mental illness. In the immigration cases I cited, Mrs. Carter had a golden opportunity to demonstrate her sincerity in doing away with psychiatric stigma and opposing political discriminations against persons identified as psychiatric patients. She could have introduced a bill—or, more modestly and precisely, she could have asked for a bill to be introduced—in Congress repealing the immigration law excluding homosexuals from America. She could have done so—but she didn't.

While still on the subject of our immigration regulations, I want to call attention here to the contrast between their unremitting hostility toward psychiatry's favorite scapegoats and their truly enlightened attitude toward those suffering from real, though contagious, diseases. On July 19, apropos of the influx of Indochinese refugees into the United States, the *New York Times* reported that San Francisco health officials found a "significant" incidence of tuberculosis and leprosy among them. However, this constituted no bar to their entry into the country. A U.S. Public Health Service official, quoted by the *Times,* commented that "tuberculosis responded quickly to antibiotics, and that leprosy was very difficult to transmit despite its biblical image."

In short, it is the state—the United States government—that produces the psychiatric stigma attached to homosexuals. And it is the state—the United States government—that produces the stigma of Americans as gasoline junkies. It is a supreme irony of history that in Germany today homosexuality is legal and gas is plentiful—while in America homosexuality is, in most states, illegal and gas is about to be rationed.

Stigmatizing the Stigmatizers

In an essay in *Inquiry* in September 1978, I predicted that President Carter's playing psychiatrist was not going to protect him from himself becoming the target of psychiatric derogation. Now my prediction has come to pass with a vengeance—and I must say it could not have happened to a more deserving person. On July 20, Senator Ted Stevens of Alaska declared, on the Senate floor, that President Carter "may be approaching some sort of mental problem . . . we are worried about his having some kind of breakdown." Questioned about his remark by reporters, he later repeated that President Carter "is acting, I think, in a very erratic manner and I do not think that's good for the country. . . ." Senator Lowell Weicker of Connecticut was more direct. "I think the President is nuts," he told the press on July 17.

Soon the *New York Times* published an article [in its *Sunday Magazine,* August 5, 1979] by Eugene Kennedy, professor of psychology at Loyola University in Chicago, suggesting that Mr. Carter was mentally ill. Kennedy speculated about "the darkness that invaded [Carter's] soul" and, in effect, diagnosed the President as suffering from depression:

> The President has spoken words that seemed to be carefully prepared, but he also invested them with the downbeat music of his own depressed attitude. For now his own immobilized spirit has been laid bare, as he almost plaintively asks the people to show him how to lead them. The enormous passivity of the man, as revealed in the last section of his speech, distresses Americans because it pulls at them like an ethnic mother in a situation comedy who battles for self-esteem and dominance through making other people feel guilty ...

Having diagnosed Carter, Kennedy called for therapy—recommending that "we offer [the President] support and sympathy along with a demand [sic] that he do something about the internal conflicts that he has so publicly advertised."

For my part, I will eschew analyzing (in the sense of psychoanalyzing) the President. Instead, I will cite evidence to show that far from being a mad person, he is just a bad president.

For example, after his Camp David domestic summit, Carter declared that "the problem [facing the nation] was not primarily political. All the legislation in the world can't fix what's wrong with America." Such statements—and Carter has made many—make it frighteningly clear that he has no concept of what an American president, the leader of a free, pluralistic society with a limited form of government, is supposed to be or do. Sometimes it seems that Carter confuses himself with, or would like to be, an Ayatollah Khomeini, or at least an Alexander Solzhenitsyn. But, luckily, Americans do not look to their president for moral leadership. They look for that to churchmen, to writers, to poets and social critics, to Supreme Court justices—and, most often, of course, to respected members of their own families. The American president is the leader of his political party. He is supposed to be a politician—and he is a politician, whether he likes it and admits it or not. Instead of listening to living socialist critics of America, President Carter might learn more by reading dead masters of political philosophy—like Aristotle, who warned that "the man who seeks to dwell outside the political relationship is either a beast or a god."

In their amateurish attempt to depoliticize politics, President and Mrs. Carter are setting a dangerous example indeed. It is unfortunate enough that the American state has as much power to meddle in our lives as it now has. It is positively alarming when the President asserts that the powers the state wields are totally insufficient for the task at hand. Such a view, however obliquely stated, can only mean an advocacy of still greater powers for the state. That such a stance should now be assumed by a man who is powerless through his own faults makes it only the more dangerous and pathetic. For an American president to plead with the American people that "We simply must have faith in each other," and that "restoring that faith . . . is now the most important task we face" is, in my opinion, both dangerous and pathetic.

A grown-up person does not whimper for faith or trust in him. He knows that there is only one way to gain such faith—by earning it through demonstrated competence, honesty, and reliability. There is no other way. But like the priests and psychiatrists he emulates, Carter believes in word magic. He prays often. That may be good for his soul, but it won't do any more for our gas supply than the Indians' rain dances did for their harvest. How deeply Carter believes in word magic is illustrated by the closing cadences of his July 15th sermon to the nation. After detailing the countless ways in which he proposes to curtail our freedoms, Carter added—as if Orwell had never written *1984:* "I do not promise you that this struggle for freedom will be easy." What struggle for freedom? The struggle to abstain from driving our own cars and setting our own thermostats?

But the most significant, and perhaps the most alarming, part of Carter's speech was yet to come. "Let your voice be heard," he said. "Whenever you have a chance, say something good about our country." Is it enough if we *say* something good? Do we also have to *mean* it, or is that not necessary? Does what we say have to be *true,* or doesn't that matter either?

That Carter is scapegoating us is really too obvious to need belaboring. Mary McGrory has also noted it. "Washington's first Citizen, Jimmy Carter, just can't stand the capital," she has written. "It's the city he loves to hate. On television, he said, 'Whenever you have a chance, say something good about our country.' But whenever he has a chance, he says something bad about us."

Carter thus blames the American people for the mistakes of their elected representatives—in particular, the president and the cabinet he appoints. Existentially, the people too are, of course, responsible for what has gone wrong. But that surely does not excuse the politicians for what they have done wrong.

Tragically, what American politicians have done wrong is too painfully obvious for words. The very simplicity of their "sins" makes their mischief seem somehow not their fault. We libertarians know that isn't so. We know that they have sinned against us and against our country by taxing too much, spending too much, wasting too much, and interfering, in every way possible, with the power of the free market to regulate the exchange of goods and services.

The Carters' evasion of these elementary facts of economics and politics is, in the end, what makes them resemble so much the modern psychiatrist and makes their performance resemble a psychodrama. The modern psychiatrist's trick of the trade has been to claim that whatever is, is really something else. A man kills someone; he didn't do it because he wanted his money or because he hated him—but because he was mentally sick. A man has sexual affairs with many women; he doesn't do it because he likes sex or sexual variety—but because he wants power. And so on, ad infinitum.

In the same way, the Carters claim that what looks like politics is really something else. Addressing the National Urban League in Chicago in July, Mrs. Carter declared that "the problems go deeper. We, as a country, are losing our confidence and our values." When Solzhenitsyn said the same thing last year, Mrs. Carter vigorously protested. But never mind that. What I want to call attention to here is her repeated use of the word "deeper"— which is pure psychobabble. To the psychobabbler, nothing is ever "more superficial." Say that someone else's "problems" are "deeper"—and presto, you appear to be a "deeper" person.

President Carter too, as I noted earlier, likes to hint darkly that our political problems are really not political at all. That, no doubt, is why of the 18 congressmen he invited to the Camp David summit, not a single one was a Republican; or why, after the summit, not a single person fired by Carter "happened," in Mrs. Carter's memorable words (spoken to the National Urgan League), "to be black." Mrs. Carter has articulated her own denial that the Camp David theatrics had anything whatever to do with "politics." "I might add," she said in her address to the National Urban League, "that none [of the guests invited to Camp David] was called to talk about politics. The matters of importance to our country today transcend politics."

If that is what happened at Camp David, what does the columnist Nick Thimmesch mean by asking: ". . . what are we to think about the prevalence of liberal economists (not known to support energy development) and other hangers-on at the Camp David revival meeting? Or was this really a political gathering?"

Is Rosalynn Carter's version of this affair rhetoric? Is it mendacity? Is it self-deception? Who is to say? It seems best to view her utterances as the lines spoken by one of the leading figures in the psychodrama the Carters are putting on in Washington. But performing in a psychodrama is—as I noted at the beginning—not the sort of thing that is likely to enhance the actors' credibility or dignity. And so it is with the President and Mrs. Carter.

Matrimonial loyalty is one thing. Deluding oneself that one's wife is an economic and political expert, when she is not, is quite another. Deputizing her to act *in loco presidentis* is going out on the proverbial limb still further.

The same considerations apply to Mrs. Carter. Her devotion to her husband (if that is what it is) is admirable. But does she really help or harm her husband's cause? She stomps the country repeating over and over again that "He [Jimmy] is healthy" (Who said he wasn't?); that "he's happy" (Who said he isn't?); that "he's confident; and he's optimistic about the future of the country."

But if President Carter is so confident about the future of the country, why does he preach the very opposite message? And if he is so happy, why doesn't he look happy?

The ACLU vs. Walter Polovchak

The case of Walter Polovchak, the twelve-year-old immigrant who has sought asylum in America though his father wants to take him back to the Ukraine, must by now be familiar to most readers. Still, a few facts—some of them overlooked, others deliberately obscured—must be underlined to permit an informed and intelligent debate about this important real-life drama in Chicago.

Michael and Anna Polovchak came to Chicago in January 1980, bringing with them their three children: Natalie, seventeen; Walter, twelve; and Michael, who was six. It took two years of pleadings and persistence—on the part of Michael, Sr., in Russia and his relatives in America—before the Polovchak family succeeded in obtaining permission to leave. According to one account, for at least eight years the Polovchaks had planned to come to America. If so, all of young Walter's life, as far back as he could remember, would be filled with memories of a family dream of settling in the United States.

But no sooner did Michael Polovchak arrive in Chicago than he decided to return to the Ukraine. Six months later he acted on his dissatisfaction. He contacted the Soviet embassy in Washington and set the wheels moving toward going home. Walter, fearing that he would be taken to Russia by force, ran away from home with his sister on July 15, to stay with a twenty-four-year-old cousin who is a computer engineer. Walter's cousin, lawyer, and clergyman all maintain that when Walter insisted on staying, Michael intended to leave him here, until the Soviet embassy told him the boy would have to return too.

Why do the Polovchaks want to go back to Russia? Anna Polovchak, 38, who had a job as a cleaning woman in a Chicago hospital, told the *Chicago Tribune* she wants to go home because "My stomach hurts. The water is bad. . . . The climate is bad." In the words of a Russian-speaking reporter for the *Tribune* who interviewed the Polovchaks: "Why he [Michael] wants to go back is unclear. In his apartment on Sunday, Polovchak blamed Chicago's climate, and then changed the subject. To friends and relatives he has talked about the 'bad air' here and complained that he was being poisoned by chemicals in the food. 'It doesn't matter why I want to go,' he said. 'Who is to say why someone comes and goes?'"

Reprinted, with permission, from *Inquiry,* October 27, 1980, pp. 6-8.

An interview with Michael Polovchak's sister, Mrs. Anastasia Junko, shed some light on this question. Mrs. Junko, who lives in Los Angeles, had been instrumental in helping her brother and his family come to the United States and has helped them financially since they arrived in January. According to her. "He [Michael] hadn't seen the light of one whole day here, and he announced that he wanted to go back. . . . I was so mad that I told him to go right ahead then." Michael Olshansky, a Chicago man from Michael's home town in the western Ukraine who was interviewed by the *Tribune,* offered this explanation for Michael Polovchak's decision to return to Russia: There "he was a bus driver. He went from station to station, stopping for a drink or a smoke. He could sell things; there is a black market where people cannot move about and buy things themselves, so they buy from people who come through. Now he works in a factory and feels like a soldier. He sees how hard people work for their money. So he wants to go back."

This, then, is how matters stood at the end of July: Michael and Anna Polovchak were going home and were taking their six-year-old son with them. Natalie, seventeen, was staying, and neither the parents nor the Soviet authorities objected. The controversy swirled around Walter; he wanted to stay but his parents wanted to take him back. Like all important moral dilemmas, the Polovchak case thus presented the courts with a conflict between two "rights": a father's right to control his son, and the son's right to protection from forced repatriation to the Soviet Union.

After Walter and Natalie ran away from their parents, they were placed in the custody of the Illinois Department of Children and Family Services. Then, at the request of a lawyer retained to represent him, Walter was granted asylum by the Immigration and Naturalization Service, which allowed him to stay in America for one year. On August 4, 1980, juvenile court Judge Joseph C. Mooney placed Walter and Natalie in the care of their aunt and uncle, Maria and Demetri Gusiev, pending further investigation and another custody trial in September. Tass, the official Soviet news agency, called these developments a "fresh provocation [and] a violation of all moral and human principles," and charged that *all* foreign families in the United States are now threatened by the same fate that befell Michael and Anna Polovchak.

One of the most remarkable aspects of this case has been the involvement of the American Civil Liberties Union in it. On the face of it, one would think that there was no reason for the ACLU to get involved. Here, at least, the state did not threaten anyone's *liberty.* All of the Polovchaks enjoyed all of the freedoms of America, and when Walter was threatened with forced repatriation, the INS promptly granted him asylum. Why, then, did the ACLU get involved? More specifically, why did the ACLU come into the case fighting for Michael Polovchak's authority to take Walter back with him to Russia rather than for Walter's right to protection from forced repatriation?

As a rule, the services of attorneys are solicited by the parties engaged in a litigation or by their representatives. This is not what happened in the case of the Polovchaks. At a press conference on July 28, 1980, Jay Miller, executive director of the Illinois Chapter of the ACLU, announced that his group *volunteered* to represent Michael and Anna Polovchak in "seeking to regain custody of their twelve-year-old son so they can take him back to the Soviet Union."

That the ACLU volunteered to intervene in this case was stupid. That it intervened on the side of the Polovchak parents was ugly. That it intervened for the reasons it gave was evil. What were those reasons? Explained ACLU staff lawyer Lois Lipton: "I don't think we can presume that a twelve-year-old knows what is best for him and then summarily withdraw his parents' rights." This position was the same, almost verbatim, as that of the Russians. "Our position," said Valentin Kamenev, a counselor at the Soviet embassy in Washington, "is that a twelve-year-old should not be able to tell his parents what he wants to do. He does what they say."

This is not the way the ACLU saw the conflict. "The real issue here," said Richard Mandel, the ACLU lawyer who represented the parents in court, "is whether the state has the right to interfere in the rights of a parent to say where his child will live. In the suburbs of Chicago, 20 percent of parents move each year. How many twelve-year-olds don't want to move? But the state doesn't intervene in those cases."

This "explanation" borders on being an outright lie. The issue involved in this case is not that Walter doesn't care to move to another city, but the brutal fact that the Soviet Union is a closed society with an emigration policy that is not like that of every other country. Thus, it is not any presumption about Walter Polovchak that needs to be demolished, but rather the ACLU's presumption that Michael Polovchak's decision to move back to Russia with his son is like any other father's decision to move to any other place. (In fact, a strong case could be made—although I will not attempt to do so here—for protecting a twelve-year-old child's right to "divorce" his parents and to choose to live with others.)

Ironically, it was a seventeen-year-old girl who left Russia only seven months ago who reminded the court of matters that the ACLU should have considered before it decided to meddle in this case. For isn't it ironic that instead of the ACLU—indeed, against the ACLU—it was Natalie Polovchak who was defending her brother's right to political asylum? "I am so scared for my brother," she said, in court. "If he is forced to go back with my parents, he will be punished there. He can have no good education or job and will be followed for the rest of his life for speaking out against the Soviet Union this way."

Do Mandel and the ACLU really believe that it is fair to equate moving from a Chicago suburb to Russia with moving from a Chicago suburb to a Los Angeles suburb? Was it fair, was it in good faith, for the ACLU attorneys to ignore the fact that this case would never have assumed the form it did were it not for the Soviet authorities' initial response to Michael Polovchak's desire to return home: They told him that since he left with Walter on his passport, he could not come back without him. After the case became headline news and the Russians had gained their propaganda advantage by highlighting the story of a poor misguided Ukranian who found out how terrible life really is in America, they magnanimously allowed him to come back without Walter. But by that time Walter had taken things in his own hands by running away.

Even after Judge Joseph C. Mooney ruled on the Polovchak case on August 4, the ACLU continued to harass Walter. The court placed Walter and Natalie in the custody of their aunt and uncle, Maria and Demetri Gusiev. Richard Lifshitz, an ACLU attorney, promptly protested this decision, claiming that the Gusievs were unfit guardians. Why? Because, said Lifshitz, the Gusievs loved the United States too much and the USSR not enough. Their unfitness was manifested by Gusiev telling a Chicago newspaper that he would urge Walter to live with him permanently if his parents continued in their efforts to move him back to the Soviet Union. Explained Lifshitz: "Gusiev has a definite bias toward Walter not returning to the Ukraine that makes him unacceptable as a foster parent for the child." Lifshitz said he was asking the judge for an emergency hearing to determine whether the Gusievs are fit as temporary foster parents.

The following week, the ACLU succeeded in its effort to pry the Polovchak children loose from the Gusievs. Reversing his earlier decision, Judge Mooney ruled that Walter should not live in the home of the aunt and uncle "because they might interfere with the family's reconciliation," and ordered that not only Walter, but also Natalie, almost eighteen, both be placed in the custody of temporary foster parents. Said Harvey Grossman, the ACLU attorney who represented the parents in this court action: "We still believe the return of the children to their parents is the only appropriate action that will serve and indicate their rights." Since the age of consent in Illinois is sixteen, and since the ACLU's dragnet has evidently been extended to recapturing Natalie as well, these ACLU-initiated court actions and the ACLU's pronouncements about the case leave one in little doubt about that organization's views on the rights of minors to protection from forced repatriation to Russia.

Sadly, the ACLU was not alone in opposing Walter Polovchak's bid for asylum in America. Support came from its faithful allies, whom it in turn supports faithfully—namely, psychiatrists.

Before Judge Mooney handed down his decision of August 4, 1980, that placed Walter and Natalie Polovchak in the custody of the Illinois Department of Children and Family Services and permitted them to live with an aunt and uncle in Chicago, the parents' lawyer called on a child psychiatrist, Dr. Ner Littner, to testify. Dr. Littner, a prominent Chicago child psychiatrist and a member of the faculty of the Chicago Institute for Psychoanalysis, testified in court, under oath, that "The boy may be displaying a rebelliousness typical of children his age and could suffer psychological harm if he gets his way." Evidently Dr. Littner was not worried about the harm Walter might suffer if he doesn't get his way.

Lest it be thought that Dr. Littner's testimony was especially stupid or unfeeling, let me assure the reader that he displayed precisely that hostility toward Walter Polovchak that child psychiatrists typically display toward their involuntary "patients." To these learned doctors the child who "runs away" is always a mentally suspect dissident against the family order. Most textbooks on child psychiatry list and discuss a mental disease called "runaway reaction" (or something like it). Richard Jenkins's textbook, *Behavior Disorders of Childhood and Adolescence* (1973), lists a disease called "The Runaway Reaction." Arthur Chapman, in his *Management of Emotional Problems of Children and Adolescents* (1974), calls "Running Away" an "Acting Out Behavior Disorder." Finally, the pretentious but influential Group for the Advancement of Psychiatry (GAP) issued a report on *Psychopathological Disorders in Childhood* in 1974 that classified "Running Away" under the heading of "Oppositional Behavior."

Unfortunately, there is nothing new about any of this nonsense. Psychiatrists have always taken a dim view of persons who oppose authorities—whether they be blacks opposing whites, women opposing men, or children opposing parents. It is no exaggeration to say that psychiatrists have always regarded, and still regard, submission to authority as a manifestation of mental health and opposition to authority as a symptom of mental illness.

The psychiatrists, like the Bourbons, never learn and never change: In a conflict between individual liberty and arbitrary authority, they unfailingly support authority and oppose liberty. I have already cited the support of one psychiatrist, Dr. Ner Littner, for the father's authority to return Walter to Russia. Like the ACLU, Dr. Littner does not stand alone: Some of the most prominent authorities on mental health in America agree with him. Here is what Dr. Alan Stone, a professor of psychiatry on the faculties of medicine and law at Harvard and the outgoing president of the American Psychiatric Association, had to say about Judge Mooney's decision: "This is totally outside the range of what family law and family courts ought to be doing. The notion that they would interfere in an ongoing, intact family boggles the mind." But the Polovchak family was not intact: both their seventeen-year-old daughter and their twelve-year-old son had clearly indicated their determination not to return to Russia with their parents, and both ran away from home to protect themselves from forced repatriation. The children's decision was, moreover, unanimously supported by the Polovchaks' many relatives in the United States—grown men and women who helped the Polovchaks leave their homeland and settle in America. This is an "intact family"? Preventing the forced return of a twelve-year-old boy from America family"? Preventing the forced return of a twelve-year-old boy from America to Russia is "interference" by a court? Isn't one *Dred Scott* decision enough for our history? Evidently not for our psychiatrists, nor for at least one prominent mental-health lawyer, Professor Joseph Goldstein of Yale Law School.

Now, it so happens that Professor Goldstein is one of the country's leading experts on laws pertaining to the welfare of children. And he too is against Walter's staying in America. "There is," he declared, "nothing that any of us would find in the current situation [i.e., the situation of the Polovchak family] to justify the state entertaining the case. We don't put someone else in the place of the parents unless they are disqualified. These parents did not abuse or neglect their children." In short, Professor Goldstein wants the court to send Walter back to Russia.

The experts supporting the ACLU's position in the Polovchak affair thus all agree that this is an "intact" family, and that Walter is the problem. Dr. Littner emphasizes Walter's "rebelliousness." Professor Stone emphasizes the Polovchaks' "ongoing, intact family." And Professor Goldstein emphasizes that the parents "did not abuse or neglect their children." In view of the published evidence about the Polovchak family, one wonders if these experts knew what they were talking about. "According to relatives [we learn from *People* magazine], the boy was brought up primarily by his grandmother, and Polovchak himself admits he has never taken his children to a movie or on vacation or attended any of their school events. 'That is for the state to provide,' he has said." If the experts knew this, then they were disingenuous, to put it mildly, in using the Polovchak affair as a vehicle for voicing their own pro-family prejudices; and if they didn't know this, then they simply didn't do their job.

There is, it seems to me, something terribly wrong with all this enthusiasm for sending Walter back to Russia, something above and beyond the arguments I have presented against it. This wrong has to do with a curious irony. On the one hand, countless individuals and groups ceaselessly labor to help Russians, including lifelong Communists who suddenly decide they don't like the system anymore, to leave their homeland. On the other, when a young, freedom-loving Soviet citizen seeks asylum in America, the civil libertarians, the lawyers, and the psychiatrists all clamor to ship him back.

The Dominion of Psychiatry

In proposing that politicians be examined by psychiatrists, and promising that this would help protect us from evil rulers, Dr. Arnold Hutschnecker (Op-Ed Page, July 4) offers another "noble lie," such as Plato considered necessary for the proper government of an ideal society. Plato looked to well-selected and well-trained guardians to protect the people from the perils of power-politics; Hutschnecker looks to politicians whose sanity is guaranteed by psychiatrists.

The psychiatric testing of politicians is, moreover, only one procedure suggested by one physician for the creation of a new Platonic state in which psychiatrists and neurosurgeons advise and assist the philosopher-king. Countless others—from Pavlov to Skinner—have labored and continue to labor on building such a Therapeutic State.

And Hutschnecker himself has contributed to it before. In 1969 he called for "a kind of mental health certificate . . . for any job of political responsibility." In 1970 he proposed that every American child between the ages of 6 and 8 be psychologically tested, and that "Corrective treatment should begin at that time for all those tested children who show delinquent tendencies." In 1971, he declared that: "[We] physicians in all countries must move to enlighten all people so that they can assert pressure on their governments to apply newer scientific methods of detecting and curing by Pavlovian methods the disposition to violence (the mass expansion of which is war)." Now he suggests that we "apply psychodynamic principles and explore possibilities other than purely political to secure that our best and brightest leaders are also our mentally and morally healthiest and soundest"; and that this be done by giving more political decision-making power to psychiatrists who are "trained in assessing human behavior objectively."

What can one say about such Orwellian debauchment of language and thought? How does one "assess objectively" the behavior of a Hitler or Stalin, or of anyone? The modern psychiatrist's and psychologist's claim to objectivity is just another "noble lie" to justify the authority of the ruler—in this case, that of the behavioral engineer or of whoever is his master.

Unfortunately, Dr. Hutschnecker's ideas are quite typical of traditional psychiatric thinking. His views may well represent those of the majority of his

Reprinted, with permission, from the *New York Times* (Op-Ed), August 5, 1973, E-15.

colleagues, and of mine. But, fortunately, Dr. Hutschnecker is an amateur: he merely proposes psychiatric horrors. His predecessors have been perpetrating such horrors, and worse, for a long time.

Dr. Benjamin Rush maintained that Negroes were black because they suffered from congenital leprosy, and became the "father" of American psychiatry. His disciples diagnosed Senator Barry Goldwater as a "dangerous schizophrenic," and got away with it. In Germany, psychiatrists murdered mental patients in gas chambers, and called it "mercy killing." In Russia, dissidents now go to mental hospitals instead of to Siberia, and the "free world" howls in protest, as if compulsory psychiatry were not more widely practiced in the U.S. than in the U.S.S.R. The ghastly history of psychiatry has been well concealed from the general public, but it can hardly be kept in the closet forever.

The problems Dr. Hutschnecker hopes to conjure away with psychiatry are, after all, the age-old problems of power. He urges us to be modern and "scientific" and entrust the job of taming the power of the politician to the behavioral engineer. Dealing with power this way is like dealing with dust by brushing it from one part of a room to another; it only increases. We have seen this over and over again in history: from Louis XVI to Robespierre; from Kaiser Wilhelm to Hitler; from Czar Nicholas to Stalin. In each case, people could no longer trust a dishonored leader and placed their faith and fate in the hands of an honest guardian. Juvenal foresaw the risk: he wanted to know who will guard the guardians?

Instead of looking ahead, to science and technology, and now especially to behavioral engineering, for solutions to our moral and political problems, I think we ought to look back, to the Greeks and the Romans, and especially to the Founding Fathers. They knew and have told us that life is a tragedy, or a comedy—in any case a drama—not a problem to be solved; that power corrupts and that the corrupt seek power; that no ruler can be trusted, and that the price of liberty is eternal vigilance. These ideas are not new, are not scientific, and are perhaps no longer very exciting. If so, that's a pity.

The choice before us is clear enough: it is between "noble lies" and ignoble truths; between trusting political power and fearing it; between looking for good, wise, benevolent or mentally healthy guardians, and looking for safeguards to protect us from our guardians. In other words, what will better protect our dignity and liberty: psychological tests—or a balance of powers among competing interests, institutions, and parties? Who will better inform us of the dangers to our dignity and liberty which perpetually threaten us from those who wield power: "psychodynamic" psychiatrists—or journalists, judges, and the politicians of opposing parties?

Our political system, like everything human, is imperfect. And it is very easy to make it even more imperfect: all we have to do is replace the controlled corruption of politicians with the uncontrolled corruption of psychiatrists.

V

PSYCHIATRY IN THE USSR

Soviet Psychiatry:
The Historical Background

For the past decade the Western press has been waxing indignant over what it calls the political misuse of psychiatry in the Soviet Union. This is a case of selective indignation with a vengeance.

The facts are not in dispute. As is usually the case with vexing political and social problems, what is in dispute is the interpretation of the facts. The Western interpretation—both in the popular press and in recent psychiatric journals—is that suppressing dissidents by incarcerating them in insane asylums is an aberration of the Soviet political system and a misuse of Soviet psychiatry. The Communist interpretation—both inside and outside Russia—is that the persons Western critics call "dissidents" are in fact schizophrenics whose hospitalization and treatment are necessitated by their psychiatric illnesses. I shall argue that both interpretations are incorrect and immoral.

Were the persecution and torture of heretics an aberration of the Inquisition and a misuse of the inquisitors' clerical powers? Were the degradation and disfranchisement of Negroes an aberration of chattel slavery and a misuse of the slaveholders' powers? Were the systematic killings of German mental patients and the concealment of these medical murders by means of false death certificates an aberration of National Socialism and a misuse of the Nazi psychiatrists' powers? The answer, with these matters safely behind us, is in each case obviously no. We now recognize each of these "aberrations" and "misuses" for what they were: integral parts of the Inquisition, of chattel slavery, and of National Socialism. The situation is the same with Institutional Psychiatry. It has no aberrations or misuses, because it is itself an aberration and misuse—of medicine.

It behooves us, then, to recognize that the modern Communist state and the modern non-Communist (or "free") state are equally hostile to those who challenge their core values: Each resorts to the psychiatric repression of the challengers. We must do so not out of any fairness toward the Communist tyrants (who do not deserve it), but for ourselves. If we deny that the practice of disposing of deviants by imprisoning them in madhouses flourished long before Khrushchev—indeed, long before Stalin or even Marx; if we deny

Reprinted, with permission, from *Inquiry,* December 5, 1977, pp. 4-5.

that the psychiatric suppression of dissent has been an integral part of all modern Western societies—then we deny ourselves the possibility of understanding the present situation in psychiatry, East and West, and thus make it impossible to assume an intelligent and responsible attitude toward it.

No recent Communist invention, the psychiatric incarceration of "dissidents" in insane asylums is actually the oldest trick in the psychiatric bag. The first step in the history of psychiatry was the building of madhouses. This development, which began in the seventeenth century, created two symmetrical populations: the keepers and the kept. Populating madhouses with madmen and mad-doctors generated the second step: It consisted of the keepers monopolizing the privilege of identifying and classifying the conduct both of themselves and their charges. The third step—the so-called "moral treatment" in psychiatry, covering approximately the first half of the nineteenth century—lay in the recognition that madmen were categorized as ill not because they were sick but because they misbehaved. However, this realization was inconsistent with the medical pretensions of the psychiatrists and the medical justifications used for confining persons innocent of law-breaking. Thus, the fourth step consisted of medicalizing madness and mad-doctoring: Everything the madman did or was accused of doing became a manifestation of his mental illness; everything the mad-doctor did or claimed to do became a method of his mental treatment. This achievement is associated with the names of Emil Kraepelin, Eugen Bleuler, and Sigmund Freud. Since the turn of the last century, then, the prestige and power of psychiatry have grown steadily throughout the world.

The now flourishing practice of involuntary mental hospitalization is no less than 300 years old. (My book *The Age of Madness,* subtitled "The History of Involuntary Mental Hospitalization Presented in Selected Texts," is a documented account of that history.) Let us look at some of the high spots in that story by way of constructing the proper historical backdrop against which to view present-day psychiatric practices on both sides of the Iron Curtain.

Philippe Pinel (1745-1826) is generally believed to have "liberated" the madman. He did nothing of the sort. He merely replaced chains with more subtle forms of restraint: He advocated "intimidation, without severity; oppression, without violence; and triumph, without outrage." How little Pinel's views on psychiatric repression differ from those popular today may be gleaned from his following recommendation concerning the proper management of madmen: "To render the effects of fear solid and durable, its influence ought to be associated with that of profound regard. For that purpose, plots must be either avoided or so well managed as not to be discovered; and coercion must always appear to be the result of necessity, reluctantly resorted to and commensurate with the violence or petulance which it is intended to correct."

Benjamin Rush (1746-1813), the father of American psychiatry—his portrait adorns the seal of the American Psychiatric Association—was also an enthusiastic advocate of psychiatric coercion. Typical of his opinions was the following: "Mankind considered as creatures made for immortality are worthy of all our cares. Let us view them as patients in a hospital. The more they resist our efforts to serve them, the more they have need of our services." As one "treatment," he advocated terror: "Terror acts powerfully upon the body, through the medium of the mind, and should be employed in the cure of madness."

If individuals incarcerated in insane asylums were, and are, so treated, it would seem obvious that such confinement would cause suffering to the inmate regardless of his mental state—that is, regardless of whether he is a "sane dissident" or an "insane patient." Nevertheless, all the victims of contemporary Soviet psychiatry—with the sole exception of Valeriy Tarsis—emphasize the "injustice" of incarcerating "sane dissidents" in mental hospitals, thus implying that the psychiatric incarceration of "insane patients" is just and proper. Even Alexander Solzhenitsyn blunders badly when it comes to this point. In 1970, protesting Zhores Medvedev's "mental hospitalization," Solzhenitsyn wrote: "The incarceration of freethinking healthy people in madhouses is spiritual murder . . . a variant of the gas chamber, and even more cruel."

But if involuntary psychiatric interventions—officially called "hospitalization" and "treatment," but actually imprisonment and torture—are moral obscenities comparable to Nazi crimes, then how could such methods be acceptably applied to any human being, well or sick, friend or foe? What is there about "mental illness" that makes a "mentally ill" person a fit victim for such crimes against humanity? We must keep in mind that when we condemn and eschew some types of human conduct as beyond the pale of morality—whether it be gassing people in rooms disguised as shower stalls, or destroying their brains by means of chemicals or electricity in prisons disguised as hospitals—we do so not only to protect the victims from torture, but also to protect those in charge of them, and society as a whole, from the barbarization inherent in and engendered by such acts. Thus, the question which we as well as the Russians must answer is whether involuntary psychiatric interventions are crimes against humanity, as I have maintained for the past 25 years—or whether they are therapeutic methods aimed at curing mentally sick patients of their diseases, as is the official view of both American and Russian psychiatry.

It is important to recall, in this connection, that the psychiatric imprisonment of sane persons was explicitly authorized by the commitment statute of the State of Illinois enacted in 1851, which stated: "Married women . . . may be entered or detained in the hospital [the state asylum at Jacksonville] at the request of the husband of the woman . . . without evidence of insanity required in other cases." No Soviet psychiatrist has ever made such a claim!

Much has been made of the fact that Soviet psychiatrists regard Russian intellectuals who oppose Communist slavery and want to escape from it as insane. In 1851, in a paper entitled "Report on the Diseases and Physical Peculiarities of the Negro Race," published in the then prestigious *New Orleans Medical and Surgical Journal,* Dr. Samuel A. Cartwright—speaking as the chairman of a committee appointed by the Medical Association of Louisiana to investigate the "diseases peculiar to the Negro race"—asserted that black slaves who refuse to work for their masters and seemingly inadvertently destroy their property suffer from the disease he called "dysaesthesia Aethiopis," while those who run away to the free states suffer from the disease he called "drapetomania." Here is how Cartwright explained his choice of the name for the disease that "causes the slave to run away": "Drapetomania is from 'drapetes,' a runaway slave, and 'mania,' mad or crazy. . . . The cause, in most of the cases, that induces the negro to run away from service, is as much a disease of the mind as any other species of mental alienation, and much more curable, as a general rule." I leave the treatments Cartwright recommended for curing these diseases to the reader's imagination.

In 1904, the Austrian satirist Karl Kraus denounced the psychiatric incarceration of a Hapsburg princess by no less prominent a psychiatrist than Julius von Wagner-Jauregg, then the professor of psychiatry at the University of Vienna and subsequently the recipient of a Nobel prize in medicine. What was the nature of the princess's mental illness? She wanted to leave her noble husband and marry a commoner!

The world has changed a great deal since those days. But psychiatry has remained much the same. "Dissidents" have always been legally and psychiatrically fit subjects for involuntary mental hospitalization, and they still are. What has changed is the contours and contents of dissidence. Before the Civil War in America, being a Negro and wanting to escape from slavery constituted dissidence. In Russia today, wanting to "reform" Marxism or escape from it by emigration constitutes dissidence.

Here are some of the criteria American psychiatrists used in the 1960s to ascertain dissidence. According to the Massachusetts commitment laws then in force, a person was a fit subject for psychiatric incarceration if, in the opinion of psychiatrists, he was "likely to conduct himself in a manner which clearly violates the established laws, ordinances, conventions or morals of the community." In 1961, Dr. Francis Braceland, one of the leading American psychiatrists and a former president of the American Psychiatric Association, offered the following criterion for commitability to a Senate committee looking into the "rights of mental patients": "If a man brings his daughter to me from California, because she is in manifest danger of falling into vice or in some way disgracing herself, he doesn't expect me to let her loose in my hometown for that same thing to happen."

I could go on. But enough! If someone wants to believe that the "abuses" of Soviet psychiatry are the misuses of a medically and morally respectable system of healing rather than the characteristic uses of a traditionally totalitarian system of social control, nothing can stop him. If someone wants to believe that the incarceration of "sane" persons in insane asylums is a peculiarly Russian practice or is a political abuse of psychiatry invented and employed only by the Soviets, evidently nothing will stop him.

Soviet Psychiatry:
Its Supporters in the West

The currently popular protest against Soviet psychiatric abuses is not only a flagrant case of selective indignation; it is, insofar as prominent American psychiatrists and the American Psychiatric Association (APA) are concerned, also a case of crass hypocrisy. Since the late 1960s, many leading American psychiatrists as well as the APA have heaped praise on the Soviet mental health system and on several leading Russian psychiatric criminals. I propose to exhume this body of American (and British) support for Soviet psychiatry and use it, much as a pathologist might use a corpse, to establish the fact that Western psychiatric totalitarians share with their Soviet colleagues the responsibility for Russian psychiatric repressions.

Western awareness of, and concern with, psychiatric abuses in the Soviet Union began in 1965, with the publication in Britain of Valeriy Tarsis's *Ward 7,* a thinly disguised autobiographical novel setting forth the psychiatric persecution, incarceration, and torture of a writer critical of the Soviet system. The title of Tarsis's book (still probably the best account of Soviet psychiatry that we have) was carefully chosen to alert the reader to the fundamental similarities between Soviet psychiatry as he exposes it and Czarist psychiatry as Anton Chekhov exposed it in 1892 in his short story, "Ward No. 6." Nevertheless, the Western press and Western psychiatrists have stubbornly ignored the historical continuity characteristic of institutional psychiatry throughout the world. Tarsis recognized that the real enemy was psychiatric power, wherever it existed and whatever shape it assumed. The result of his book, however, was the unleashing of a journalistic and professional criticism of coercive psychiatry that is, in fact, doubly selective. It is aimed only at Russian psychiatry and ignores the parallel problems and practices in Western countries; and it is aimed only at protecting so-called "sane intellectuals" or "political dissidents" from psychiatric imprisonment and torture, and ignores the predicament of "insane nonintellectuals" or "nonpolitical dissidents" subjected to identical persecutions and punishments. I shall remark on each of these matters presently. Before doing so, however, I want to deliver the exhumed body I promised.

Reprinted, with permission, from *Inquiry,* January 2, 1978, pp. 4-5.

In the November 1969 issue of the *International Journal of Psychiatry,* Mike Gorman, then the celebrated executive director of the National Committee Against Mental Illness, published a report entitled "Soviet Psychiatry and the Russian Citizen." To call Gorman's article adulatory would be an understatement. A single quotation from it should suffice to illustrate his views: "Leaving aside the paramount virtue of a psychiatric system that brings a high quality of care to all those in trouble without any invidious economic distinctions, it is my considered opinion that the tailoring of psychiatric care in all kinds of settings—in the school, in the factory, in the dispensary, in the emergency services, in the home—to the individual needs of each patient is the crowning achievement of Soviet psychiatry."

Gorman's own crowning achievement as a mental health propagandist was, of course, that in listing all the "settings" in which Russian psychiatrists dispense their cures, he managed to omit the two most important ones: the courtroom and the psychiatric concentration camp called "special hospital." In addition, it was no doubt also an achievement, testifying to Gorman's own mental health, that he could sleep at night while deliberately covering up for the crimes of the psychiatric Robespierres and Marats of his beloved Soviet mental health system.

Accompanying Gorman's article was a "critical evaluation" of it by Zigmond Lebensohn, a card-carrying institutional psychiatrist and longtime spokesman for APA policies. "As a Gorman-watcher of many years standing," wrote Lebensohn, "I read his paper and could hardly believe my eyes! Gone were the sharp barbs and telling innuendoes, which have characterized so many of his diatribes on practically all aspects of psychiatry in the United States. Instead, we find him in a mellow and expansive mood, describing Soviet psychiatry in roseate terms with enthusiasm, eulogy, and panegyrics."

In the late 1960s, Gorman was, of course, articulating the then "correct" American psychiatric position on Russian psychiatry. His voice was in perfect harmony with the views of leading American psychiatrists and the APA. For example, in 1968 Dr. Ari Kiev, a recognized expert on Soviet psychiatry, edited and contributed two chapters to a book entitled *Psychiatry in the Communist World,* in which there is not a single reference, however oblique, to the psychiatric incarceration of political dissenters. (Both the Tarsis case and the case of General Petro Grigorenko had at that time already been widely reported in the newspapers.) In 1969, Dr. Kiev published an article in the magazine *Attitude* reviewing Soviet psychiatric theory and practice, again without any reference to the psychiatric abuses.

I should like to pause here in my presentation of the evidence against American psychiatry's posture vis-à-vis Soviet psychiatry and note that, even before 1970, the American mental-health establishment's hypocrisy on this subject was glaringly obvious. When American newspapermen then looked at Soviet psychiatry, they saw its horrors clearly and reported them honestly. In December 1969, for example, *Time* magazine ran a piece entitled "Dissent

= Insanity," reporting on General Grigorenko's psychiatric persecution. On February 2, 1970, *Parade* magazine published a long essay by Lloyd Shearer denouncing Soviet psychiatric atrocities. However, when American psychiatrists and mental health experts looked at the same scene, all they saw was a Russian psychiatric paradise, which Americans could not emulate fast enough.

To appreciate fully the APA's support of Soviet psychiatric practices, it is necessary now to name two of the leading Soviet psychiatrists responsible for them. The highest-ranking, best-known, and most influential psychiatrist in the Soviet Union is Professor Andrei V. Snezhnevsky, director of the Institute of Psychiatry of the Academy of Medical Sciences. All Russian critics of Soviet psychiatry identify Snezhnevsky as the person most responsible for the psychiatric persecution of dissidents. In 1970, at the annual meeting of the APA held in San Francisco, the association honored Snezhnevsky by naming him a "distinguished fellow" for his "outstanding contribution to psychiatry and related sciences." Also named as a "distinguished fellow" was Dr. Boris Lebedev, the director of the World Health Organization's project on "Psychiatric Diagnosis, Classification, and Statistics," who has also been identified as a leading figure in the psychiatric disposition of dissidents.

Viewed against this background, it is not surprising that something less than resounding success has met the efforts of some groups to secure the condemnation of Soviet psychiatric abuses by official Western psychiatric bodies. One of the earliest such attempts was a January 1971 report by a committee of the Canadian Psychiatric Association, which condemned "the alleged wrongful detention in mental hospitals in the USSR of seemingly healthy individuals whose views and attitudes are in conflict with those of the regime." That report became the nucleus of a more broadly based effort to pass a resolution at the fifth congress of the World Psychiatric Association (WPA), meeting in Mexico City in November 1971. The attempt was foiled by the Russian and pro-Russian forces in the WPA, led by its secretary-general, the British psychiatrist Dr. Denis Leigh, whose concluding report declared: "Nowhere in the statutes is there any mention of the WPA making itself responsible for the ethical aspects of psychiatry."

Dr. Leigh did not have long to wait for his reward for that intervention. The following year, both Dr. Leigh and Professor Linford Rees, the treasurer of the WPA, were made honorary members of the All-Union Society of Neurologists and Psychiatrists. According to Sidney Bloch and Peter Reddaway (about whose book *Psychiatric Terror* more later), Leigh at that time asserted "that in his opinion the campaign against Soviet abuse was a sophisticated and expensively organized operation, with CIA participation; that he doubted the authenticity of the evidence; and that [Vladimir] Bukovsky [one of the psychiatrically incarcerated dissidents] was indeed a schizophrenic, or at any rate had a history of the condition." Professor Snezhnevsky concurred:

"It [the attempt to condemn alleged Soviet psychiatric abuses] is a 'cold war' maneuver carried out by expert hands."

In 1973, in an interview in the *Observer*, Leigh explained his position in this way: "We [the WPA] are not concerned with political matters. . . . Schizophrenia is the most important topic in psychiatry. It's the scourge of the world. The Russians have about 200 people researching it and they have a good chance of solving it. That's all there is to it."

Sean MacBride, chairman of Amnesty International at the time, supported Leigh and the Russians, declaring: "I think there has been a good deal of exaggeration in the foreign press reports in regard to the extent, if any, to which psychiatric hospitals are being used in dealing with political prisoners."

During the years since then, the popular as well as the psychiatric press have continued their campaign of selective indignation and protest. Typically, articles in the popular press would condemn Soviet emigration policies preventing Russian Jews from leaving the country; the writers of such articles must believe that it is quite proper for the Soviet government to prevent Russian Christians from leaving their country. Similarly, articles in both the popular press and in psychiatric journals would condemn Soviet mental health policies preventing Russian dissidents from leaving mental hospitals; the writers of such articles must likewise believe that it is quite proper for the Soviet government to prevent Russian nondissidents from leaving mental hospitals. That the Soviet Union is a police state—that it is, as it were, one big prison, concentration camp, or mental hospital—is a fact at once too simple, obvious, and unpalatable for many observers of the contemporary political and psychiatric scene to admit.

At long last, on September 1, 1977, Western psychiatry won a Pyrrhic victory over Soviet psychiatry. At the sixth congress of the WPA, meeting in Honolulu, the British Royal College of Psychiatrists introduced a resolution condemning "the systematic abuse of psychiatry for political purposes in the USSR." The General Assembly of the WPA passed that resolution by a vote of 90 to 88.

In August 1977, I was on a lecture tour in Australia. Anticipating just such an outcome in the tragi-comic struggle between the forces of psychiatric good and evil, I repeatedly called attention to the basic similarities between institutional psychiatry on both sides of the Iron Curtain. After the resounding victory of the forces of good over evil in Honolulu, Frank Knöpfelmacher, professor of psychology at Melbourne University, offered the following comments on the crucial similarities, and differences, between the political-psychiatric situation in Russia and America:

> In a strict sense there is not much difference between Soviet and American psychiatry in terms of moral rectitude and intellectual probity, as Szasz was fully justified in pointing out. As professions, they are both much of a muchness. This may very well be the reason why the Western psychiatric profession

showed its now notorious reluctance to condemn Soviet psychiatry, and why they had to be shamed from without, sometimes by the most elaborate methods, to "protest." The difference between our own and Soviet uses of psychiatry lies elsewhere.

It is a very complex difference but its gist can be indicated thus. Unlike General Grigorenko and the psychiatrist [Semyon] Gluzman, who revealed the uses of Soviet psychiatry, Senator Goldwater and Thomas Szasz are not in concentration camps. And they certainly do not depend for their physical survival on pleas and protests from the psychiatrists of the Serbsky Institute [one of the notorious Soviet "special hospitals"].

However obvious they might be, certain elementary facts about Soviet society must be stated and restated, lest one succumb to the temptation to engage in the debate between Soviet psychiatrists and their Western critics on their own false terms. Russia is a closed society: One cannot leave it at will. In Russia, the state is the psychiatrist's only employer. Soviet psychiatrists work for the state—or get out (if they can), or get locked up (as insane). In Russia, rejecting the moral and political principles of Marxism and Communism is regarded as a characteristic symptom of schizophrenia; the Russian psychiatrist may be quite "sincere" in believing that dissidents are demented.

It is clear, then, that from a libertarian viewpoint the line between the Soviet uses and abuses of psychiatry is an invisible one. *All* of Soviet psychiatry is an instrument of the political power of the Soviet state, just as *most* of our psychiatry is an instrument of the political power of the American state. Wrenching analyses of psychiatric practices out of their historical, economic, and political contexts is an exercise not only in futility but also in foolishness.

Soviet Psychiatry:
Winking at Psychiatric Terror

In previous essays, I reviewed the history of psychiatric coercion and showed why any effort to confront the problems it poses without considering the economic and political context in which such coercion is practiced is an exercise in futility. Obviously, this caveat applies especially to psychiatric practices in the Soviet Union.

It is, nevertheless, possible to write about Soviet psychiatry without observing the intellectual and moral decencies. The results of such an effort will predictably be that those who attempt it will look knavish and foolish, and their work will be intellectually feeble and morally repugnant. Sidney Bloch, lecturer in psychiatry at Oxford University, and Peter Reddaway, senior lecturer in political science at the London School of Economics, are the authors of just such a book.

The American edition of their work is titled, somewhat grandiosely and misleadingly, *Psychiatric Terror,* and is subtitled, "How Soviet Psychiatry Is Used to Suppress Dissent." In fact, the book is not about psychiatric terror in general, but only about psychiatric terror in Russia and only as it affects a very small part of the psychiatrically terrorized population. For as the subtitle indicates, Bloch and Reddaway are not concerned with psychiatric terror used to suppress those not formally defined as dissidents. Moreover, the subtitle itself is also curiously misleading. The book is not about "how Soviet psychiatry is used to suppress dissent," but about how "psychiatry is used to suppress dissent in the Soviet Union"— which is an important distinction. To my knowledge, Soviet psychiatry has not been used to suppress dissent (or to defame living or dead persons) outside the Soviet Union, whereas Western psychiatry has been. From Jesus Christ to Mary Baker Eddy, from Abraham Lincoln to Woodrow Wilson, from Hitler, Stalin, and Idi Amin to Marilyn Monroe and Barry Goldwater—countless persons, foreign and American, living and dead, have been and continue to be diagnosed and discredited by Western psychiatrists.

The original British edition of the Bloch-Reddaway book was published under a different, and more precise, title: *Russia's Political Hospitals: The*

Reprinted, with permission, from *Inquiry,* February 6, 1978, pp. 3-4.

Abuse of Psychiatry in the Soviet Union. However, what that title gains in accuracy, it loses in self-incrimination. That title implies, it seems to me, that in the authors' opinion the sort of psychiatry the Soviet mad-doctors practice on the ordinary civilian population—on the toiling masses that do not qualify as "dissidents"—is not an "abuse." This is a "use" of psychiatry that Bloch and Reddaway couldn't be more pleased with.

The impression that Bloch and Reddaway have no principled objection to psychiatric coercion—quite the contrary—is reinforced by the book's dedication and confirmed by what is included in and excluded from their work. The dedication reads: "To Vladimir Bukovsky, Semyon Gluzman, and all defenders of humane psychiatry in the Soviet Union." What "humane psychiatry in the Soviet Union" is remains a mystery. Bloch and Reddaway never discuss it. Among the appendixes, however, they include a short narrative titled "Life in an Ordinary Psychiatric Hospital," written by a Soviet psychiatrist who has defected to the West. That brief account is the only glimpse we get of the "use" of ordinary Russian psychiatry to "treat" ordinary Russians in ordinary mental hospitals. It is enough to make the dedication of the book an obscene mockery.

The foreword, written by Vladimir Bukovsky, himself a victim of Soviet psychiatry, fits the text perfectly. Bukovsky is insensitive to the fact that one does not have to be a victim of the Soviet's system to understand it and to oppose it. "For most Western people," he writes, "it is psychologically difficult to grasp the atmosphere of a country in which phenomena like those described in this book have become routine." This opinion is inconsistent with some plain facts. Thousands, perhaps even millions, of persons in the West, and especially in the United States, seem to be, and claim to be, bitterly dissatisfied with their lot in life. Many attribute their dissatisfaction to the political system under which they live. They are, however, free to leave. Few emigrate to Russia. Maybe they know more than Bukovsky gives them credit for.

About the history of psychiatry, Bukovsky is as ignorant as are the authors. "The Soviet psychiatrist," he observes, "is a part of the Soviet system. He cannot say, 'I find no symptom of illness in this person.'" That is a fine statement. What is wrong with it is that Bukovsky offers it as if it were true only for the Soviet psychiatrist. In fact, it is true for any psychiatrist who is an employee of a bureaucracy. Moreover, the identical observation and complaint was made about psychiatry a long time ago by the very person who invented the concept of schizophrenia. In 1919 Eugen Bleuler wrote:

Almost as difficult as saying "I can't give any help," or "I don't know," or at any rate much too hard for a great number of doctors, is the statement "I find nothing wrong," when he makes an examination of a patient. When a doctor feels duty-bound to find something, yet without sufficient grounds or evidence, and only to please, a ticklish problem is posed.

As I have remarked elsewhere, in this way a "ticklish problem" is not so much posed as it is bypassed, and ticklish new problems—that is, new "diseases," new "medical interventions," and new complications caused by such interventions—are created. The psychiatrist as a physician who diagnoses nonexistent diseases and tortures the patients so created is not a fresh historical figure created by the Soviet psychiatric system. He is what psychiatry is all about.

After some brief and quite inadequate remarks about the nature of psychiatry and the problem of mental illness, Bloch and Reddaway plunge into their subject. They never raise their heads above it until they surface for air at the end. In between they offer what they consider to be the evidence for psychiatric abuse in the Soviet Union, its nature and victims, and the opposition to it both in Russia and in the West. On the narrow subject of the psychiatric repression of dissidents in the Soviet Union, the authors' research has been reasonably thorough. In tracing the Western reaction to it, however, their bias renders their account incomplete and selective. Finally, in their interpretation of the events reported and in the recommendations they suggest for how to respond to them, Bloch and Reddaway are wrong and wrong-headed.

Although Bloch and Reddaway do not discuss what constitutes "mental illness," their views about it emerge from some of their passing comments, like the following: "One can easily imagine what it is like for a healthy person to be interned indefinitely with disturbed patients. In the SPH [special psychiatric hospital] the latter are suffering from severe forms of mental illness and many have committed acts of violence—murder, assault, rape." Like their "humane" colleagues throughout the civilized world today, Bloch and Reddaway accept it as perfectly obvious that men and women who commit violent crimes are patients rather than criminals. They also accept as perfectly proper that, for example, husbands should be able to sentence their depressed wives, or wives their alcoholic husbands, to indefinite internment in regular psychiatric hospitals, both East and West. They do not actually say so, since they never discuss the psychiatric terrorization of ordinary people; but I believe that is a reasonable inference to draw from their tacit acceptance of involuntary psychiatric interventions not only in Russia but also in Britain and the United States.

I have remarked already on the dedication of *Psychiatric Terror* to the "defenders of humane psychiatry" in the Soviet Union. Instead of defining what they mean by it, Bloch and Reddaway repeat the phrase several times. For example, in the epilogue they write: "If humane psychiatric values should ultimately gain the upper hand in the Soviet Union, one result would indeed be that all imprisoned dissenters would be held in labour camps and none in mental hospitals."

That is an imbecilic and immoral statement. Bukovsky correctly asserts that the Soviet psychiatrist is a part of Soviet society. Bloch and Reddaway agree with that. How, then, could Soviet psychiatry become "humane" unless Soviet society itself became humane? But if Soviet society were humane, dissidents would not be locked up *at all.* In fact, there would be no "dissidents," since that very concept and phenomenon is a product of the totalitarian mind and the totalitarian system. Bloch and Reddaway do not seem to notice that contradiction. They hope to contribute to the creation of a Soviet society in which dissidents are incarcerated in labor camps instead of in mental hospitals—and call that society one in which "humane psychiatric values" would prevail. I submit that their own values are perilously close, politically as well as psychiatrically, to those of the Soviet psychiatrists they criticize.

Jesus said: "Why beholdest thou the mote that is in your brother's eye, but perceivest not the beam that is in thine own eye? . . . Thou hypocrite, cast first the beam out of thine own eye, and then shalt thou see clearly to pull out the mote that is in thine brother's eye." Bloch and Reddaway stubbornly ignore psychiatric coercion in the West, and only want to correct psychiatric "abuses" in the Soviet Union. "The main burden of opposing the [Soviet] abuse now falls," they conclude, "on Western psychiatrists."

The apparatus of psychiatric coercion in the Soviet Union is certainly no mere mote. Nor is the apparatus of psychiatric coercion in the West a mere beam. It is more like a vast forest. Facts and figures are important in this connection. Bloch and Reddaway state that they have reliable information about only 210 persons "who have been interned in mental hospitals since 1962 for reasons connected with their beliefs." Even if the actual figure is twice that, or three times, or 10 times, it is still a small fraction of the hundreds of thousands of persons who are compulsorily hospitalized in the West—not since 1962 but *annually*—for their "beliefs." Why should we close our eyes to the predicament of these ordinary men and women and children, whose lives are forcibly controlled by a psychiatric and parapsychiatric police, and try to save only the most intellectually, economically, and politically favored victims of Soviet psychiatry?

To be sure, intellectuals, writers, critics of the prevailing political fashions and of the dominant social ethic need protection from psychiatric repression, in the East as well as the West. But so does everyone else. For those of us who cherish the rule of law rather than a "humane psychiatry," psychiatric terror will remain a brutal wrong not because its victims are "sane dissidents" in the Soviet Union, but because they are human beings wherever they happen to be.

``More Cruel Than the Gas Chamber''

Without going into the semantic or technical intricacies of psychiatry, it is necessary to clarify a few basic issues before a book like *A Question of Madness* can be sensibly discussed.

The most important of these has to do with the concept of illness. When a person claims to be ill, he usually means: first, that he suffers (or believes he suffers) from an abnormality or malfunctioning of his body; and second, that he wants (or is at least willing to accept) medical help for it. Should the first of these conditions be absent, we would not consider the person to be physically ill; should the second be absent, we would not consider him to be a medical patient. The practice of modern Western medicine rests on the *scientific* premise that the physician's task is to diagnose and treat disorders of the human body, and on the *ethical* premise that he can carry out these services only with consent of his patient. In other words, physicians are trained to treat bodily ills—not economic, moral, racial, religious or political "ills." And they themselves (except psychiatrists) expect, and in turn are expected by their patients, to treat bodily illnesses—not envy and rage, fear and folly, poverty and stupidity, and all the other miseries that beset man.

To understand psychiatry, we must also understand the concept of mental illness, which arises in part from the fact that it is possible for a person to act *as if* he were sick without really having a bodily illness. How should we react to such a person? Should we treat him as if he were ill, or as if he were not ill? Today, it is considered shamefully uncivilized and naively unscientific to treat him as if he were not, everyone regarding such a person as *obviously* sick—that is, as "mentally sick." I believe this is a serious error. I hold that mental illness is a metaphorical disease.

Such considerations lead to two diametrically opposed points of view about mental illness and involuntary psychiatry (i.e., psychiatry over which the patient has no control): according to the one, mental illness is like any other illness, and psychiatric treatment, like any other treatment; according to the other, there is no such thing as mental illness, and involuntary psychiatric intervention is not treatment but torture. Western and Communist

---

A review of *A Question of Madness*, by Zhores A. Medvedev and Roy A. Medvedev, reprinted, with permission, from *New Society* (London), December 16, 1971, pp. 1213-15.

psychiatrists alike are united in their commitment to the former view. The differences between them come down to what constitutes mental illness, who should be involuntarily hospitalized, and how he should be treated once so confined.

On 29 May 1970, Zhores Medvedev, an outspokenly anti-Lysenkoist biologist, was, like many another Russian intellectual, incarcerated in a mental hospital. As a result of protests by prominent scientists and writers, both in and outside Russia, he was released less than three weeks later. What makes his account of interest is, in my opinion, not that it proves that the Communists have prostituted psychiatry for political purposes, as the Medvedev brothers claim and as most commentators on this affair agree: for *all* involuntary psychiatric interventions are political—in every such case the police power of the state is employed for the control of persons deemed troublesome by society. What seems to me of interest, instead, is the view that the Medvedevs and their Russian supporters have of Soviet psychiatry, and the reactions of Western journalists and psychiatrists to the Medvedev affair and to Soviet mental-health practices generally.

To begin with, then, Zhores Medvedev is neither critical of, nor even particularly thoughtful about, involuntary psychiatry. On the contrary, he is a true believer in it: he *knows* that some men are sane and others insane; that the sane should be free and the insane psychiatrically confined; and, although he is not a physician or psychiatrist, that *he* can tell the sane from the insane. Insisting that ". . . in the ordinary everyday sense I was normally adapted to the environment," he ceaselessly protests the "illegality" of his commitment. But he hastens to assure us that he is not against psychiatry; that his views on this subject, as on everything else, are perfectly normal: "Now, at the end of this account, I want to stress that it certainly has not been written because I feel there is anything shameful about mental illness. Illness is not a vice but a misfortune which calls for sympathy and compassion. For both patient and doctor, the struggle with mental illness may be arduous and heroic. Mental illness is widespread . . . Of course nobody can consider himself exempt from the possibility of falling prey to mental illness—there simply can be no guarantee against illness of any kind."

In support of this view, he cites the "cases" of Gogol, Dostoyevsky and Chekhov, Huxley and Darwin, Tolstoy, Jack London, Hemingway and several others, mental patients one and all. In short, Medvedev spouts psychiatric propaganda indistinguishable from the official line of the American Medical and Psychiatric Associations.

The sincerity of Medvedev's psychiatric beliefs is, however, above reproach. His faith in involuntary psychiatry is so firm and unshakable that he unhesitatingly employs it in dealing with his own beloved eldest son. When his boy showed behavior Medvedev himself characterized as "hippie"—this we learn at the very beginning of the book—"we felt compelled to turn to a psychiatrist for advice: that is, we took the natural steps for parents baffled by unacceptable changes in the character of their teenage child."

Did Medvedev not know then what he knew when, later in the book, he writes that: "Psychiatrists are playing an increasingly important role in all this [referring to the social and political uses of medical dossiers]—they may secretly veto a young person's entry to an academic institution, or a trip abroad—even only as a tourist—or pronounce on his suitability for many categories of employment. The medical record kept in a clinic or outpatient department may cause a man as much trouble as a court conviction or Jewish origin."

This suggests that Medvedev understands the nature of institutional psychiatry (by which I refer to psychiatric services paid for and controlled by the state) perfectly well, for he describes it here correctly as a system of social controls resting on the placing of stigma. But he never admits this, insisting that psychiatry is just another form of medical practice "abused" by bad bureaucrats. He, of course, would use it correctly. Here is how: "We know only too well, of course, that there have been maniacs and fanatics with 'reformist delusions' who have been capable of carrying out mass murder, terror, genocide—the list includes Nero, Hitler, Himmler, Yezhov, Beria, Stalin." It is really all too pathetically absurd and ridiculous, except for the fact that it is precisely this unwavering belief in the mythology of mental illness and all that it implies that has caused such misery not only to Medvedev but to countless others.

Long ago, Chekhov and Zamiatin recognized the psychiatric institution for what it was. And, more recently, so has Valeriy Tarsis. But not Zhores Medvedev. Though himself a victim of this medical crime against humanity, he is as repellent as those who have victimized him: for he never claims that all those subjected to involuntary psychiatry are tortured unjustly—but only that *he* was (and a few others with whom he sympathizes).

Moreover, the protests of Russian intellectuals against Medvedev's psychiatric incarceration, so enthusiastically hailed in the Western press, are not nearly as encouraging as they seem at first glance. For, like the Medvedevs themselves, the protesters profess their loyalty to coercive psychiatry. What they tried to do, or so it would seem, was simply to protect one of their own.

Among those who protested Zhores Medvedev's commitment was Alexander Solzhenitsyn, who wrote: "It is time to understand that the imprisonment of sane persons in madhouses because they have minds of their own is *spiritual murder,* a variation on the gas chamber and even more (Solzhenitsyn's emphasis). But why does Solzhenitsyn object only to the psychiatric imprisonment of *sane* persons? And what makes him so sure that Medvedev was not "insane?" It so happens that, according to the mental-hygiene laws of the Commonwealth of Massachusetts, Medvedev was certifiably insane, the applicable standard there being that the person be "likely to conduct himself in a manner which clearly violates the established laws, ordinances, conventions, or morals of the community." It would, in fact, be difficult to imagine *anyone* who would not qualify under this statute as certifiably mentally ill.

It would be a mistake to attribute this to the stupidity of the legislators who draft such laws. On the contrary, it proves that they are clever, for the vagueness and all-inclusiveness of all standards for commitment serve the purpose intended—to give discretionary powers to those who administer the mental-hygiene laws.

This, then, is the inconsistency in Solzhenitsyn's otherwise admirable plea. What is there about "mental illness" that makes one "afflicted" with it and—solely because he is so afflicted—a fit victim of such crimes against humanity? If involuntary mental "hospitalization" and "treatment" are moral obscenities on a par with the medical crimes of the Nazis, then it is not clear how such methods could be acceptably applied to *any human being,* well or sick, friend or foe.

Why, in other words, protest only against burning innocent persons at the stake? Why not protest against burning heretics as well? If we believe that involuntary psychiatric interventions are crimes, then we must abolish involuntary psychiatric interventions; if we believe they are treatments, then we must be vigilant that the people subjected to such interventions be indeed "mentally sick" and thus deserving of the "help" so solicitously given them.

Solzhenitsyn's plea, and especially the language in which it is couched, is, however, important. It is only strange, and more than a little saddening, that he, as well as the journalists and psychiatrists who have rallied to his protest, do not press his argument further: that they do not see, or refuse to see, the striking similarities between a state-controlled press and a state-controlled psychiatry. When the state controls the press, as it does in Russia, it prints what it wants the people to read. What the people themselves want to read, but which the state does not want them to read, they either cannot obtain at all, or must read in *samizdat* (that is, privately printed or reproduced) copies. The same goes for psychiatry: when the state controls psychiatry, as it does in Russia, it gives the people the "treatment" it wants them to have. If the people were to have the kind of mental health services they want for themselves (not for their "loved ones"), they would have to get it from a *samizdat* psychiatry. But that, of course, would be politically impossible. Hence it is that all psychiatry in totalitarian countries, and all institutional psychiatry in non-totalitarian ones, is in the service of the state.

There is, moreover, bitter irony in the prominent display given in the Western press to the predicament of a Zhores Medvedev, and of other prominent Russians so "treated," and to the protests of Soviet intellectuals against it. All this creates the impression that such psychiatric practices are peculiar aberrations of the Soviet political or mental health systems. To be sure, the kinds of people Americans repress by means of psychiatry may not be exactly the same as those the Russians repress. But the fact is that

Americans repress *more* of them, and more savagely, than do the Russians.

There are approximately three times as many people incarcerated in mental hospitals in the United States as in Russia. Ezra Pound was locked up for 13 years, Zhores Medvedev for only 19 days. James Forrestal, Ernest Hemingway, Marilyn Monroe, and Earl Long are but a few of the more notable Americans whom institutional psychiatrists have stigmatized as insane, locked up in the madhouse, and thus helped to destroy, physically or spiritually, or both. And where were, where are, the American or British Solzhenitsyns to protest on *their* behalf?

This, then, may at least be said for Soviet scientists and writers: they recognize the inquisitorial alliance between psychiatry and the (Russian) state when they see it. Whereas American scientists and writers stand by and applaud the massacre of the victims as if it were the model of modern mental healing its perpetrators claim it is.

Concealed behind the rhetoric of contemporary politics ("capitalism," "communism," "socialism," "democracy") and psychiatry ("diagnosis," "hospitalization," "treatment"), there remains a simple and forever inescapable issue: in the daily life of the citizen, what does the state control, and what does the individual? In Russia, the state controls employment and housing, transportation and medicine, industry and agriculture, education and the press. In Britain and the United States, some of these activities still remain under private control. But not institutional psychiatry; in both Communist and non-Communist societies, such psychiatric interventions are initiated, continued, and terminated at the will of the institutional psychiatrist and his superiors.

Institutional psychiatry thus constitutes a type of client-expert relationship in which, ostensibly, something is done *for* the client, while actually something is done *to* him. How could it be otherwise? When the expert can, by means of the police power of the state, impose himself and his services on an unwilling client, and when the client is deprived of the power to reject the ministrations of such an expert—then the client has had it.

In the old days, this arrangement was regarded favorably by the church and the faithful, and was called the Inquisition. Now, the same sort of arrangement is regarded favorably by science and intellectuals—and is called the Mental Health Movement.

Toward the Therapeutic State

Valeriy Tarsis is a literary critic, translator, and writer. In 1960 he sent an English publisher a manuscript which was highly critical of life in Khrushchev's Russia. This work, *The Bluebottle,* appeared in England in October, 1962, under the pseudonym Ivan Valeriy. Actually, Tarsis had opposed the use of a pseudonym and made no secret in Russia of having sent his book abroad. In August, 1962, two months before the appearance of *The Bluebottle* in London, Tarsis was arrested and committed to the Koschchenko Psychiatric Hospital in Moscow. News of his fate soon reached the West, and an article about it by the British journalist Edward Crankshaw appeared in the *Observer* for February 1963. In March, Tarsis was released.

Ward 7 is Tarsis' account of what happened to him in the "mental hospital." It was written shortly after his release and smuggled to England in the summer of 1964. In this autobiographical novel, Valentine Alamazov, a Russian writer, is arrested and incarcerated in a psychiatric institution for the same offense as Tarsis had been; he is held in the notorious Russian insane asylum, the "Villat Kanatchikov," the nickname in Moscow for the Koschchenko Hospital; and he is released after protests from the West.

This, in bare outline, is the plot of *Ward 7* and the story of the events behind it. The question is: What shall we make of it?

I have seen many English and American comments on this book; all deal with it as political criticism. Nearly a year before the book's American publication, such an interpretation was offered by C. L. Sulzberger, in the *New York Times* for October 28, 1964:

> "Khrushchev . . . conducted a running battle with writers who felt sufficiently revitalized by his reforms to fight for total freedom. Khrushchev struck back by restraining some of the boldest of these spirits—not in prisons or concentration camps, but in mental homes and sanatoriums.

After briefly reviewing the book, and noting that "The material conditions of Ward 7 are not too bad. . . . All they [the 'patients'] lack is freedom," Sulzberger concluded:

Review of *Ward 7: An Autobiographical Novel,* by Valeriy Tarsis, reprinted, with permission, from the *New Republic,* December 11, 1965, pp. 26-29.

When contemplating this strange book one cannot but wonder if in any way the system that invented *Ward 7* under Khrushchev as a halfway house to prison might now be affecting Khrushchev himself. In Stalin's day, political disgrace terminated in torture cells, execution cellars or Siberian barbed wire enclaves. Khrushchev, to his enduring credit, virtually did away with all that. . . .

The supposition that *Ward 7* should be read as political commentary on contemporary Soviet society is further borne out by Elliott Graham of E. P. Dutton & Co. Tarsis was eager to have *Ward 7* published in the West, writes Graham, "because although the Soviet government claims that there are no political prisoners in the Soviet Union, the practice of putting inconvenient citizens into lunatic asylums seems to have become fairly widespread and is all the more shocking because this can be done without putting them on trial and because the term of their detention is indefinite."

These comments do not, in my opinion, penetrate to the significant lessons in this book. Approached as a piece on psychiatric hospitalization—as an exposé, as it were, of the Soviet mental-hospital system—what do we find? The same claim—that they have been incarcerated improperly and unjustly—is made by people in mental hospitals all over the world. How do we judge whether such a claim is valid or not?

The irony of *Ward 7* will elude those who do not mentally substitute a German, a Frenchman, or an American for Valeriy Tarsis. Suppose an American poet were committed to a mental hospital and were to claim that he is sane; who would believe him? Valeriy Tarsis was confined for 6 months; Ezra Pound, for 13 years.

Our logic concerning involuntary mental hospitalization is evidently this: If a Russian is committed as insane, it is because he is sane but loves liberty too much; if an American is committed as insane, it is because he is insane but loves liberty so little that by depriving him of it we provide him with a "therapeutic milieu." "This is the only court," said a judge in Chicago, "where the defendant always wins. If he is released, it means he is well. If he is committed, it is for his own good." Pity the poor Russians, deprived of such guarantees of the "civil rights of the mentally ill."

Actually, Tarsis' comments about psychiatry and psychiatrists are far more detailed and damaging than his observations about Soviet society or the Soviet political system. Here are a few examples.

The hero, Alamazov, has been taken to the hospital by force: "In the morning Alamazov was examined by the head city psychiatrist, exactly as a prisoner is examined by a magistrate. He was brought to Dr. Yanushkevich's consulting room under guard. The doctor made no attempt to treat him as a patient; illness was never mentioned. Pink and smug, he seemed to take his role as prosecutor for granted."

Alamazov's view of the situation is this: "I don't regard you as a doctor. You call this a hospital, I call it a prison to which, in a typically fascist way,

I have been sent without trial. So now, let's get everything straight. I am your prisoner, you are my jailer, and there isn't going to be any nonsense about my health or relations, or about examination and treatment. . . ." Clearly, Alamazov has no insight into his condition: the poor fellow does not even realize he is sick!

Then there is this revealing exchange between Alamazov and Professor Stein, one of the nastier psychiatric types in the hospital:

"We shall get acquainted, Valentine Ivanovich. . . . Tell us why you are here—what are your symptoms?"—Alamazov glared at him with such contempt that Stein looked uncomfortable. "I have not the slightest wish to get acquainted with you, but evidently I must. The reason I am here is that I was brought in by the police. My health is excellent. It's your job to make me ill. But I warn you, you won't succeed."—"How you actually got here is irrelevant. The point you should keep in mind is that healthy people are not in hospitals." —"That's exactly what the Cheka interrogators used to say to their victims: 'Innocent people are not in prison. You say you are innocent, that means you are anti-Soviet, so prison is the place for you.' The only difference is that now it's the madhouse."

It would be a grave mistake to believe that *Ward 7* is populated only by political dissenters. Many of the inmates are ordinary people, like the elderly husband who stood in the way of his wife's fuller sexual life. This is Tatyana speaking to her friend Anna:

"It's quite simple. You write to the clinic. You tell them that your husband, who is much older than you are and beginning to be impotent, is insanely jealous and has been threatening your life."—"It's true. He said 'I'll kill you.'"

I was intrigued, and pleased, by the views Tarsis put in the mouth of Professor Nezhevsky. Nezhevsky is an elderly psychiatrist, at odds with the police methods of his Soviet colleagues. In a conversation with a French psychiatrist, René Gillard, Nezhevsky says: "I told them at the Ministry that you avoid drugs. . . . your staff are forbidden to talk about 'illness,' the patients . . . are free to come and go. . . ." Replies Gillard: "So you stick to happiness pills?" "Yes, exactly," says Nezhevsky. "Happiness pills. Andaxin, aminodin, and the rest of the muck—our doctors think the world of it." And so on, until at the end, Gillard says: "I must say, the idea of compulsory treatment really revolts me. We'd never stand for it."

On the day I write this—responding partly to CORE demonstrations and draft-card burning by a Syracuse youth—Mayor William F. Walsh of Syracuse offered a "six-point legislative program aimed at reducing youthful crime and *civil disobedience*. . . ." Walsh asked that "a treatment and research center for juvenile delinquents be included in the new multi-million dollar *mental health center* to be built here."

No, *Ward 7* is not only in Moscow. Nor is *Ward 7* a recent phenom-enon. Psychiatric sanctions have been with us for centuries. Successors to the witch hunts, they are one of the manifestations of a passage, in Western societies, from theological to secular, and from magical to "scientific," methods of *social control.* However, only through the creation of vast psychiatric bureaucracies in modern mass societies has involuntary mental hospitalization become a major force in the police powers of the state. To attribute this evil to communism, or to capitalism, would thus be both an oversimplification and an evasion.

Indeed, by alluding to Chekhov's *Ward No. 6,* Tarsis admits that he knows this. Chekhov, himself a physician, had as his protagonist not a patient, but a psychiatrist—Dr. Andrei Yefimich. The psychiatrist is honest and soon cannot tolerate the task he has unwittingly assumed. He then commits the fatal mistake of actually engaging a patient in *conversation*—as if such a thing were possible with one who is insane! The dramatic end follows swiftly: the psychiatrist is declared insane, is committed to the hospital, and following a near-fatal beating by an attendant, dies of a stroke. Before he is declared insane, Chekhov's psychiatrist has this to say:

> I am serving an evil cause, and receive my salary from people whom I dupe; I am not honest. But then I, by myself, am nothing; I am but a particle of a necessary social evil: all the district bureaucrats are harmful and receive their salaries for nothing. Therefore it is not I who am to blame for my dishonesty but the times.

It is necessary to be absolutely clear about two points, lest *Ward 7* be misread: 1. Neither involuntary mental hospitalization as such, nor its politi-cal uses and abuses, was discovered by the Soviets. 2. The fundamental logic behind commitment has been accepted throughout the world for several centuries, and is still widely accepted today: according to it, it is "humane" and "helpful" to deprive a person of his *liberty*—a right second only to his right to his life—on the ground of "mental illness" (or because such "illness" renders him "dangerous to himself and others"); if so, the only question is to define and determine what mental illness is or who is mentally ill.

Thus, Tarsis explains, it is "assumed, by doctors and politicians, writers and ideologists, that anyone dissatisfied with the socialist paradise must be a lunatic. . . ." Every one of the modern nation-states has, in the course of the last century-and-a-half, produced its own definitions and theories of lunacy. It is in this way that both a political and a psychiatric analysis of *Ward 7* must come to the same thing: a better understanding of secular society, its bureaucracies, and its methods of social control – among them, institutional psychiatry.

The list of famous persons deprived of liberty by means of psychiatric incarceration would run to several pages; for example, Secretary of State

Forrestal, Governor Earl Long, General Edwin Walker, Ezra Pound, Ernest Hemingway, and Mary Todd Lincoln in the United States; in Germany— Marga Krupp, the wife of Fritz Krupp, committed by the Kaiser for making a nuisance of herself with complaints about her husband's homosexual orgies; and, in Austria-Hungary, Ignaz Semmelweis, discoverer of childbed fever, for upsetting his colleagues and the public with the view that the disease was caused by the doctors' dirty hands.

Only a short time ago, men believed that slavery was a good institution, so long as only the proper people were enslaved: in historical order, the proper persons were the enemy vanquished in battle, the heathen, and the Negro. At long last, mankind concluded that slavery was a basic human wrong, regardless of who was placed in the class of slaves or why. I consider involuntary mental hospitalization also a basic human wrong. No adult should ever be cast in the sick role through the power of the state. The only deviance of which a person should be accused by the government is law-breaking; and once so charged, he should, of course, enjoy all the protections of the Constitution.

Many years ago, Bertrand Russell predicted that the Communist East and the free West will, under the pressure of the forces of collectivism, drift ever closer together until the differences between the two will be indistinguishable. Years later, Orwell warned of the same dismal future in *Animal Farm*. The concluding paragraph reads thus: "Twelve voices were shouting . . . and they were all alike. No question, now, what had happened to the faces of the pigs. The creatures outside looked from pig to man, and from man to pig, and pig to man again; but already it was impossible to say which was which."

The nature of the "machine" that homogenizes man and pig now seems clear: it is the modern state, regardless of whether it is the police state of the East or the bureaucratic state of the West. By substituting "private happiness" for "public happiness," all modern societies tend to wean the individual from the *polis,* and thus deprive him of a voice in the decision of all but his most trivial interests. The result is depoliticized man. It is small wonder, then, that the "Psychological Man" of today is more interested in mental health than in liberty. Thus it is inevitable that the individual seems less a citizen and more a patient.

But not only is the nature of modern bureaucratic mass society as a depoliticizing apparatus clear. It is also clear that institutional psychiatry is an important cog in it: the Russians call it Ward 7 and Villat Kanatchikov; we call it the state hospital and the community mental-health center. Totalitarian tyranny and popular (non-constitutional) democracy thus rush to meet each other in the Therapeutic State.

VI

DRUGS

Bad Habits Are Not Diseases

Morris E. Chafetz, M.D., director of the National Institute of Alcohol Abuse and Alcoholism, has announced the promulgation of a "Bill of Rights for Alcoholic People," drafted for them by the Commissioners on Uniform State Laws at their annual meeting in August 1971. This bill, Dr. Chafetz explains, removes "the crime of public intoxication and the illness of alcoholism from the criminal codes and places them in the public health area where they rightfully belong." Since some people who drink do not consider themselves alcoholics and hence decline medical care, Dr. Chafetz adds that the Uniform Alcoholism and Intoxication Treatment Act adopted by the Commission "guarantees, in those few instances where civil commitment is necessary, a right to treatment 'which is likely to be beneficial.'"[1] A subsequent editorial warmly endorsed the creation of the Institute headed by Dr. Chafetz, and concluded with this ringing exhortation:

> It is hoped that through government incentives, the support of medical students throughout the country, and the efforts of local medical societies together with the American Medical Association and other professional organizations, the medical schools will become much more aware of the need to equip tomorrow's physicians with the ability and imagination to cope with two of the most pressing problems of medical care facing the nation—alcoholism and drug dependence.[2]

I submit that the foregoing views consist of an approximately equal mixture of mendacity and nonsense. As a teacher in a medical school, I believe it is my duty to teach facts and theories as I see them, and not as the state, the American Medical Association, Alcoholics Anonymous, the Women's Christian Temperance Union, the liquor industry, or any other group of special interests see them. In my judgment, the view that alcoholism is a disease is false; and the programs sponsored by the state and supported by tax monies to "cure" it are immoral and inconsistent with our political commitment to individual freedom and responsibility.[3]

It is impossible, of course, to discuss what is and is not illness, without agreement on how we shall use the word "illness." First, then, we must

---

Reprinted, with permission, from the *Lancet*, July 8, 1972, pp. 83-84.

distinguish—as do both physicians and patients, and as our language does—between bodily and mental illness.

When a person asserts that he is ill, he usually means two things: first, that he suffers, or that he believes he suffers, from an abnormality or malfunctioning of his body; and, second, that he wants, or is at least willing to accept, medical help for it. Should the first of these conditions be absent, we would not consider the person to be physically ill; should the second be absent we would not consider him to be a medical patient. This is because the practice of modern Western medicine rests on the scientific premise that the physician's task is to diagnose and treat disorders of the human body; and on the moral premise that he can carry out these services only with the consent of his patient. Strictly speaking, then, disease or illness can affect only the body. Accordingly, there can be no such thing as mental illness. The term "mental illness" is a metaphor.

With the foregoing definition in mind, I offer the following observations about alcoholism and its relation to the medical profession.

1. Drinking to excess may cause illness, but in itself is not a disease—in the ordinary sense of the word "disease." Excessive drinking is a habit. According to the person's values, he may consider it a good or a bad habit. If we choose to call bad habits "diseases," there is no limit to what we may define as "disease"—and "treat" involuntarily. The misuse of alcohol—whatever the reason for it—is no more an illness than is the misuse of any other product of human inventiveness, from language to nuclear energy.

2. Every individual, the alcoholic included, is capable of injuring or killing himself. This potentiality is a fundamental expression of man's freedom of action. Such conduct may be regarded as immoral or sinful or undisciplined, and penalized by means of informal sanctions. But it should not, in a free society, be regarded as either a crime or a disease, warranting the use of the police powers of the state for its control or suppression.

3. Every individual, the alcoholic included, is also capable of injuring or killing others—both while under the influence of alcohol and while not under its influence. This potentiality, too, is a fundamental expression of man's freedom. Such conduct not only justifies self-defense by those attacked, but also often requires the formalized protection of society from the harmful individual by means of criminal laws and sanctions. In other words, the alcoholic should be left free to injure himself; those who wish to help him should be left free to offer their services to him, but should not be allowed to use force or fraud in their efforts to "help"; at the same time, the alcoholic should not be left free to injure others; nor should his alcoholism be accepted as an excuse for any criminal act he may have committed.

4. It is one thing to maintain that a person is not responsible for being an alcoholic; it is quite another to maintain that he is not responsible for the interpersonal, occupational, economic, and legal consequences of his actions. The former proposition implies only an unwillingness to punish a person for

excessive drinking; the latter implies either giving the alcoholic an excuse for injuring others, or justifying legislation for controlling his alcoholism rather than his illegal behavior.

5. If we regard alcoholism as a bona-fide disease—"like any other"— then we ought to let the alcoholic accept or reject treatment for it. Venereal diseases are now said to be of epidemic proportions. They are, moreover, genuine, bodily diseases for which we now possess efficacious and safe methods of treatment—yet such treatment is not compulsory. Advocating the compulsory "treatment" of alcoholics (and other "addicts") through what is euphemistically called "civil commitment," and calling such involuntary interventions a "Bill of Rights for Alcoholic People," are, in my opinion, the manifestations of a state of affairs in American medicine and government far more alarming than the "diseases" against which such "cures" and their sordid justifications are invoked.[4]

By a curious coincidence, in one of his most important short pieces, George Orwell compared the abuse of language with the abuse of alcohol. "A man may take to drink," he wrote, "because he feels himself to be a failure, and then fail all the more completely because he drinks. It is rather the same thing that is happening to the English language. It becomes ugly and inaccurate because our thoughts are foolish, but the slovenliness of our language makes it easier for us to have foolish thoughts."[5]

When Dr. Chafetz asserts that alcoholism is an illness—without telling us what "alcoholism" is and what "illness" is; that "it is the task of the practicing physician to take the initiative in acting to provide adequate medical and follow-up care for alcoholic persons . . .",[6] when in fact his task is to offer care only to those persons who want it; when he calls giving physicians the power to imprison alcoholics a "Bill of Rights" for the victims; and when the American Medical Association uncritically and unqualifiedly endorses such humbug—we then stand before the very phenomenon Orwell described.

But, of course, Orwell did more than describe; he warned that ". . . if thought corrupts language, language can also corrupt thought."[7] And he concluded that political language—and to this we may here add medical language—"is designed to make lies sound truthful and murder respectable, and to give an appearance of solidity to pure wind."[8]

As an academician and a teacher, I believe our duty now is to stand up against the Lyshenkoism that is sweeping the country. Whether we may want to dub it "Jaffeism," or "Chafetzism," or the "Crusade Against Alcoholism and Addiction," or by some other catchy phrase hardly matters; what matters is that as physicians and teachers we resist politically motivated and mandated redefinitions of (bad) habits as diseases; that we condemn and eschew involuntary medical and psychiatric interventions; and that, instead of joining and supporting the "holy war" on alcoholism and drug abuse, we actively repudiate this contemporary version of "popular delusion and crowd madness."[9]

In the past half-century, the medical sciences have advanced as never before in history; yet, morally, the medical profession has fallen upon bad times. Everywhere, it has allowed itself to be enslaved by the state; at the same time, it has encroached on the liberties of the patients, making them, in turn, the slaves of the doctors. But, as Montaigne, quoting Apollonius, observed: "It is for slaves to lie, and for free men to speak the truth."[10] Where are the free men of medicine?

Notes

1. M. E., Chafetz, *J. A. M. A., 219* (1972), p. 1471.

2. Ibid., p. 1757.

3. T. S. Szasz, *West. Med., 7,* 1966, p.15.

4. T. S. Szasz, *Harper's Magazine,* April 1972, p. 74.

5. George Orwell, "Politics and the English Language" (1946), in *The Orwell Reader* (New York, 1956), p. 355.

6. Chafetz, op. cit.

7. Orwell, op. cit., p. 364.

8. Ibid., p. 366.

9. C. Mackay, *Extraordinary Popular Delusions and the Madness of Crowds* (1841), (New York, 1962).

10. Michel de Montaigne, *Essays* (1580), trans. by J. M. Cohen (Harmondsworth, England, 1967), p. 208.

A Dialogue on Drugs

In constructing this imaginary dialogue between Socrates and Hippocrates, I have of course taken certain liberties with historical events. However, these two immortal Athenians were contemporaries, and the sap of the poppy was known and used by the ancient Greeks. The following facts may be of interest to the reader in this connection.

Socrates lived from about 470 B.C. till 399 B.C.; Hippocrates, from about 460 till 377 B.C. The word "opium" is derived from the Greek word for juice, the drug being obtained from the juice of the poppy capsules. The term "codeine" comes from the Greek word for poppy head. Although opium was used before recorded history, the first undisputed reference to poppy juice is in the writings of Theophrastus (371-287 B.C.).

Hippocrates: My dear Socrates, I am so relieved I found you here. I must seek your advice about the terrible plague that has struck our beloved Athens.

Socrates: Come, sit by me and rest. You are like all physicians: you work too hard and do not take proper care of yourself. You say you need my advice about a plague. But what do I know about diseases and treatments?

Hippocrates: This plague is unlike most others, dear friend. Despite our efforts—and you know how wondrously skillful our Athenian physicians have become—we can do nothing to halt it.

Socrates: Tell me more about it. I fear I must be getting old and out of touch with things, for though I have been mingling and talking with my fellow citizens, as has been my custom for longer than I care to think, I have not seen any sign of a plague. Indeed, our people seem to me to be more robust than ever.

Hippocrates: I feel more rested now. And I see I assumed you knew more about our medical problems than you do. No matter. I can explain my mission easily enough. And I say "mission" advisedly: for, much as I love to converse with you, dear Socrates, I come not just of my own accord, but at the request of our Senate. Some of our senators believe that the very survival of Athens is at stake. And, I must say, I quite agree with them.

Reprinted, with permission, from *Psychiatric Opinion, 14* (March/April 1977), pp. 44-47.

Socrates: Dear friend, you keep on exciting yourself. You tell me how very serious the problem is that you want to talk about, but you do not tell me what that problem is. Is it possible that part of your difficulty lies in this exaggerated importance you attach to it?

Hippocrates: Please, Socrates, save your skepticism until you have heard me out.

Socrates: Forgive me. I will try.

Hippocrates: First, then, let me tell you something about the dire effects of this plague. It disables many of our young men, men in the prime of their physical and mental powers. Instead of working, defending their city, taking care of their wives and children, they loaf and sponge off others.

Socrates: You must explain this to me more fully, Hippocrates. You know I am not familiar with the details of your craft. But are you not describing men who are lazy rather than sick?

Hippocrates: They only seem lazy. They are ill, I can assure you, dear Socrates. Perhaps I should tell you about how this plague kills; then you will understand what a serious disease we have to contend with. It amazes me, in fact, that you seem so unaware that, among our young adults, this plague has become a leading cause of death. Don't you read the newspapers? Don't you know that not a day passes in Athens without such a death?

Socrates: I am getting more and more confused. Of course I read the newspapers. But, as you know, I don't believe anything they print. Besides, they don't know how to use the Greek language our gods gave us. You keep talking about a terrible plague, but you don't tell me just what it is. Instead, you now tell me that it kills a lot of young people. But people die of all sorts of things. For example, they get killed in war. Now, you don't mean to tell me that war is a plague? What, my dear Hippocrates, do you call this plague, this disease?

Hippocrates: We call it "drug addiction," of course.

Socrates: Do you physicians know how a person acquires this illness?

Hippocrates: Yes. By contagion: one person catches it from another.

Socrates: And how do you physicians know that a person has caught it?

Hippocrates: That is a good question, my dear Socrates. I am glad our Senate finally decided to solicit your views on this problem; though, I must say, our senators are so frantic, I think they no longer know how to listen to anyone but themselves. But I should answer your question. The fact is, we physicians often don't know whether a person has this disease. The patients often prefer not to come to us. I am ashamed to confess, we usually discover the disease only after our policemen take the patients into custody and bring them to us.

Socrates: You mean to tell me that if our law enforcers would not make these arrests, you would not know that these citizens were ill? Don't they complain of feeling ill? Don't they want your help?

Hippocrates: It's not so simple, Socrates. Does a wounded warrior lying unconscious on the battlefield complain of being ill? Does he ask for our help? Of course not. But you will have to admit he is nevertheless sick and will be grateful to us for binding his wounds. It's just the same with the drug addict.

Socrates: Perhaps so.

Hippocrates: Let me tell you more about the nature of this disease, about how it affects the person, his body and his mind, and what we are trying to do to cure it. In the first place, the person who develops this affliction acquires an irresistible urge to take certain drugs, which, in small doses, make him feel especially well, but in larger doses may kill him. Extracts made from the sap of the poppy are very popular, as you know.

Socrates: Yes, I know that. But no one has to use the poppy in this way.

Hippocrates: But that is just the point. The addict has an irresistible craving for it, a craving like the feverish man has for water.

Socrates: So let him eat poppy.

Hippocrates: But it's illegal to do so. It's illegal even to have it, much less to use it.

Socrates: Dear Hippocrates, either you are confused, or you are trying to confuse me. First, you compare the addict's need for the extract of poppy—I think you doctors call it opium—to the feverish man's need for water, and then you tell me that it is illegal to possess and use opium. What, then, is the problem: the craving or the difficulty to satisfy it?

Hippocrates: You are right, of course. But opium is unlike water. It can kill you if you take too much of it.

Socrates: But why should you worry about that? Surely you know that killing oneself is not against our morals or laws?

Hippocrates: Dear Socrates, you are not letting me put the problem before you—the problem as the Senate sees it, and as our physicians see it.

Socrates: All right, please state it, and I will keep quiet.

Hippocrates: The problem with drug addiction is that large numbers of young people, and even children, take illegal drugs—opium is just one of the substances they use—and, as a result, do not study in school, neglect their civic duties, and infect others with their drug habit. And this is just a small part of the problem. These patients also become economically dependent on others—on their families, on the state. And, last but not least, many of them rob and steal to get the money to buy the drugs they want. Do you see now what the problem is, and that it is like a veritable plague?

Socrates: Wait, dear friend. Are you asking me if this *is* a plague, or if it is *like* a plague?

Hippocrates: What is the difference?

Socrates: It is the difference between a thing and something else that resembles it. Like the difference between water and opium, in your own example.

Hippocrates: But what difference does it make, as a practical matter?

We want people to stop taking opium. Don't you?

Socrates: Why should I? That's their affair. But you are getting excited again, dear Hippocrates. Let us go back to the beginning. Why did you come to talk to me: to get my help to make our fellow Athenians to do this or that thing, or to discuss the plague which you say has afflicted our city?

Hippocrates: The latter, of course.

Socrates: Good. Because you know that's all I am competent to do, if indeed I am competent to do that.

Hippocrates: You have listened patiently to my complaints, dear Socrates. Perhaps you should ask me some questions now. I know that is how you reason things out.

Socrates: Yes. Let us proceed. And I know I can be direct with you, because you are both honest and courageous. You say that the addicts—the patients who, you say, are addicted to various things—take drugs. If they didn't take them, they would not be ill. Is that correct?

Hippocrates: Yes, of course.

Socrates: What, then, makes them ill? Why do you say they suffer from a disease?

Hippocrates: Isn't it obvious? Suppose your enemies poison your food or drink—with hemlock, or with any of the numerous poisons we have— and you fall sick. Will you not be suffering from an illness? And if you die, will you not have died of the poisoning?

Socrates: Yes, of course. But young people who use drugs want to please themselves, not to poison themselves. Is that not so?

Hippocrates: Yes, that is so. When taken in proper amounts, the poppy—and many other drugs our noble physicians have developed—do indeed have a pleasant effect. Don't you see, Socrates, that is precisely what makes our problem so difficult: our patients feel well so long as they take the drugs to which they have become accustomed.

Socrates: It seems, then, that these drugs satisfy some sort of appetite— much as food satisfies hunger, and a handsome maiden, or boy as the case may be, satisfies lust.

Hippocrates: Those are apt comparisons, dear Socrates.

Socrates: But bear with me, then, Hippocrates. For if the effect of the poppy is of this kind, why trouble yourself about it? What our people eat or with whom they bed is no concern of yours or of other doctors. Why, then, concern yourself with whether they take poppy?

Hippocrates: Because if they take too much, they die.

Socrates: If they eat too much, they die, too.

Hippocrates: That's sophistry, dear Socrates, and you know it.

Socrates: Perhaps you are right. But if you want to reason along with me about whether or not the use of the poppy consitutes an illness and is something that you physicians ought to worry about, then you must not simply base your claim on the fact that its misuse may be fatal. You must think more clearly than that. You know perfectly well that the misuse of countless things may prove to be fatal. If you swim out too far into the sea, you may drown. Will that make you conclude that swimming is an illness?

Hippocrates: But our Senate has seen fit to prohibit the use of the poppy. It has decreed that those who use it are addicts and must be treated.

Socrates: So next they'll prohibit swimming in the sea.

Hippocrates: Don't jest, Socrates. This is a serious matter.

Socrates: I know it is serious. But it is also silly. You are a wise and compassionate physician, Hippocrates, beloved in all of Athens. And you let our senators, about whose wisdom the less said the better, tell you that young people in the best of health are sick, just because they put something into their bodies the senators don't think they should?

Hippocrates: Sometimes you use words, Socrates, as we physicians use the poppy: you, to soften the pain of truth; we, to soften the pain of illness and old age.

Socrates: Thank you, my friend. And our people who use the poppy without being ill, without the permission of you doctors, use it perhaps to soften the pain of boredom, of futility, of life itself.

Hippocrates: Of course, that is so. We have always known that.

Socrates: It is clear now, dear Hippocrates, that you have two quite separate problems. One is the effects of the poppy on those who use them, and what, if anything, physicians ought to do about it. The other is the effect of its prohibition, and what, if anything, physicians ought to do about it. By combining these two problems, you only make each the more difficult to solve.

Hippocrates: So it is. Will you please tell me, Socrates, your views on each?

Socrates: How to resolve such dilemmas is your responsibility, and the responsiblity of your colleagues and patients. For it is you, much more than I, who are affected thereby. I neither use nor prescribe drugs. Were I to use the poppy myself, it would only becloud my powers of reasoning; and were I to recommend its use, I would be guilty of beclouding the powers of reasoning of others.

Hippocrates: I understand that. It is just this detachment which makes your judgment so valuable. So please do answer my question. I understand that I am solely responsible for how I use your words. As you seem to believe that those who want to use the poppy should be allowed to do so, will you grant me the same privilege with your words?

Socrates: Well argued, dear Hippocrates! All right, then. Here is my answer to your first question—that is, about the effects of the poppy and the physicians' moral duty in this matter. Physicians ought to study the effects of the poppy and explain their findings to the people. If they misuse it and, as a result, fall ill, physicians ought to treat them, they desire such treatment. But I really should not tell you all this, dear friend: You are justly sought after because you insist on putting the interests of your patients above all other considerations. In short, if a person misuses the poppy, or any other drug, with the result of what we might call "self-poisoning," and if he seeks medical help, then it is right and proper that you and your colleagues should help him. Otherwise, you should leave him alone. And you should certainly leave alone those who use the poppy in moderation. They are neither sick, nor are they your patients or the patients of any other physician.

Hippocrates: I am afraid to hear your answer to the second question, Socrates, for I can surmise it now. But I would like to hear it in your own words.

Socrates: All right. That is the question about the effects of the prohibition of the poppy, and what the physician ought to do about this problem. Do you remember the time when our senators prohibited the use of wine? That was before your time and mine. But you have read Herodotus. You have talked to people who lived then. It's the same now. Except it's worse. Much worse. Why? Because no Athenian took seriously the idea that drunkenness was an illness that you physicians ought to cure.

Hippocrates: How true! Our people were wise enough to see through that ruse. The cure for gluttony and drunkenness is self-discipline, not medicines.

Socrates: But our people have forgotten all this. And so have our senators and physicians. They now all believe that just because something is called "drug abuse" and "drug addiction" that makes them diseases. And to justify legislating about them, they call them "contagious diseases."

Hippocrates: That is all so. But what shall the physician do?

Socrates: I must repeat: that is for him to decide. In any case, he must make a choice: he will serve either the Senate or his own conscience.

Hippocrates: What about serving the patients?

Socrates: There you go again, Hippocrates. I thought you were with me, but I guess you have lost me. There are no patients. Didn't you tell me at the beginning that your "patients" are brought to you by the police? That they feel perfectly well after taking the extract of the poppy?

Hippocrates: What are we doing, then, trying to fight the use of the poppy?

Socrates: I am afraid the answer to that is too simple. You are trying to impose the will of the Senate on the citizens of Athens.

Hippocrates: But is that wrong, if it helps them?

Socrates: You must be the judge of that. But don't be discouraged, dear friend. It seems to me that our discussion has at least dissipated one of your problems—the problem you have created for yourself by using poisoning as an analogy for the voluntary use of drugs.

Hippocrates: Please, can you go over this again for me? You always treat people as if they knew more than they do.

Socrates: No, I only treat them as if they knew what in fact they know.

But no matter. The point I thought we had managed to clarify was your failure to distinguish between what *my enemies do* and what *happens to me* as a result. You must admit that what *they do* has nothing to do with your business, which is healing. Let us suppose that my enemies try to poison me, to kill me. Whether they do it with drugs, or daggers, or by pushing me off a cliff is beside the point here. If they succeed partially, I shall be sick; and if they succeed completely, I shall be dead. That much is clear. In other words, what they *do* we should call poisoning; what *happens* to me we may call falling ill. Is that clear?

Hippocrates: Yes. And it's the same for the addict.

Socrates: Is that a fact? Or is it an analogy which you use to try to understand your problem? Or is it one of the ways you confuse yourself?

Hippocrates: Please, Socrates, you know I am just a humble physician, not a philosopher.

Socrates: Everyone is a philosopher. No one can help it. Some are just better at it than others, as in any other craft. Forgive my sarcasm, dear friend. But my patience has its limits, too.

Hippocrates: All right, then, I am using an analogy when I say that the addict poisons himself, and that we should prevent him from poisoning himself just as we prevent criminals from poisoning peace-loving citizens. But I think it's a useful analogy.

Socrates: Yes, it is useful if you want to wax indignant over what the addict does. But it does not seem to me useful otherwise, for your analogy flies in the face of the most glaring difference between these two acts.

Hippocrates: And what is that, pray tell me?

Socrates: Well, the fact that the victim of a poisoning does not want to be poisoned, whereas the drug addict wants very much to be "poisoned," to use your term.

Hippocrates: Yes, that is quite true. But we physicians are scientists. We know that a person may be poisoned, whether he wants to be or does not want to be.

Socrates: I am afraid we are getting stuck on the word "poisoned," my dear Hippocrates. You are not using it in the sense that the gods gave it, but in the sense that you physicians have given it. You must remember that when you ask an ordinary Athenian what he means by poisoning, he will have no trouble telling you. He will mean that someone has put some substance, some chemical, into his food or drink to make him sick or to kill him. Or he will mean that he has himself taken poison in order to kill himself. In either case, the purpose of the poisoning is to injure or kill him. Is that not so?

Hippocrates: Yes, it is. Go on.

Socrates: Then we are agreed that this is what we usually mean by "poisoning." We Athenians use many things not just because we need them as a source of food but because we like their effects on our minds, on how we feel. Wine is a good example. Now, if a man drinks wine in moderation, would you say he is poisoning himself?

Hippocrates: Of course not.

Socrates: And if he drinks wine to excess?

Hippocrates: It would depend on how often he does so. If he drinks excessively on occasion, that won't hurt him; but if he does so habitually, it will.

Socrates: All right, just so we understand each other.

Hippocrates: So you agree that the result of habitual drunkenness is illness?

Socrates: It would be foolish of me if I did not agree with you on that point. But, you see, we have only come back to our starting point: namely, to the question of what is the "illness" in this case—the drinking or its effects?

Hippocrates: What's the difference? You can prevent the effect only by preventing the cause, which is the drinking.

Socrates: That is true. But you confuse understanding drinking with stopping it. Since you are so intent on stopping it, let us now approach our problem from that angle. Tell me, my dear Hippocrates, what do you think you and your medical colleagues should do about preventing the harmful consequences of drinking?

Hippocrates: We should tell people to drink in moderation or not at all.

Socrates: They know that anyway. They don't need you for that.

Hippocrates: But many people drink immoderately, anyway. Perhaps they don't know how harmful it is.

Socrates: Perhaps so. Or perhaps they prefer to indulge themselves. In any case, you do not prohibit the use of wine; nor do our senators.

Hippocrates: It would be folly to do so.

Socrates: More than folly. It would be wicked. It would be punishing the many who use drink moderately to make their life more pleasant—and it's good for the digestion, too, is it not?—by depriving them of drink altogether, to protect the few from their own bad habit.

Hippocrates: I see what you are getting at. But opium is much more habit-forming than drink.

Socrates: If that is indeed true—and I think you should be a little more skeptical about these things—it would only make it more important for those who use it to use it carefully, or perhaps not at all.

Hippocrates: Everyone is not as calm and reasoned as you are, dear Socrates. That's why the Senate has long ago decided that the sale and the use of opium should be illegal, except when dispensed by physicians.

Socrates: Yes, I know. That was long ago, when I was a child. My father talked about it, and, I must tell you, although he was a simple, uneducated man, he said it made no sense to him.

Hippocrates: Why did it make no sense to him?

Socrates: Do you want me to tell you what he told me? Or at least what I remember of it? For, as you know, although you and the Senate are all excited about this business, and you call it a "plague," people have been using the poppy for a long, long time.

Hippocrates: I am waiting to hear what your father thought about the prohibition of the poppy.

Socrates: Yes, excuse me. I am getting old. What he told me was something like this: "Son, I am ashamed of my Senate. They are beginning to treat us as if we were stupid children. The Spartans grow poppy. They don't use it. They just use it as a flower—it is very pretty you know. (I had never seen any.) And they sell it to traders who carry it to all parts of the world. We also grow poppy. And our Senate now tells us we must stop growing it, and must stop buying it—they will punish us harshly if we so much as trade in it!—because we are using it to our own detriment. So they tell us, in effect, that the Spartans know how to take care of themselves, but that we Athenians, their own people, do not know how to take care of ourselves. It is a sad day for Athens."

Hippocrates: I wish my father had told me that. Our medical society never mentions the Spartans—except to disparage their poor surgical practices.

Socrates: I never forgot that story, but you were the first one who ever asked me about it. I suppose everyone now knows that drug addiction is an illness and no one bothers to ask why it afflicts Athens but not Sparta.

Hippocrates: That is so. And yet we physicians are taught to make comparisons, to ask why one person or group is afflicted with an illness, but not another.

Socrates: It seems, then, dear Hippocrates, that the fact that some of our people take drugs which some others of our people do not want them to take is not an illness at all. Of course, it may be undesirable that so many people take drugs and that so much of the Senate's time and effort is wasted on trying to make them stop. But the first thing we must do, if we want to understand all this, is to stop assuming that this is some sort of "plague."

Hippocrates: I see your point now. After all, illness is something that usually happens to a person. Addiction is something a person does to himself.

Socrates: Exactly. Instead of comparing drug use to illness, I would suggest a quite different analogy. When a person is given drugs without his knowledge or against his will, and the drugs injure or kill him, that is like attempted murder or successful murder. Whereas, when a person takes drugs, and the drugs injure or kill him, that is like attempted suicide or successsful suicide.

Hippocrates: It would follow, then, that our Senate would rightly condemn the one, but not the other. And that it should prohibit "giving" poison, but not "taking" it.

Socrates: That would be consistent with our moral beliefs, as Athenians. But you see, these are problems for the philosopher and for the statesman, not for the physician.

Hippocrates: Do not be so easy on us doctors, Socrates. It seems to me we have let ourselves be fooled into believing that some things are diseases that are not, perhaps because it flattered our vanity—and our pocketbooks—to be called upon to "save" our people from all kinds of predicaments. But what do I tell the Senate?

Socrates: I am afraid you have to decide that. But do not worry about it. Senators have power and are therefore not curious. They'll hear only what they want to hear.

Hippocrates: I cannot afford to be so skeptical. Anyway, I am grateful for your counsel. I will tell them there is no plague. I will tell them that our problem is that some men are immoderate in their use of drugs, and others in their use of laws; and that the immoderateness of the one stimulates the immoderateness of the other.

Socrates: Thank you, my friend. I hope the senators will listen. But it does not matter. Maybe one of the pages or visitors will. And the truth will be burned into his heart. That is how it survives.

A Dialogue
About Drug Education

Socrates and Hippocrates are presently in a heaven reserved for noble rhetoricians. The following dialogue, reproduced here with their permission, was recorded on a sophisticated radio-telescope atop Mount Olympus.

Hippocrates: Dear Socrates! It is good to see you again. And to see you looking so well.

Socrates: It is good to see you, too, Hippocrates. But you look troubled. Your brow is furrowed.

Hippocrates: You could always read my face. Dear friend, may I treat myself to a draught of your healing words?

Socrates: My plain speech deserves no such flattery. Don't you remember that your colleagues considered my words more toxic than therapeutic?

Hippocrates: They were timid men. They destroyed our beloved Athens. But let us not reminisce. We have an infinite present to savor, unless we upset ourselves, as I have done. Can you surmise the cause of my furrowed brow?

Socrates: I only know what can no longer be its cause—your concern about your patients and your duties as guardian of the public health. I warned you, back in Athens, that to conquer illness you must conquer life itself.

Hippocrates: Tease me if you will. You know well enough that each person's strength is also his weakness. I had to overcome the effects of my training in our medical academies.

Socrates: Yes, there are things mere mortals cannot change. Your devotion to healing and your prominence in the Athenian Medical Association made it impossible for you to value clear thinking more highly than respectable healing. Now that you need no longer be a good doctor, you can be a good philosopher.

Hippocrates: I hope so. But let us not waste time contemplating the effects of childhood and youth on later life. That is the favorite subject of the base rhetoricians from whose semantic pollutions we are spared up here,

Reprinted, with permission, from *Psychiatric Opinion,* October 1978, pp. 10-14.

unless we watch them practicing their ignoble craft down below.

Socrates: Is that what you have been doing? Hence your furrowed brow?

Hippocrates: Yes. I have been studying our successors in the great experiment in freedom.

Socrates: Oh, the Americans.

Hippocrates: Yes, of course. And it troubles me to see them repeating our mistakes.

Socrates: Are they already overcome by the base rhetoric of their politicians?

Hippocrates: That, like most of your questions, is not one for which there is an easy answer. You no doubt remember our friend Plato recommending that politicians strive to be like physicians. I'm sure he never dreamed of physicians behaving like politicians.

Socrates: But he should have. Doctors have always had to resist the temptation of treating their patients like children—to be guided rather than enlightened.

Hippocrates: How true! In fact, I myself was barely able to join you. Of course, base rhetoric was foreign to my nature. But my ceaseless concern for health framed a context which depressed rather than elevated my patients' self-esteem and self-control. That was held against me, and rightly so.

Socrates: I know. Luckily, you were known by some influential friends up here, me among them. Can you imagine spending the rest of your death with all those quacks—phlebotomists and phrenologists? Rush and Cerletti and Moniz?

Hippocrates: I am grateful to you. But you keep distracting me. May I get on with what's on my mind?

Socrates: My apologies, dear Hippocrates. I suppose I did so deliberately. I rarely watch geovision. I stopped watching it after Flexner and Freud retired. I hear, by the way, that they are having a grand time in their heaven: everyone is sick—and some of the patients double as doctors.

Hippocrates: What a joy it is to talk to you! By the way, have you seen our friend Mark Twain lately? I had the most delightful dinner with him recently.

Socrates: I love Clemens as much as you do. But please, pray tell, who is distracting whom now?

Hippocrates: All right. Obviously, I want to talk to you about a certain matter, and yet I find it distasteful to do so. In a moment you will see why.

Socrates: Why?

Hippocrates: Because it concerns a decent American family—the Fords.

Socrates: You mean the automaker?

Hippocrates: Can't you stop jesting for a moment? You are Socrates, not Clemens.

Socrates: The former president, then?

Hippocrates: Yes. And his wife. His whole family.

Socrates: Well, get on with it. What's happened to them? What have they done?

Hippocrates: Mrs. Ford has taken to drink.

Socrates: That is a problem? Americans have always had a love affair with alcohol.

Hippocrates: Of course. Please hear me out. I have barely begun.

Socrates: I will do that, patiently. But may I ask you a question?

Hippocrates: Certainly.

Socrates: How do you know that Mrs. Ford drinks too much?

Hippocrates: I learned of it through geovision—looking at American newspapers, listening to their radios, watching their television screens.

Socrates: You mean it's in the American newspapers that Mrs. Ford drinks too much! How do *they* know that?

Hippocrates: She said so herself.

Socrates: You jest!

Hippocrates: No. I am quite serious.

Socrates: Why did she say so? To humiliate her husband? To ruin his political future?

Hippocrates: So it might seem to us. But that is not what she says. It's not what her husband says. It's not what the newspapers say. They all say she did it to educate the American public.

Socrates: Now I *know* you are jesting. To educate them? In what? In the art of liberal libation? By Bacchus, they don't need any lessons in that.

Hippocrates: No, they don't. But I must tell you how Mrs. Ford has justified making her "drinking problem"—which to us would seem quintessentially private—a public affair.

Socrates: I am curious to hear this.

Hippocrates: Mrs. Ford wants to *teach* the American public that her "alcoholism," which is now being "cured," is a disease—just as her breast cancer, which was cured, was a disease.

Socrates: Surely you are teasing me, now.

Hippocrates: No. You noticed the sick look on my face. I am telling you the reason for it. It is assuredly no joke.

Socrates: All right. Give me some facts. I see your pockets bulging with newspaper clippings.

Hippocrates: Facts will be best. I shall summarize these accounts for you, indicating where I quote, as I know how much importance you attach to the use of certain words.

Former First Lady Betty Ford was admitted to the alcohol and drug rehabilitation center of Long Beach Naval Hospital Monday [April 10, 1978] for treatment of what officials described as a "problem with medication. . . . She has developed a dependence she is trying to overcome," said Dr. James Zimble, commanding officer of the hospital. He denied that Mrs. Ford, 60, was in any way addicted to drugs.[1]

Socrates: There is nothing here about alcohol or alcoholism.

Hippocrates: That comes later. This was the initial announcement. Mrs. Ford supposedly had become dependent on certain drugs prescribed to alleviate her arthritic discomfort.

Socrates: But isn't that a private matter?

Hippocrates: Yes and no. Obviously, you haven't heard about controlled substances.

Socrates: Controlled *what?* Dear friend, watch your language, lest you confirm the judgment of our purist brethren that you don't belong in the company of noble rhetoricians.

Hippocrates: Please, dear Socrates, I know there are no "controlled substances"—there are only "controlled persons." But you interrupt me. You didn't give me a chance to explain that this is an American term. You must understand it in order to comprehend this sad affair I'm reporting.

Socrates: I am relieved to know that the term isn't of your own making. Please explain.

Hippocrates: Until not long ago, American doctors and patients managed diseases and drugs much as we did in our beloved Athens. But then they decided that the state should take a greater interest in medical matters—as our city did in the health of our slaves.

Socrates: That is a strange way for a free people to behave.

Hippocrates: It is strange for you to say that. We were free, too, before our nerve failed us. The same thing seems to be happening to the Americans. We wanted political security. They want medical security. To gain that security, they have created drug laws. Americans now divide their drugs into three classes: those anyone can buy, just like food; those only patients can buy with a doctor's prescription; and those no one can buy, because their sale and use are strictly prohibited.

Socrates: That's pretty stupid.

Hippocrates: There is worse to come.

Socrates: Please go on.

Hippocrates: There is even more arbitrariness in this American drug classification. Their so-called prescription drugs are subdivided into drugs whose consumption is not monitored or "controlled" (as they put it) by the government, and those whose consumption is. This latter subgroup, the "controlled substances," contains many drugs that make people feel better—happier—whether they are sick or well. When people who are not sick take these drugs, or when sick people take them in what the government regards as excessive amounts, the Americans consider that "drug abuse."

Socrates: I can see now what you are getting at. First they treat the patients like children. Then the doctors. So the doctors worry about prescribing certain useful drugs lest they be suspected of wrongdoing by the government.

Hippocrates: Precisely. And thus Mrs. Ford's "problem" with alcohol and overmedication. For us, the use of drink and drugs was a moral matter. For Americans, it is a medical matter.

Socrates: Haven't they learned anything from what they called their Noble Experiment?

Hippocrates: This is different. They enacted the Prohibition Amendment to repudiate indulgence and pleasure. They were, or so they thought, against vice.

Socrates: And now they are against disease.

Hippocrates: Or so they think.

Socrates: All right, please go on. I begin to understand the gravity you've attached to all this.

Hippocrates: On April 21, in a hospital statement, Mrs. Ford declared: "I am addicted to alcohol."[2]

Socrates: Thus making the commanding officer of the Long Beach Naval Hospital into a liar.

Hippocrates: Yes. It used to be a Navy rule that only enlisted men had alcoholism. Officers and other VIPs had gastroenteritis or some other dignified disease. That went with the rank.

Socrates: And everyone knew that drinking was not a disease.

Hippocrates: Yet "disease" is just what Mrs. Ford is calling her use of drink—in what she says is an attempt to educate the public about alcohol.

Socrates: But if she wants to educate people, she ought, above all, to be truthful. Doesn't she know that?

Hippocrates: I am sure she does. But, you see, it seems that in regard to drinking alcohol, the Fords—perhaps most Americans—are unable to distinguish truth from falsehood.

Socrates: I cannot believe that. Any four-year-old can see that drinking alcohol is like drinking water. The only difference is what is in the glass.

Hippocrates: That is beside the point. The point is that the Americans want to believe, and to convince each other, that "alcoholism is a disease."

Socrates: And just how do they propose to accomplish that?

Hippocrates: By endlessly repeating what our poor Plato called "noble lies." Except that the Americans have convinced themselves that they are telling "medical truths." The Ford family spokesman asserted that alcoholism "is just like any other disease."[3] The National Council on Alcholism praised Mrs. Ford, saying that she "gave alcoholism's stigma a devastating blow by stating that she is addicted to alcohol. There is no question that many of these people will now seek treatment as a result of Mrs. Ford's action."[4] And, predictably, Ann Landers lost no time declaring that Mrs. Ford's "admission that she had grown dependent on both drugs and alcohol has made it easier for others to come forward and get the help they need."[5]

Socrates: By Zeus, our friend Ibsen would love to hear that. It provides new proof for his theorem about the sociology of compact majorities.

Hippocrates: Do you want to hear more?

Socrates: Frankly, I have heard enough. But I suppose I should hear you out.

Hippocrates: I will be brief. Mrs. Ford's son Steve said that he was "proud" of his mother.

Socrates: Of her drinking? Maybe he wants to be another Billy Carter?

Hippocrates: You can't stay serious very long, I am afraid.

Socrates: Yes I can. But not when I have to listen to such humbug.

Hippocrates: You haven't heard the worst of it yet.

Socrates: Well, then, tell me and be done with it.

Hippocrates: It is Mrs. Ford's own press release explaining to the public why she didn't treat her drinking and drug-taking as a private affair. Here it is, verbatim:

"I have found that I am not only addicted to the medication I have been taking for my arthritis, but also to alcohol, so I am grateful for this program of recovery. . . . I expect this treatment and fellowship to be a solution for my problems and I embrace it not only for me, but for all the many others who are here to participate."[6]

Socrates: Do you think anyone will believe Mrs. Ford?

Hippocrates: I am afraid so.

Socrates: Even though her own words belie her claims? You noticed, no doubt, the verb she used to describe her feelings about her hospital care: she "embraces" her anti-alcoholism treatment.

Hippocrates: Yes. You taught me to heed such things. When Mrs. Ford had cancer of the breast, she did not "embrace" anesthesia or histopathology or mastectomy.

Socrates: I fear that this good woman has set out to teach regarding matters about which she has much to learn. She seems herself a victim of the base medical rhetoric American politicians have for so long used to dupe the people. Evidently she believes the unspeakable nonsense she utters. What wretched foolishness!

Hippocrates: You must be right, dear Socrates. Else she would not have announced that she was "cured" as soon as she embarked on her efforts to overcome her bad habits.

Socrates: That would have amused our friend Clemens.

Hippocrates: He had some theories about drinking?

Socrates: Not exactly. I was recalling his marvellous remark about how easy it is to stop smoking. He had done it, he said, a thousand times.

Hippocrates: That hits the mark. In those days, Americans were level-headed people. They knew the difference between a habit, like drinking or drug-taking, and a disease, like cancer or rheumatism. Now they prattle about "alcoholism" and "drug abuse" as diseases. What nonsense!

Socrates: It's worse than nonsense. It's an outright lie. But you must remember that lies like these keep people from killing themselves. They stay alive by killing others.

Hippocrates: Yes. And you spoiled their sport. For that they dishonored you.

Socrates: You, of course, were always ready to help them without insisting that they help themselves. And for that they honored you.

Hippocrates: I feel sorry for the Fords. And for the Americans. But thank Zeus, we can do nothing for, or to, them.

Socrates: Don't despair. Perhaps they'll reject this folly and reaffirm their dedication to individual dignity. Perhaps.

Notes

1. "Betty Ford Gets Treatment for Overmedication," *Syracuse Post-Standard,* April 11, 1978, p. 1.

2. R. Lindsey, "Mrs. Ford, in Hospital Statement, Says: 'I'm Addicted to Alcohol,'" *New York Times,* April 22, 1978, p. 6.

3. "Mrs. Ford Spends Weekend at Home," People, *International Herald-Tribune,* May 2, 1978, p. 16.

4. Notes on People, *New York Times,* April 26, 1978, p. 22.

5. Ann Landers, "Real Crazies Won't Admit the Problem," *Charlotte* [S.C.] *Observer,* May 29, 1978, p. 11-A.

6. "Betty Ford Admits She's an Alcoholic," *Syracuse Post-Standard,* April 22, 1978, p. 2.

Might Makes the Metaphor

Recently, I participated in one of those now-fashionable symposia, in which a group of well-known (at least among their colleagues) psychiatrists enact the drama of Babel: each in his own jargon (largely incomprehensible to others) sets forth, in utter seriousness, the character, cause, and cure of mental illness. The meeting was heavy on biology, with elegant graphs and tables projected onto expensive screens demonstrating, with irrefutable scientific evidence, the genetic basis of alcoholism and antisocial personality.

My presence there was, I suppose, a symptom of the "schizophrenia" now affecting the psychiatric establishment itself. I refer to the fact that mental health professionals now display an equally intense interest in the view that mental illnesses are baffling brain diseases, and in the view that their names are malicious medical metaphors.

I do not smoke and usually do not mind if others do. However, as I was coming down with the flu and my throat was dry, I was undoubtedly more sensitive than I might otherwise have been to what I was being exposed to—both through my ears and my nostrils. The intellectual fare was not my dish. However, I felt that my colleagues were entitled to their opinions. What I felt they were not entitled to was to proclaim that alcoholism and antisocial personality were genetically determined mental diseases, and at the same time to produce smoke by steadily puffing on cigars, cigarettes, and pipes.

When my turn came to speak, I asked why, if alcoholism is a mental disease, is *nicotinism* not also a mental disease, and whether filling a room with tobacco smoke might not be viewed as an antisocial act by those who don't smoke. The response was a ripple of applause from a small contingent of nonsmokers in the audience, and a rising wave of anger and clouds of smoke directed toward me by my colleagues. Since the audience was composed mainly of psychiatrists and other mental health professionals, and since the members of these disciplines are especially fond of smoking, we nonsmokers were greatly outnumbered. As to my fellow panelists, they evidently felt that my remark did not deserve to be taken seriously: they did not answer my question and continued to smoke.

"Might," Plato asserted, "is right," thus offering one of the earliest and

---

Reprinted, with permission, from the *Journal of the American Medical Association, 229* (September 2, 1974), p. 1326.

most often endorsed justifications of political justice. Since medicine, and especially psychiatry, is now even more politicized than law, it is time that we realize that might is also the power to make medical metaphors—called "psychiatric diagnoses." Psychiatrists thus speak of "alcoholism," regard it as a mental illness, and offer cures for it, but they do not speak of "nicotinism" and do not regard it as a disease. Indeed, there is now, in a Washington suburb, a much ballyhooed National Institute of Alcohol Abuse and Alcoholism, but there is no National Institute of Nicotine Abuse and Nicotinism. Isn't this because psychiatrists disapprove of alcoholism, but approve of— and indeed encourage, by the most potent means of moral teaching in the world, namely example—nicotinism? I submit that this inconsistency provides more insight into and understanding of what psychiatrists really mean by mental illness than the fakery and foolishness they now foist on the public under the guise of discoveries into the genetic causes and chemical cures of this "illness."

Drug Prohibition

Americans regard freedom of speech and religion as fundamental rights. Until 1914, they also regarded freedom of choosing their diets and drugs as fundamental rights. Today, however, virtually all Americans regard ingesting certain substances—prohibited by the government—as both crimes and diseases.

What is behind this fateful moral and political transformation, which has resulted in the rejection by the overwhelming majority of Americans of their right to self-control over their diets and drugs in favor of the alleged protection of their health from their own actions by a medically corrupt and corrupted state? How could it have come about in view of the obvious parallels between the freedom to put things into one's mind and its restriction by the state by means of censorship of the press, and the freedom to put things into one's body and its restriction by the state by means of drug controls?

Censorship

The answer to these questions lies basically in the fact that our society is *therapeutic* in much the same sense in which medieval Spanish society was *theocratic.* Just as the men and women living in a theocratic society did not believe in the separation of church and state but, on the contrary, fervently embraced their union, so we, living in a therapeutic society, do not believe in the separation of medicine and the state but fervently embrace their union. The censorship of drugs follows from the latter ideology as inexorably as the censorship of books followed from the former. That explains why liberals and conservatives—and people in that imaginary center as well—all favor drug controls. In fact, persons of all political and religious convictions, save libertarians, now favor drug controls.

Liberals tend to be permissive towards socially disreputable psychoactive drugs, especially when they are used by young and hairy persons; so they generally favor decriminalizing marijuana and treating rather than punishing those engaged in the trade of LSD. They are not at all permissive, however, toward nonpsychoactive drugs that are allegedly unsafe or worthless and

---

Reprinted, with permission, from *Reason,* January 1978, pp. 14-18.

thus favor banning saccharin and Laetrile. In these ways they betray their fantasy of the state—as good parent: such a state should restrain erring citizens by mild, minimal, and medical sanctions, and it should protect ignorant citizens by pharmacological censorship.

Conservatives, on the other hand, tend to be prohibitive toward socially disreputable psychoactive drugs, especially when they are used by young and hairy persons; so they generally favor criminalizing the use of marijuana and punishing rather than treating those engaged in the trade of LSD. At the same time, they are permissive toward nonpsychoactive drugs that are allegedly unsafe or worthless and thus favor free trade in saccharin and Laetrile. In these ways, they too betray their fantasy of the state—as the enforcer of the dominant ethic: such a state should punish citizens who deviate from the moral precepts of the majority and should abstain from meddling with people's self-care.

Viewed as a political issue, drugs, books, and religious practices all present the same problem to a people and its rulers. The state, as the representative of a particular class or dominant ethic, may choose to embrace some drugs, some books, and some religious practices and reject the others as dangerous, depraved, demented, or devilish. Throughout history, such an arrangement has characterized most societies. Or the state, as the representative of a constitution ceremonializing the supremacy of individual choice over collective comfort, may ensure a free trade in drugs, books, and religious practices. Such an arrangement has traditionally characterized the United States. Its Constitution explicitly guarantees the right to freedom of religion and the press and implicitly guarantees the right to freedom of self-determination with respect to what we put into our bodies.

Why did the framers of the Constitution not explicitly guarantee the right to take drugs? For two obvious reasons. First, because 200 years ago medical science was not even in its infancy; medical practice was socially unorganized and therapeutically worthless. Second, because there was then no conceivable danger of an alliance between medicine and the state. The very idea that the government should lend its police power to physicians to deprive people of their free choice to ingest certain substances would have seemed absurd to the drafters of the Bill of Rights.

This conjecture is strongly supported by a casual remark by Thomas Jefferson, clearly indicating that he regarded our freedom to put into our bodies whatever we want as essentially similar to our freedom to put into our own minds whatever we want. "Was the government to prescribe to us our medicine and diet," wrote Jefferson in 1782, "our bodies would be in such keeping as our souls are now. Thus in France the emetic was once forbidden as a medicine, the potato as an article of food."

A Therapeutic State

Jefferson poked fun at the French for their pioneering efforts to prohibit drugs and diets. What, then, would he think of the state that now forbids the use of harmless sweeteners while encouraging the use of dangerous contraceptives? that labels marijuana a narcotic and prohibits it while calling tobacco an agricultural product and promoting it? and that defines the voluntary use of heroin as a disease and the legally coerced use of methadone as a treatment for it?

Freedom of religion is indeed a political idea of transcendent importance. As that idea has been understood in the United States, it does not mean that members of the traditional churches—that is, Christians, Jews, and Muslims—may practice their faith unmolested by the government but that others—for example, Jehovah's Witnesses—may not. American religious freedom is unconditional; it is not contingent on any particular church proving, to the satisfaction of the state, that its principles or practices possess "religious efficacy."

The requirement that the supporters of a religion establish its theological credentials in order to be tolerated is the hallmark of a theological state. In Spain, under the Inquisition, there was, in an ironic sense, religious tolerance: religion was tolerated, indeed, actively encouraged. The point is that religions other than Roman Catholicism were considered to be heresies. The same considerations now apply to drugs.

The fact that we accept the requirement that the supporters of a drug establish its therapeutic credentials before we tolerate its sale or use shows that we live in a therapeutic state. In the United States today, there is, in an ironic sense, pharmacological tolerance: approved drugs are tolerated, indeed, actively encouraged. But drugs other than those officially sanctioned as therapeutic are considered worthless or dangerous. Therein, precisely, lies the moral and political point: governments are notoriously tolerant about permitting the dissemination of ideas or drugs of which they approve. Their mettle is tested by their attitude toward the dissemination of ideas and drugs of which they disapprove.

The argument that people need the protection of the state from dangerous drugs but not from dangerous ideas is unpersuasive. No one has to ingest any drug he does not want, just as no one has to read a book he does not want. Insofar as the state assumes control over such matters, it can only be in order to subjugate its citizens—by protecting them from temptation, as befits children; and by preventing them from assuming self-determination over their lives, as befits an enslaved population.

Controlling Danger

Conventional wisdom now approves—indeed, assumes as obvious—that it is the legitimate business of the state to control certain substances we take into our bodies, especially so-called psychoactive drugs. According to this view, as the state must, for the benefit of society, control dangerous persons, so it must also control dangerous drugs. The obvious fallacy in this analogy is obscured by the riveting together of the notions of dangerous drugs and dangerous acts: as a result, people now "know" that dangerous drugs cause people to behave dangerously and that it is just as much the duty of the state to protect its citizens from dope as it is to protect them from murder and theft. The trouble is that all these supposed facts are false.

It is impossible to come to grips with the problem of drug controls unless we distinguish between things and persons. A drug, whether it be heroin or insulin, is a thing. It does not do anything to anyone unless a person ingests it or injects it into himself or administers it to another. Obviously, a drug has no biological effect on a person unless it gets into his body. The basic question—that is logically prior to whether the drug is good or bad—is, therefore: How does a drug get into the person's body? Although there are many ways for that to happen, we need to consider here only a few typical instances of it.

A person may take an accepted nonprescription drug like aspirin by way of self-medication. Or, he may be given an accepted prescription drug like penicillin by way of medication by his physician. Neither of these situations disturbs most people nowadays. What disturbs the compact majority is a person taking a drug like LSD or selling a drug like heroin to others.

The most cursory attention to how drugs get into the human body thus reveals that the moral and political crux of the problem of drug controls lies not in the pharmacological properties of the chemicals in question, but in the characterological properties of the persons who take them (and of the people who permit, prescribe, and prohibit drugs.)

The true believer in conventional wisdom might wish to insist at this point—not without justification—that some drugs are more dangerous than others; that, in other words, the properties of drugs are no less relevant to understanding our present-day drug problems than are the properties of the persons. That is true. But it is important that we not let that truth divert our attention from the distinction between pharmacological facts and the social policies they supposedly justify.

Prohibition

Today, ordinary, "normal" people do not really want to keep an open mind about drugs and drug controls. Instead of thinking about the problem, they tend to dismiss it with some cliche such as: "Don't tell me that heroin or LSD aren't dangerous drugs?" Ergo, they imply and indeed assert: "Don't tell me that it doesn't make good sense to prohibit their production, sale, and possession!"

What is wrong with this argument? Quite simply, everything. In the first place, the proposition that heroin or LSD is dangerous must be qualified and placed in relation to the dangerousness of other drugs and other artifacts that are not drugs. Second, the social policy that heroin or LSD should be prohibited does not follow, as a matter of logic, from the proposition that they are dangerous, even if they are dangerous.

Admittedly, heroin is more dangerous than aspirin, in the sense that it gives more pleasure to its user than aspirin; heroin is therefore more likely than aspirin to be taken for the self-induction of euphoria. Heroin is also more dangerous than aspirin in the sense that it is easier to kill oneself with it; heroin is therefore more likely to be used for committing suicide.

The fact that people take heroin to make themselves feel happy or high—and use other psychoactive drugs for their mind-altering effects—raises a simple but basic issue that the drug-prohibitionists like to avoid, namely: What is wrong with people using drugs for that purpose? Why shouldn't people make themselves happy by means of self-medication? Let me say at once that I believe these are questions to which honest and reasonable men may offer different answers. Whatever the answers, however, I insist that they flow from moral rather than medical considerations.

For example, some people say that individuals should not take heroin because it diverts them from doing productive work, making those who use the drugs, as well as those economically dependent on them, burdens on society. Others say that whether individuals use, abuse, or avoid heroin is, unless they harm others, their private business. And still others opt for a compromise between the total prohibition of heroin and a free trade in it.

There is, however, more to the prohibitionist's position than his concern that hedonic drugs seduce people from hard labor to happy leisure. If prohibitionists were truly motivated by such concerns, they would advocate permission to use heroin contingent on the individual's proven ability to support himself (and perhaps others), rather than its unqualified suppression. The fact that they advocate no such thing highlights the symbolic aspects of drugs and drug controls.

Drugs, Fun, and Sin

The objects we now call "dangerous drugs" are metaphors for all that we consider sinful and wicked; that is why they are prohibited, rather than because they are demonstrably more harmful than countless other objects in the environment that do not now symbolize sin for us. In this connection, it is instructive to consider the cultural metamorphosis we have undergone during the past half-century, shifting our symbols of sin from sexuality to chemistry.

Our present views on drugs, especially psychoactive drugs, are strikingly similar to our former views on sex, especially masturbation. Intercourse in marriage with the aim of procreation used to be the paradigm of the proper use of one's sexual organs; whereas intercourse outside of marriage with the aim of carnal pleasure used to be the paradigm of their improper use. Until recently, masturbation—or self-abuse, as it was called—was professionally declared, and popularly accepted, as both the cause and the symptom of a variety of illnesses, especially insanity. To be sure, it is now virtually impossible to cite a contemporary medical authority to support this concept of self-abuse. Expert medical opinion now holds that there is simply no such thing: that whether a person masturbates or not is medically irrelevant, and that engaging in the practice or refraining from it is a matter of personal morals or life style.

On the other hand, it is now impossible to cite a contemporary medical authority to oppose the concept of drug abuse. Expert medical opinion now holds that drug abuse is a major medical, psychiatric, and public-health problem: that drug addition is a disease similar to diabetes, requiring prolonged (or life-long) and medically carefully supervised treatment; and that taking or not taking drugs is primarily, if not solely, a matter of medical concern and responsibility.

Like any social policy, our drug laws may be examined from two entirely different points of view: technical and moral. Our present inclination is either to ignore the moral perspective or to mistake the technical for the moral.

A Medical Problem?

An example of our misplaced overreliance on a technical approach to the so-called drug problem is the professionalized mendacity about the dangerousness of certain types of drugs. Since most propagandists against drug abuse seek to justify certain repressive policies by appeals to the alleged dangerousness of various drugs, they often falsify the facts about the true pharmacological properties of the drugs they seek to prohibit. They do so for two reasons: first, because many substances in daily use are just as harmful as the substances they want to prohibit; second, because they realize that dangerousness alone is never a sufficiently persuasive argument to justify the prohibition of any drug, substance, or artifact. Accordingly, the more they ignore the moral dimensions of the problem, the more they must escalate their fraudulent claims about the dangers of drugs.

To be sure, some drugs are more dangerous than others. It *is* easier to kill oneself with heroin than with aspirin. But it is also easier to kill oneself by jumping off a high building than a low one. In the case of drugs, we regard their potentiality for self-injury as a justification for their prohibition; in the case of buildings, we do not. Furthermore, we systematically blur and confuse the two quite different ways in which narcotics can cause death: by a deliberate act of suicide and by accidental overdose.

I maintain that suicide is an act, not a disease. It is therefore a moral, not a medical, problem. The fact that suicide results in death does not make it a medical problem any more than the fact that execution in the electric chair results in death makes the death penalty a medical problem.

Hence, it is morally absurd—and, in a free society, politically illegitimate—to deprive an adult of a drug because he might use it to kill himself. To do so is to treat people as institutional psychiatrists treat so-called psychotics: they not only imprison such persons but take everything away from them— shoelaces, belts, razor blades, eating utensils, and so forth—until the "patients" lie naked on a mattress in a padded cell, lest they kill themselves. The result is one of the most degrading tyrannizations in the annals of human history.

Death by accidental overdose is an altogether different matter. But can anyone doubt that this danger now looms so large precisely because the sale of narcotics and many other drugs is illegal? Persons buying illicit drugs cannot be sure what they are getting or how much of it. Free trade in drugs, with governmental action limited to safeguarding the purity of the product and the veracity of labeling, would reduce the risk of accidental overdose with so-called dangerous drugs to the same levels that prevail, and that we find acceptable, with respect to other chemical agents and physical artifacts that abound in our complex technological society.

In my view, regardless of their dangerousness, all drugs should be "legalized" (a misleading term that I employ reluctantly as a concession to common usage). Although I realize that some drugs—notably, heroin, amphetamine, and LSD among those now in vogue—may have dangerous consequences, I favor free trade in drugs for the same reason the Founding Fathers favored free trade in ideas: in a free society it is none of the govern- ment's business what ideas a man puts into his mind; likewise, it should be none of its business what drug he puts into his body.

"Heresy"

Clearly, the argument that marijuana—or heroin, methadone, or morphine— is prohibited because it is addictive or dangerous cannot be supported by facts. For one thing, there are many drugs, from insulin to penicillin, that are neither addictive nor dangerous but are nevertheless also prohibited: they can be obtained only through a physician's prescription. For another, there are many things, from poisons to guns, that are much more dangerous than narcotics (especially to others) but are not prohibited. As everyone knows, it is still possible in the United States to walk into a store and walk out with a shotgun. We enjoy that right, not because we do not believe that guns are dangerous, but because we believe even more strongly that civil liberties are precious. At the same time, it is not possible in the United States to walk into a store and walk out with a bottle of barbiturates or codeine or, indeed, even with an empty hypodermic syringe. We are now deprived of that right because we have come to value medical paternalism more highly than the right to obtain and use drugs without recourse to medical intermediaries.

I submit, therefore, that our so-called drug-abuse problem is an integral part of our present social ethic that accepts "protections" and repressions justified by appeals to health similar to those which medieval societies accepted when they were justified by appeals to faith. Drug abuse (as we now know it) is one of the inevitable consequences of the medical monopoly over drugs—a monopoly whose value is daily acclaimed by science and law, state and church, the professions and the laity. As formerly the church regulated man's relations to God, so medicine now regulates his relations to his body. Deviation from the rules set forth by the church was then considered heresy and was punished by appropriate theological sanctions, called penance; deviation from the rules set forth by medicine is now considered drug abuse (or some sort of "mental illness") and is punished by appropriate medical sanctions, called treatment.

The problem of drug abuse will thus be with us so long as we live under medical tutelage. That is not to say that, if all access to drugs were free, some people would not medicate themselves in ways that might upset us or harm them. That, of course, is precisely what happened when religious practices became free. People proceeded to engage in all sorts of religious behaviors that true believers in traditional faiths found obnoxious and upsetting. Nevertheless, in the conflict between freedom and religion, the American political system has come down squarely for the former and against the latter.

If the grown son of a devoutly religious Jewish father has a ham sandwich for lunch, the father cannot use the police power of American society to impose his moral views on his son. But if the grown son of a devoutly alcoholic father has heroin for lunch, the father can, indeed, use the police power of American society to impose his moral views on his son. Moreover, the penalty that that father could legally visit on his son might exceed the penalty that would be imposed on the son for killing his mother. It is that moral calculus—refracted through our present differential treatment of those who literally abuse others by killing, maiming, and robbing them as against those who metaphorically abuse themselves by using illicit chemicals—which reveals the depravity into which our preoccupation with drugs and drug controls has led us.

Self-Medication

I believe that just as we regard freedom of speech and religion as fundamental rights, so we should also regard freedom of self-medication as a fundamental right; and that, instead of mendaciously opposing or mindlessly promoting illicit drugs, we should, paraphrasing Voltaire, make this maxim our rule: "I disapprove of what you take, but I will defend to the death your right to take it!"

Sooner or later we shall have to confront the basic moral dilemma underlying the so-called drug problem: Does a person have the right to take a drug, any drug—not because he needs it to cure an illness, but because he wants to take it?

The Constitution and the Bill of Rights are silent on the subject of drugs. That would seem to imply that the adult citizen has, or ought to have, the right to medicate his own body as he sees fit. Were that not the case, why should there have been a need for a constitutional amendment to outlaw drinking? But if ingesting alcohol was, and is now again, a constitutional right, is ingesting opium or heroin or barbiturates or anything else not also such a right?

It is a fact that we Americans have a right to read a book—any book— not because we are stupid and want to learn from it, nor because a government-supported educational authority claims that it will be good for us, but simply because we want to read it; because the government—as our servant rather than our master—hasn't the right to meddle in our private reading affairs.

I believe that we also have a right to eat, drink, or inject a substance— any substance—not because we are sick and want it to cure us, nor because a government-supported medical authority claims that it will be good for us, but simply because we want to take it; because the government—as our servant rather than our master—hasn't the right to meddle in our private dietary and drug affairs.

It is also a fact, however, that Americans now go to jail for picking harmless marijuana growing wild in the fields, but not for picking poisonous mushrooms growing wild in the forests. Why? Because we Americans have collectively chosen to cast away our freedom to determine what we should eat, drink, or smoke. In this large and ever-expanding area of our lives, we have rejected the principle that the state is our servant rather than our master. This proposition is painfully obvious when people plaintively insist that we need the government to protect us from the hazards of "dangerous" drugs. To be sure, we need private voluntary associations—or also, some might argue, the government—to *warn* us of the dangers of heroin, high-tension wires, and high-fat diets.

But it is one thing for our would-be protectors to *inform* us of what they regard as dangerous objects in our environment. It is quite another thing for them to *punish* us if we disagree with them.

Prescription for Control

"The patient has no rights." That phrase sounds like a quotation from one of my jeremiads against the Therapeutic State, but it is not. It is a quotation from a county medical society newsletter. The precise context in which it appears is important.

On April 1, 1978, a new law became effective in New York state, requiring the physician to indicate on his prescription blanks whether or not the pharmacists may substitute a generic drug for the proprietary, or brand name, drug he has prescribed. I have before me a copy of the Onondaga County Medical Society's *President's Newsletter,* which explains this law to physicians and offers a model prescription form for their use. At the bottom of the prescription form are two entries, reading: "Dispense as written" and "Substitution permissible." According to the new law, prescription forms without these two "signature lines" cannot be honored by pharmacists. To make the prescription valid, the physician must sign above one or another of these "orders" to the pharmacist. Unless the physician orders the pharmacist to "Dispense as written," the law requires that the prescription be filled generically. In fact, at the bottom of the blank, the model prescription form carries this legend, stipulated by the new law: "This prescription will be filled generically unless the physician signs on the line stating 'Dispense as written.'" If the physician indicates that a substitution is permissible, then, according to the law, the pharmacist must provide a less expensive drug product than the one prescribed.

The New York state "drug substitution law" is not the first of its kind in the nation. On the contrary, its enactment probably heralds the dawn of a new age and style of drug dispensing in America. Thus, on March 16, 1978, according to an Associated Press report, "The Carter administration proposed overhauling prescription drug laws to encourage the sale of less expensive generic drugs. [This] would make it easier for physicians to prescribe generic drugs regardless of brand names." Remaining silent about whether the proposed legal changes would make life easier or more difficult for the patient, the report emphasized that "many states now require pharmacists to substitute the cheapest generic drug available unless the physician insists on a specific brand name."

Reprinted, with permission, from *Inquiry,* May 1, 1978, pp. 4-5.

So much for the relevant facts. What are the motives behind this law? What will be its actual consequences? Ostensibly, the principal motive behind the law is to allow and encourage the patient to save money. How? By giving him access to the less expensive generic equivalents of proprietary preparations. Such generic equivalents are, as a rule, just as good as the proprietary preparations whose trade names are protected by copyright. Depending on the drug, such substitution can reduce the cost of a prescription by as much as several hundred percent. It must be noted, however, that there is considerable controversy among clinicians and pharmacologists about whether all generic preparations are as effective as their brand-name equivalents. Although generics have the same chemically active ingredients as their equivalent proprietary products, the inert substances used to bind or otherwise prepare the ingredients may differ. Thus, one preparation may dissolve more quickly in water or stomach juices than another. The point is that however slight the demonstrable differences between proprietary and generic preparations might be, such differences do exist. Moreover, name brands inspire confidence in many people, a psychological fact of no trifling importance in the healing arts. I emphasize these seemingly elementary facts and considerations because the New York state "drug substitution law" rides roughshod over them.

The existence of a two-tier system of pharmaceutical preparations—comprising brand name and generic drugs—has been with us for a long time. It betokens, for good or ill, our commitment to competition and a free market (however much "regulated") in pharmaceuticals, as opposed to a single government-run monopoly. For example, every time a person walks into a drugstore to buy aspirin, he must choose between Bayer (or some other brand name) and a less expensive generic aspirin (distributed over the labels of various drug chains). People now have such a choice in a wide variety of over-the-counter products.

With prescription drugs, the situation is different. As a rule, such drugs are dispensed either as ordered by the physician or as determined by the pharmacist. For example, if a physician writes a prescription for "Achromycin" (Lederle brand tetracycline, a broad-spectrum antibiotic), then that is what the pharmacist must give the patient unless he obtains the physician's permission to substitute another manufacturer's product. On the other hand, if the physician writes a prescription for "tetracycline," then the pharmacist can choose—depending on which brand he has in stock and on the cost to him of the various products—whether to dispense a proprietary or generic tetracycline. Until now, the customer—assuming that he was knowledgable and wanted to exercise a choice—could choose to buy tetracycline carrying the Bristol or Lederle or Parke-Davis label rather than the Rexall label.

The ostensible purpose of the New York law is to save the patient money by making generic drugs freely available to him. However, if that were the law's true purpose, it would give the choice between brand name and generic drug *to the patient;* actually, the law deprives the patient of just that choice. (And whether it will save him money at all remains to be seen.)

Anticipating questions about the interpretation of the new "drug substitution law," the *Newsletter* includes a two-page legal interpretation of it, cast in a question and answer format. Significantly, only two of the 11 questions and answers deal with the law's effects on patients. They deserve to be quoted in full:

> Q: What does a pharmacist do when the patient insists upon a brand name when the physician writes "substitution permissible"?
> A: The patient has no rights.
> Q: If a patient prefers to pay for a brand name, does he have this option?
> A: No. The patient has no rights.

This is a wonderfully revealing example of the language of medical totalitarianism, in both its covert and overt forms. The phrase "substitution permissible" evidently means "substitution required." The phrase, "The patient has no rights" means just what it says.

Assuming that the interpretation given in the *Newsletter* is correct, patients in New York state will be deprived of a certain choice they previously possessed. (That few persons exercised their right to choose does not alter the significance of its abolition. If the freedom to exercise that right was an insignificant issue, why should the new law deliberately abolish it?) In the final analysis, our politicians—and the people who elect them—must decide whether to permit or prohibit competition within the drug industry: in the former case, pharmaceutical manufacturers must be allowed to appeal to the brand names of drugs and the good names of their companies; in the latter case, the manufacture and sale of drugs must be turned into a government monopoly, with pharmacies becoming chemical post offices.

Furthermore, if politicians believe that there is something inherently evil in brand names, why do they pick on brand-name drugs? In free societies, people buy countless supposedly identical products on the basis of brand names. That is how we buy appliances and automobiles, furniture, and frozen foods. Such freedom in the marketplace is considered to be an integral part of what we mean by individual liberty. Hence, it is important—both practically and symbolically—what happens when, allegedly to protect the citizen's pocketbook, the state legislates a choice between brand name and generic prescription drugs. The question is, is the result more or less freedom for the individual?

Nearly a half a century ago, Ortega y Gasset correctly diagnosed our malady as precisely that statism which we now embrace as therapy. "Society, that it may live better," he wrote in *The Revolt of the Masses,* "creates the State as an instrument. Then the State gets the upper hand and society has to begin to live for the State. . . . This is what State intervention leads to: the

people are converted into fuel to feed the mere machine which is the State."
When, as now, the state is therapeutic, it is only to be expected that the
physician should be simultaneously executioner and victim: he supports and
implements the disfranchisement of the patient, in the name of health and
treatment, while he himself is disfranchised, in the name of economy and
equality.

Is there a way to stop these self-mutilations of our liberties that we seem
so glad to suffer in exchange for the promise of perfect therapeutic paternalism and egalitarianism? There is indeed. In fact, the area of prescription
drugs is one which today offers perhaps the best case for the abolition of
government controls and the restoration of the free market.

Prescription drugs could—and should—be available in the same way as
over-the-counter drugs are available. As a result, the physician's prescription
would be restored to its rightful role: a recommendation to the patient about
what drug he should take and how he should take it, rather than permission
to purchase an otherwise legally prohibited and medically mystified product.
In such a free pharmaceutical market, the patient would have the combined
benefits of medical advice, of an economically competitive pharmaceutical
industry, and of his own legally unfettered choice in the selection of the drugs
he buys and takes.

New Addictions for Old

Everyone must surely know by now that Joseph Califano, secretary of Health, Education, and Welfare, formerly a confirmed cigarette addict, has become an anti-cigarette addict. (For the sake of brevity I am using the terms "addict" and "addiction" in their conventional senses. The reader who is interested in my linguistic and moral objections to these terms may consult my book *Ceremonial Chemistry.*) Although smoking and anti-smoking are now much in the news, two aspects of this business seem to have been somewhat neglected—namely, the dependence of both the supporters and the opponents of smoking on government subsidies, and the lesson implicit in the history of the promotion and prohibition of smoking. Herewith are some observations about each.

At present the government is looting the citizenry (smokers and non-smokers alike) to the tune of $65 million annually in agricultural subsidies for the tobacco industry. While such price supports do not subsidize smokers by making cigarettes less expensive (indeed, they have the opposite effect), they do support the smoking habit indirectly. By guaranteeing a price floor for tobacco, the government symbolizes its approval—something more important than a direct subsidy—of the cultivation of that crop and its determination to guarantee the continuing prosperity of that segment of agriculture.

Now that Secretary Califano is an avid anti-smoker, his habit is subsidized by the taxpayer directly. Moreover, Califano's new addiction is far more dangerous to society at large than was his old one—for no one is as fanatical as an ex-addict high on abstinence. While a tax on cigarettes loots only the smokers, a tax for a campaign against cigarettes loots everyone. Intoxicated with the righteousness of his cause, Califano has already announced the creation of an Office of Smoking and Health with an appropriation of $23 million for the 1979 campaign against smoking. No doubt, he will try to funnel ever-larger chunks of tax monies into supporting his new habit.

Secretary Califano emphasizes that he considers the tobacco subsidy "political" and has no intention of interfering with it. Neither does the current president of the American Cancer Society, Dr. R. Wayne Rundles. When Dr. Rundles, professor of medicine at Duke University (in the heart of tobacco

Reprinted, with permission, from *Inquiry,* May 29, 1978, pp. 4-5.

country) was elected last November, he declared that the Society "will continue to stress education and research rather than try to end federal price supports for tobacco." Even the National Cancer Institute is subtly pro-smoking: it spent $25 million of the taxpayers' money on a program to develop a "safer cigarette." Although such a program would appear to be the responsibility of private individuals or voluntary groups, or of the tobacco industry, that is not the view of Dr. Gio Gori, the head of NCI's "safe cigarette program." Explained Gori: "Our efforts to develop cigarettes with less tar and nicotine may help the tobacco industry, but it will benefit the country's 55 million smokers more."

With that project, the American government has assumed the burden of mitigating the bad effects of a specific bad habit. But why stop with the effort to develop a safer cigarette? Why not also develop safer booze—a drug that simulates the psychophysiological effect of alcohol but does not cause cirrhosis of the liver? Clearly, the technological—and political—possibilities of making the unsafe habits of some people safe at the expense of everyone else are virtually limitless.

The campaign against smoking has created the widespread impression that physicians are solidly against the habit. That is not so. Mental health professionals not only continue to smoke in large numbers, they also continue to support smoking as "therapeutic." Dr. Norman Tabachnick, a psychiatrist at the University of California School of Medicine in Los Angeles, asserts that smoking relieves anxiety and helps the patient maintain an identity. Dr. Walter Menninger, of the famed Menninger Clinic, states that smoking relieves tension. Dr. Peter Bourne, the President's personal psychiatric expert on drugs, emphasizes that there are known and unknown beneficial effects from smoking. In this connection, it is important to recall that the surgeon general's celebrated 1964 report acknowledges that "the significant beneficial effects of smoking occur primarily in the area of mental health." Perhaps in order to be consistent with their beliefs, mental health workers smoke significantly more than do other professionals. For example, a study reported at the 1976 meeting of the American Cancer Society revealed that among high school personnel, "guidance counselors smoke the most."

The promotion-use and the prohibition-avoidance of various mind-altering substances (described in detail in *Ceremonial Chemistry)* constitute an integral—albeit a remarkably neglected—part of cultural and political history. I list below, without comment, some of the highlights of the history, especially recent American history, of the campaign for and against smoking:

1493. The use of tobacco is introduced into Europe by Columbus and his crew returning from America. By the middle of the seventeenth century, efforts to stamp out the habit—in Europe and the Ottoman Empire—are ferocious but fruitless. Sultan Murad IV decrees the death penalty for smoking. According to a contemporary observer, "Wherever the Sultan went on his travels or on a military expedition, his halting places were always distinguished by a terrible increase in the number of executions . . . Nevertheless the passion for smoking still persisted."

1912. Many (alcohol) prohibitionists extend their campaign to cigarettes. A writer in *Century* magazine declares: "Morphine is the legitimate consequence of alcohol, and alcohol is the legitimate consequence of tobacco. Cigarettes, drink, opium, is the logical and regular series." A physician warns: "There is no energy more destructive of soul, mind, and body, or more subversive of good morals, than the cigarette. The fight against the cigarette is a fight for civilization."

1921. The sale of cigarettes is illegal in 14 states; 92 anti-cigarette bills are pending in 28 states. Wherever cigarettes are illegal, the sale of bootleg cigarettes flourishes.

1963. Tobacco sales in the United States total $8.08 billion, of which $3.3 billion go to federal, state, and local governments. A news release from the tobacco industry proudly states: "Tobacco products pass across sales counters more frequently than anything else—except money."

1964. The surgeon general's famous warning about tobacco smoking is issued. The American Medical Association accepts $10 million from a group of tobacco companies; coincidentally, the AMA opposes the Federal Trade Commission's order requiring that cigarettes be labeled as a health hazard.

1966. The Agriculture Department spends $210,000 to subsidize cigarette commercials in Japan, Thailand, and Austria, and pays $106,000 to Warner Brothers to insert scenes designed to stimulate cigarette smoking in a travelogue that will be distributed in eight countries.

1976. The Agriculture Department reports that Americans smoked 620 billion cigarettes, almost 13 billion more than in 1975, and 84 billion more than in 1970. America's cigarette production for the year was 700 billion, of which 62 billion were for export, and 10 billion (tax-exempt) went to American servicemen stationed overseas. Exports grew by more than 20 percent, from 50.2 billion in 1975 to 62 billion in 1976.

1977. Former Surgeons General Dr. Luther Terry and Dr. Jesse Steinfeld, together with a group of prominent anti-smokers, petition the FDA, requesting: "That the agency recognize its authority over cigarettes as a drug . . . under the broad definition in the Food and Drug Act. . . . and that the agency restrict the sale of cigarettes to pharmacies." The FDA replies that "nicotine is not a drug because the sellers of tobacco have never claimed it is a drug."

1978. According to a survey published in the *New England Journal of Medicine,* the cost of smoking and alcohol abuse in the United States is $60 billion a year, or about 25 percent of the total cost of all illnesses. In 1976, direct health-care costs attributable to smoking amounted to $8.2 billion.

1978. According to a study published by the Worldwatch Institute of Washington, D.C., "Consumers the world over spend . . . $85 billion to $100 billion each year on tobacco." The Institute's report identifies the "Peking [mainland Chinese] government monopoly" as the world's largest cigarette manufacturer, and notes that "in the United States, cigarette smoking now causes 320,000 premature deaths a year and $20 billion in such hidden social costs as medical expenses, lost working time, and fire damage."

All societies make use of various substances for ceremonial as well as medicinal purposes. In primitive societies, these two aims and functions are indistinguishable. The witch doctor's mask, dance, and herbal medicine combine and conflate the ostensibly empirical and overtly religious dimensions of healing. In modern societies, these two aims and functions are distinguishable, but the distinction is usually repressed: in the physician's prescription of tranquilizers, the ceremonial aspect of healing is repressed; in the politician's promotion of tobacco, the medicinal aspect is repressed. This situation is at once consequence and cause. It is the consequence of modern man's having lost touch with the significance of community and communion—that is, with the ceremonial and religious aspects of life; in turn, it is the cause of his attributing absurd powers of good or evil to his officially nonmedicinal drugs (and even to the paraphernalia associated with their use, like lighters, pipes, syringes, and so forth).

People in Western societies, and especially the American people, are playing a dangerous game. They preach political freedom and personal responsibility, but they practice medical despotism and medicinal irresponsibility. If anything is a drug, then nicotine—the mendacity of the FDA and the entire American government notwithstanding—is a drug. Whether it is considered therapeutic or toxic depends on who uses it, on how it is used, and on who has the power to define what constitutes a desirable or undesirable drug.

Should the FDA Ban Water?

People have always been prey to popular fallacies and our age is no exception. One such fallacy, long popular in America, is that doctors, being faced with a host of crippling and fatal diseases, try to find cures for them. Some still do. But the work is hard and its outcome uncertain. Worse, physicians who discover the "wrong" cure or prevention—for example, as Ignaz Semmelweis did for puerperal fever—may be scorned and punished, rather than praised and rewarded. This is why many American physicians are now idolized, not for having discovered cures, but for having invented diseases.

The main reason why treating (or alleviating) disease has been downgraded in our society is that the only people who really care about cures are the patients. But patients no longer pay the doctor, they don't license him, and they don't give him grants or put his picture in *Time* magazine. Hence, they don't count for much. The way to get ahead in medicine today—on both sides of the Iron Curtain—is to please the state.

However, since the state doesn't suffer the pains and terrors of illness, it doesn't care about cures. What it does care about is diseases. The more diseases the state has at its disposal, the more it can display its phony solicitude toward the citizen-patient. This tragic fact is one of the pillars on which the therapeutic state rests. It also explains why the modern "scientific" physician has rediscovered the classic stock-in-trade of the medical "quack"—namely, "discovering" (inventing) new diseases. "My function," explains Jules Romain's immortal Dr. Knock, "is to direct [people] into a life of medical care. . . . Nothing gets on my nerves like that indeterminate nonentity called the healthy man." That ambition, harnessed to the service of the modern state, has yielded, and continues to yield, a harvest of diseases never before seen on the face of this earth. I offer the following observations as a brief review of some of these recent medical triumphs.

With betting parlors and casinos spreading across the nation, the American Medical Association is sounding the alert for a new disease—gambling. In the January 5, 1979, issue of *American Medical News,* the association devoted a feature article to this subject. Quoting a psychiatric expert on the disease, the AMA explains to doctors—who, in their ignorance,

First published as "Should the FDA Ban H$_2$O?" in *Inquiry,* April 2, 1979, pp. 5-6. Reprinted with permission.

might not have known this—that "self-destruction, not winning, is the goal of compulsive gamblers." The "compulsive gambler"—not otherwise defined, but no doubt diagnosable from his disposition to lose rather than win—"shares a common goal with those who exhibit other forms of destructive behavior, such as alcoholics and drug abusers."

The fakery involved in this method of discovering diseases requires and results in two additional pieces of fakery. The first consists of labeling certain ordinary human interactions—for example, individual or group discussions—"treatments." The second consists of using the existence (or effectiveness) of the "treatment" as evidence that the conduct it is intended to alter is an illness.

True to form, in Brecksville, Ohio, the Veterans Administration Hospital has established a "treatment program" for gamblers. "We've had to bootleg the gambling program in with alcoholism-treatment," explains Dr. Alida Glen, the chief of the hospital's alcoholism-treatment program. Why was such subterfuge necessary? Because, says Glen, "Our chief psychiatrist and several others don't believe compulsive gambling is a treatable disorder. We think we can prove that." For the medical profession, therefore, the question has now become, not whether gambling is a disease, but whether it is treatable.

Before science discovered the mind, prescientific people actually believed that individuals played roulette or the stock market for the excitement or the prospect of gain, rather than because mental diseases made them do so. People used to entertain such primitive notions even about sex, believing that individuals decided to engage in, or refrain from, certain sexual acts because of their individual desires, tastes, or values. Modern medical sexology has dispelled that notion too. Although William Masters and Virginia Johnson are generally considered to be the discoverers of new sexual treatments, they have discovered some new sexual diseases as well—among which the most important seems to be "masturbatory orgasmic inadequacy." It is a malady that afflicts only women. According to Masters and Johnson, "A woman with masturbatory orgasmic inadequacy has not achieved orgasmic release by partner or self-stimulation in either homosexual or heterosexual experience. She can and does reach orgasmic experience during coital connection." In plain English, what Masters and Johnson are saying is that women who have satisfying sexual experiences in heterosexual intercourse but neither masturbate nor engage in masturbatory acts with men or women are, because they abstain from the latter acts, sick. They claim to have "treated" eleven women suffering from this disease, and to have cured all but one.

Clearly, disease is one of the most promising growth industries in America. State-licensed quacks never had it so good. Just imagine what lies over the horizon: thousands of orthodox Jews, able to relish kosher food, suffering from "alimentary inadequacy" with respect to roast pork and lobster

Newburg; millions of Americans, with unimpaired powers to enjoy whiskey and vodka, suffering from "psychopharmacological inadequacy" with respect to opium and marijuana. The possibilities are mind-boggling, which, no doubt, is why psychiatrists are the main bogglers in advancing these scientific frontiers.

Although psychiatric cures are notoriously ineffective (perhaps because it is so very difficult to treat diseases that do not exist), psychiatrists excel in discovering new (mental) diseases. One of the most notable recent discoveries of this type, authenticated by the American Psychiatric Association, is the disease called "Tobacco Use Disorder." Tobacco Use Disorder differs from smoking in roughly the same way as an agricultural implement for soil penetration differs from a spade. Actually, the official description of the "diagnosis" is even more labored and ludicrous: "In this manual [that is, in the proposed new diagnostic manual of the APA] the use of tobacco is considered a disorder either when the use of the substance is directly associated with distress at the need to use the substance repeatedly; or there is evidence of a serious tobacco-related physical disorder in an individual who is judged to be currently physiologically dependent upon tobacco." Some of the most distinguished American psychiatrists actually wrote that. These psychiatrists predict that "social acceptability for tobacco use will decrease [and] restrictions on public use will become more widespread"; "therefore," they conclude gleefully, "the prevalence of Tobacco Use Disorder will increase."

While still on the subject of tobacco—and perhaps remembering the cigars and cigarettes which until recently they smoked so avidly—the soul-doctors extended their discovery to a closely related but nevertheless distinctly different disease, namely, "Tobacco Withdrawal." That is the disease people get when they try to quit smoking: "The diagnosis is usually self-evident and the disappearance of symptoms upon resumption of smoking is confirmatory." Sounds like the Mark Twain syndrome to me.

Contrary to popular impression, psychiatrists have in fact fallen on hard times—financially as well as in terms of academic prestige. Now they seem to be getting desperate and in desperation, like gamblers, they have raised their stakes and risk losing everything. But instead of blowing the whistle, some former victims rush to the support of their former victimizers.

Psychiatrists have long been in the habit of calling certain types of prejudice "mental diseases." Thus, for example, did racism in post-World War II America become a disease. And now the leaders of the National Gay Task Force have embraced the psychiatric rhetoric. For them it is not enough to call the traditional Judeo-Christian abhorrence of homosexuality—reinforced by two centuries of psychiatric persecution—what it is: prejudice or bigotry. Instead they defame anti-homosexual bigots as mentally sick. In a letter to the *New York Times* (Nov. 22, 1978) the co-executive directors of the organization declare: "Mental health professionals have identified the condition known as homophobia, which is defined as irrational fear and hatred of homosexuals and homosexuality. We suggest that this 'flawed personality trait' is a genuine ground for exclusion from police work." With a little more imagination, these leaders could have discovered that their adversaries displayed the "manfestations" of a full-fledged eponymous medical disorder: the "Anita Bryant syndrome."

Farfetched? In the October 7, 1978, issue of *Lancet,* one of the most prestigious medical journals in the English language, a physician reports his discovery of a new disease, which he calls the "Oblomov syndrome." This "condition," he says, is characterized by "wakeful and sociable apathy or laziness not associated with any other evident mental or physical disturbance or subnormality." He cites the "case" of a woman ordered to bed by a doctor in the 1930s, when she had the flu, who stayed in bed for forty years.

However, as Ivan Goncharov knew so well, laziness has its advantages. Among other things, it protects the "Oblomov patient" from the disease due to excessive enthusiasm for drinking water. Since this behavior can cause death, doctors are convinced that it is a disease. They call it "psychogenic polydipsia." Two cases of it are reported in the December 1, 1978, issue of the *Journal of the American Medical Association.* These tragic deaths dramatize the persistently irresponsible attitude of the medical profession and the government toward what must surely be one of the commonest hazardous substances in our environment—namely, hydrogen monoxide. How many more innocent Americans must lose their lives to psychogenic polydipsia before the medical profession recognizes its duty to dispense water by prescription only? In view of the incontrovertible evidence that the ingestion of hydrogen monoxide can be fatal, why has the Food and Drug Administration failed to place this dangerous chemical on its list of "controlled substances"? And why is the American government wasting the taxpayers' money trying to develop a safe cigarette instead of launching a crash program to develop a type of nonlethal water?

The afflictions I have discussed are only a few of the conditions that physicians have recently discovered to be diseases, and that medical organizations and government agencies have recently recognized as such. There are many others to which I may devote later columns if interest merits it—such as "workaholism" (working too much and liking it), the "emancipation disorder" ("internal conflict over increased independence from parental control," afflicting teenagers), and the "Huckleberry Finn syndrome" (persistent truancy).

In the old days—the days of John Hunter and William C. Gorgas and the great microbiologists—doctors made medical discoveries by giving themselves dangerous diseases. Now, that would be considered a sick way of pursuing health. Today, under carefully controlled conditions of intellectual sterility, the physician invents diseases—and gives them to others (who are often more useful to the state sick than healthy). The result is the medicalization of everyday life, which stupefies the people, glorifies the doctors, and bedazzles the media.

Peter Bourne's
Quaalude Caper

On July 19, 1978, Dr. Peter G. Bourne, special assistant to the president and director of the White House Office of Drug Abuse Policy, was publicly incriminated as a "drug abuser" and exposed as a "drug pusher." The allegation that the nation's highest-ranking drug-prohibition agent not only uses illegal drugs but also dispenses "controlled" drugs to the White House staff sent shock waves of surprised indignation across the columns of America's political commentators. As I shall show, however, Bourne's dual role—as simultaneously both supporter and opponent of drug controls—is consistent with his previous activities and the means by which he rose to prominence and power.

Bourne has long been a Carter family friend. By all accounts, he was very influential in persuading Carter to seek the presidency. As a physician, however, Bourne has no medical or pharmacological achievement to his credit; he is not even a board-certified psychiatrist. Making Bourne America's chief drug-prohibition agent was Carter's repayment of a personal obligation and political debt. But Carter went much further: by presidential declaration, Bourne was elevated to the rank of "the world's foremost expert on drugs." To appreciate the absurdity of this claim, imagine a newly elected American president declaring his doctor-friend, bereft of any demonstrable achievement in cancer research or heart disease, the world's greatest oncologist or cardiologist. Physicians would laugh at such arrogance. No one, however, challenged Carter's claim that Bourne knew more about "drugs" than pharmacology professors or research chemists. In my opinion, that relatively harmless mendacity about Bourne was an integral part of countless not so very harmless mendacities that permeate the drug-prohibition industry.

Indeed, Carter's praise of Bourne was coupled with a statement that should have warned anyone alert to English usage about the grave danger inherent in Carter's vision of the American drug problem. I refer to Carter's linking Bourne's alleged *knowledge* about drugs with his supposed expertise in *controlling* them. Bourne, declared the President, is "the world's foremost expert on drugs—their origin, their processing, their sale, their use, their

---

Reprinted, with permission, from *Inquiry,* October 30, 1978, pp. 4-7.

effect on the human body, how they might be controlled." A most odious non sequitur. Surely, a person need not be an authority on African history to excel as a slave trader or slaveholder. Nor need a person be an authority on Jewish theology to excel in persecuting and killing Jews. Nor, to use a less dramatic example, need a person be an authority on ballistics to excel in advocating or enforcing gun controls. After all, the term "drug control" is merely a modern American euphemism for prohibiting certain drugs and persecuting those who sell and use them. As everyone knows, the American government now permits and promotes the use of certain drugs, while it prohibits and persecutes the use of others. Whether a particular drug falls into one class or another is only marginally related to its pharmacological properties.

The adage "the higher they rise, the harder they fall" seems to apply to Bourne. Carter raised him up, and Bourne allowed himself to be raised up, as America's supernarc. When Bourne let his ambivalence about this job get the better of him, his downfall was inevitable.

Whether President and Mrs. Carter will also suffer from the Quaalude caper depends partly on their complicity (if any) in the drug-law violations committed by Bourne and other members of the White House staff, and partly on whether the press and other influential critics of the administration call for an investigation and prosecution of these law violations as vigorously as the critics of the Nixon administration rightly pushed for an investigation and prosecution of Watergate.

When Bourne resigned from his lofty position, he was politically the most powerful physician in the nation. How did a 38-year-old psychiatrist achieve such prominence? Who, exactly, is Peter Bourne?

Bourne received his M.D. degree from Emory University in Atlanta in 1962. Before his psychiatric residency at Stanford, he was drafted and received a remarkably high-level assignment in Vietnam. Ostensibly, Bourne's task was to study and evaluate the morale and stress reactions of Green Berets in combat. However, according to a report in the magazine *State and Mind* (July-September 1976), "the reality was that this work required a high security clearance and active involvement with military intelligence. . . . Bourne was given this assignment even though he'd only graduated from Emory University Medical School in 1962, three years earlier, and had virtually no qualification to do this work. He had a carte blanche air-pass for travel anywhere in the country. He received a Bronze Star, Air Medal, and Combat Medics badge after being sent overseas for one year."

Clearly, Bourne showed an early talent for influencing men in power, for living well—and for working both sides of the street. While still a captain in the army, Bourne testified on behalf of Dr. Howard Levy in his trial for refusing orders to train Green Berets. Thus, Bourne was working with the Green Berets one day, was testifying against them the next, and was, at the same time, able to convince both sides that he was their agent. "Bourne identified himself as a friend and political sympathizer of Levy and other war resisters [according to *State and Mind*]. At large anti-war gatherings at Stanford University, Bourne spoke about the Levy case and took a clearly anti-war position. . . . He gave a taped interview to Gisele Halimi as evidence in the War Crimes Tribunal, held in Stockholm, Sweden." These and other similar activities of Bourne's "created the impression that Bourne changed from being a Bronze Star-winning Green Beret advisor to a top-level anti-war advisor in a few months time." Perhaps as long as he was "top-level," Bourne didn't really care which side he was on. This assumption is supported by the fact that before his downfall, Bourne enthusiastically endorsed the paraquat war against marijuana and at the same time hobnobbed with the leaders of the marijuana-legalization lobby.

Bourne's meteoric rise to the role of the world's foremost expert on drugs began in earnest in 1971 with his appointment by then-Governor Jimmy Carter, as director of the Georgia Drug Abuse Services. At Carter's insistence, he was chosen by the Food and Drug Administration to be the only man in Georgia with a license to dispense methadone. Soon, Carter pointed with pride to his—and Bourne's—methadone-maintenance program as the "best in the country." What was so good about it? Supposedly that all persons on methadone maintenance had to come to Atlanta regardless of where they lived in the state, to be registered on computerized tapes. (Nevertheless, Bourne justified the felonious prescription-writing that brought him down by appealing to his passionate commitment to protecting his "patient's" privacy.)

Having solved the drug problem in Georgia, Bourne was ready to solve it for the rest of America. In September 1972, barely a year after assuming his Georgia drug job, Bourne moved to Washington as assistant director of President Nixon's Special Action Office for Drug Abuse Prevention. The next phase of his career is described in an article in *Science* (August 1977) this way: "In March, 1974, Bourne, who never stays terribly long doing the same thing in the same place, left that office to romp around the world as a high-priced health and drug-abuse consultant as president of the one-man Foundation for International Resources. He also served as a consultant to his friend, Atlanta lawyer and physician Tom Bryant" (who subsequently served as chairman of President Carter's Commission on Mental Health).

"All this travelling," we are assured by *Science,* "does not mean Bourne has forgotten about drugs. Actually, his global focus is extended to efforts to bring worldwide trafficking in illegal substances under control." To say that Bourne had not forgotten about drugs was clearly an understatement. Drugs were, indeed, never far from Bourne's mind—or the minds of those on whose shoulders he rose to power. "Those of us from Georgia," remarked Bourne smugly not long before his exposure, "have a kind of longevity [in the White House] that is secure." Bourne's sense of security may have been supported not only by Carter's political debt to him, but also by his secret role as the

Georgians' drug dispenser. "He endured in the affection of the Carters," explained a story in *Newsweek*, "and an ad hoc role as family doctor to the Georgians dating to statehouse days in Atlanta—a source of routine medication . . . and, in those days, as one old hand remembered, 'something to make you sleep or help keep you awake' in high-stress political situations."

In short, in our day of pharmacological prohibition, Bourne was at once the White House's chief drug-prohibition agent and its most trusted bootlegger. Moreover, Bourne was not only supplying "controlled" drugs to his friends, he was also scheming to deprive Americans of one of the most useful sedatives and anticonvulsants. "Barbiturates," explained Bourne to the reporter for *Science*, "are contributing to more deaths than any other drug except heroin. Ergo, maybe we ought to consider taking them off the market."* Some logic. Barbiturates contribute to death. Ergo, prohibit them. But barbiturates contribute only to the deaths of those persons who decide to take them, and pose no more danger to those who wish to live than do countless other drugs. Automobiles contribute to many more deaths than barbiturates—including the deaths of innocent bystanders. So why not ban automobiles? Despite the patently political nature of Bourne's position on barbiturates, his prohibitionism was labeled by Mathea Falco, the State Department's senior adviser on narcotics matters, as "very courageous." It is really not surprising that Bourne came to believe that he could get away with anything.

On July 20, the day after the *Washington Post* exposed his illegal prescription, Bourne was forced to resign. The acts and events that led to his resignation were, at least as we now know them, briefly the following.

On July 11, 1978, a young woman named Toby Long took a prescription to a shopping-mall drugstore in Prince William County, Virginia, 35 miles south of Washington. The prescription, made out to the name of Sarah Brown for 15 Quaaludes (a brand of sedative with the worst reputation for "abuse" among all the legally available drugs on the American market), was signed by Peter G. Bourne, M.D. A state pharmacy inspector who happened to be in the drugstore at the time noted that the prescription failed to include directions for the potency of the capsules. She called Bourne's number as it appeared on the form and got a recorded message that the number had been disconnected. The inspector located Bourne's new number and got no answer. She thereupon called the county narcotics squad, who arrested Long and charged her with passing a fictitious prescription, a felony

---

*Bourne, as I shall describe later, has been an enthusiastic supporter of the government's program of spraying Mexican marijuana with the toxic chemical paraquat. Ironically, just as the story of Bourne's shenanigans was unfolding, a medical magazine reported that in Ireland paraquat has emerged as the leading poison used by persons committing suicide (*Medical World News*, July 19, 1978). The parallels between the American government's poisoning ethyl alcohol with methyl alcohol during Prohibition and poisoning marijuana with paraquat now are too obvious to require further comment here.

carrying a sentence of one to five years. So much for the uncontested facts. All else is claim and conjecture.

The *Washington Post* learned of the story soon after Long's arrest but did not print it until a week later. Bourne and the White House remained silent until the *Post* broke the story on July 19.

According to the federal code, as well as Virginia law, a prescription for a controlled substance must contain the name and address of the patient, as well as the name, address, and narcotics registration number of the physician. Writing a prescription to a fictitious person is a felony. Despite these facts, Bourne's first official statement was to assert his complete innocence: "I have consulted legal counsel and believe that what I have done was neither legally nor morally wrong." He claimed that he wrote the prescription that Toby Long had tried to pick up for his aide, Ellen Metsky. Metsky had, according to Bourne, sought his help for insomnia after her boyfriend left her. Bourne contended that he used a "pseudonym" to protect her privacy and that he prescribed Quaaludes partly because he considered this drug to be medically indicated and partly because, in view of his widely publicized opposition to barbiturates, he wanted to avoid prescribing a drug belonging to that chemical family. He told a reporter that he recalls thinking: "Good Lord, I can't write a prescription for barbiturates and have that out there, floating around." Bourne justified writing a prescription for a nonexistent person this way: "It's no secret that hard-liners in the Drug Enforcement Administration are highly displeased with my approach to the subject. They could easily get into the controlled-substances files and find out who on my staff or on the White House staff has been taking such drugs—and they could use it. Ellen knew that and didn't want to create any record of a possible link between us."

To believe this story one would have to be high indeed—on misplaced trust in mendacious psychiatrists. Consider, once more, some of Bourne's claims and certain questions about them:

—Bourne claims, and Metsky acknowledges, that the fake prescription was for Metsky. But Metsky did not pick up the prescription—allegedly because she was too busy—delegating the job of committing the felonious act to Long. What, precisely, was the relationship between Bourne and Metsky, and Metsky and Long? Was Long merely a fall girl? Bourne's claim, moreover, that he wanted to avoid barbiturates and therefore prescribed methaqualone is, to put it charitably, a self-deception. As he must have known, he could have prescribed chloral hydrate, or Dalmane, or Valium (or several other drugs) without attracting suspicion.

—Bourne claims that he wrote a fake name on the prescription solely out of concern for his "patient." Specifically, he contends that he wanted to protect Metsky's confidentiality "with regard to her taking medication and to the creation of a record anywhere that she has been seen by a psychiatrist." That claim is unpersuasive. According to Bourne's own account, Metsky wanted two things: to confide her troubles to someone she could trust and to obtain some sleeping pills. Bourne could have listened and talked to her, and no one would have been the wiser. And he could have referred her to a family physician, internist, or gynecologist (assuming that Metsky did not have an established patient-doctor relationship with such a physician), who could have prescribed a sleeping pill for her. There was simply no medical need—as against personal need—for Bourne to dispense a drug, especially one as notorious as Quaalude.

In a statement issued on July 19, Bourne asserted that he took "legitimate precautions" to protect the confidentiality of his patient and that "one way" of doing so was by the use of what he called a "pseudonym." In support of his conduct, he cited a part of Section 9 of the American Medical Association's Principles of Medical Ethics which states that "a physician may not reveal confidences entrusted to him in the course of medical attendance . . ." With the same arrogance that characterized his prescribing methaqualone to a nonexistent patient, Bourne simply omitted the second half of that statement which qualifies the first half as follows: ". . . unless he [the physician] is required to do so by law." Bourne's attempt to hide behind the skirt of medical confidentiality has the stench of hypocrisy squared. More than any other prominent physician in America, Bourne was, in the words of a *Medical World News* article (August 7, 1978), "the driving force behind the President's most definitive campaign speech on National Health Insurance . . ." The same publication characterizes him as the administration's "most committed advocate of a cradle-to-grave national health insurance plan." What would be the status of medical confidentiality for persons seeking psychiatric help or sleeping pills under such a collectivized, computerized system of medical care? It is safe to predict that were such a plan to come into being, our present situation with respect to patient confidentiality would seem utopian.

In leaving the White House, Bourne proved, once and for all, the depth of his devotion to the cause of confidentiality: He gratuitously incriminated his "patients" and colleagues, asserting that there was a "high incidence of marijuana use" and "occasional use of cocaine" by members of the White House staff. On July 22, seven junior members of the White House staff admitted to a *New York Times* reporter that "they smoked marijuana regularly . . . and were directly and indirectly aware of the use of cocaine by some of their colleagues."

Predictably, neither Bourne nor anyone else connected with alleged drug abuse in the White House has so far been prosecuted. On August 22, Paul Ebert, the prosecutor in Prince William County, announced he was dropping the Bourne case because "I don't think Virginia law applies to a drug violation outside the state." In Washington, a spokesman for the U.S. attorney's office said: "We originally deferred to Virginia authorities to decide whether to prosecute or not in this case. They've made their decision and, as far as this office is concerned, that's the end of the matter." And of the successful sealing of the Quaalude cover-up?

When Jimmy Carter became president, he and Rosalynn Carter self-righteously announced that no hard liquor would be served in the White House. Bourne's Quaaludes, and God knows what else "prescribed" in the White House, make that practice a gesture at once comic and contemptible.

More About Peter
Bourne's Quaalude Caper

As we have seen, Dr. Peter Bourne, Carter's deposed chief drug-prohibition agent, is a man of many faces: adviser to the Green Berets and antiwar activist; supporter of national health insurance and defender of traditional medical confidentiality; drug abuseologist and drug abuser [*Inquiry,* Oct. 30, 1978]. Such behavior can be called by many names: dishonesty, hypocrisy, opportunism, two-facedness, working both sides of the street. Whatever it might be called, this aspect of Bourne's personality—dramatized by his conduct with respect to marijuana—helps to dispel much of the mystery surrounding the events that precipitated his downfall.

Bourne rose to prominence as a personal friend of, and political adviser to, Jimmy Carter, and as a drug-prohibition agent—that is, as a psychiatrist condemning illegal drugs and their users. In this latter role, Bourne supported the American program of spraying Mexican marijuana with paraquat, rendering it toxic for human consumption.

The paraquat program, initiated in 1975, consists of spraying Mexican marijuana and poppy fields with a toxic herbicide. The idea behind this program was that it would reduce the flow of marijuana and heroin across the border. "It did," according to a report in the *Los Angeles Times,* "but there is also evidence that some marijuana contaminated with chemicals has been reaching the United States." Bourne was then quoted as having commented: "It is true we provided them with helicopters and trained pilots, but it was their decision to use herbicides and spray." That sounds quite a bit like Adolf Eichmann saying that he supplied only the railroads for transporting Jews to the death camps. Then, as if two immoral excuses were better than one, Bourne added: "We are very happy they are doing it, because the program has been dramatically successful in reducing the flow of heroin in the United States. But the paraquat does not come from us. The Mexican government buys it in Europe. It is a Mexican program not a U.S. program."

According to an article in the *Nation,* Bourne's claim that the paraquat spraying was a Mexican idea is simply not true. "It took a lot of convincing to get Mexico to agree to spray," wrote Leslie Danoff. "In the fall

First published as "Bourne's Quaalude Caper," *Inquiry,* November 27, 1978, pp. 4-6. Reprinted with permission.

of 1969, the United States first offered Mexico herbicides and airborne sensors like those used in Vietnam . . . But the Mexicans turned down the spraying plan in October. . . . Six years later, U.S. negotiators made their breakthrough when Mexico finally agreed to give up its ineffectual field burnings."

After endorsing the policy of toxifying marijuana with paraquat, Bourne denied that paraquat-sprayed marijuana was dangerous. Confronted with the fact that 6 out of 45 samples of marijuana confiscated by the Drug Enforcement Administration (DEA) in November 1977 and analyzed by the National Institute on Drug Abuse were found to be "tainted with paraquat," Bourne remained unperturbed. "The risk from paraquat," he declared, "may be overblown." That is quite a twist. The risk from barbiturates (sedatives of proven safety and anticonvulsants indispensable for some epileptics) is not overblown—but the risk from paraquat (the sole use of which is as a toxic herbicide) is overblown. Bourne's hypocrisy in relation to marijuana and paraquat seems to have been boundless. According to the *New Republic*, "Bourne was adamant in his refusal to sympathize with people who might suffer permanent lung damage by smoking Mexican marijuana laced with paraquat. 'If the risk exists the guy still has the option not to smoke the grass to begin with.'"

While Bourne's very office symbolized opposition to the use of marijuana, and while he shamelessly fronted for paraquat, one of his best friends was Keith Stroup, head of the National Organization for the Reform of Marijuana Laws (NORML), a registered Washington lobby for promoting the decriminalization of marijuana. In December 1977, Bourne was the keynote speaker at the annual meeting of NORML. He also accepted an invitation to a large party given by NORML; it was at that party that he was allegedly seen, by several reporters, to be smoking marijuana and sniffing cocaine.

The 1977 annual meeting of NORML was a fateful occasion for Peter Bourne in more than one way. At that conference, Aaron Kaye, a man characterized by *New Times* magazine as a "Yippie pie-assassin," threw a lemon meringue pie at Joe Nellis, chief counsel of the House Select Committee on Narcotics Abuse and Control. Accused of having masterminded the pie plot, Stroup admitted that the "meringuecide" was his idea.

On February 3, 1978, Bob Angarola, White House general counsel to the Office of Drug Abuse Policy, wrote an angry letter on White House stationery to Stroup, protesting the pie-throwing incident. News of this reprimand leaked and made Stroup angry. He called Bourne, demanding "an apology." To stress to Bourne that the Angarola matter was of "mutual concern," Stroup, according to *New Times*, told "Bourne aides to pass on to their boss . . . that he [Stroup] might know too much about the recreational drug preferences of certain senior White House aides." The threat of blackmail worked: On February 11, 1978, Bourne wrote Stroup telling him of "the very high personal regard in which I hold you."

In the end, it was not so much writing a fake prescription that led to Bourne's resignation as the suddenly increasing tempo of public disclosures about his alleged drug habits. After the Quaalude caper hit the headlines, Bourne took a leave of absence with pay and vowed to vindicate himself. Even on July 20, less than two hours before his resignation, Bourne told *Washington Star* columnist Mary McGrory "that he had no intention whatever of quitting and that he was determined to prove his innocence of any wrongdoing." Then Bourne was told that Jack Anderson, the syndicated columnist, had announced on the ABC morning news that Bourne used cocaine at a party given in Washington by NORML in December 1977. Bourne denied the cocaine charge, but quickly resigned. The sequence of events suggests that, up to the last minute, Bourne was planning to brazen it out; and that the reports about Bourne's drug-related activities made public thus far have probably barely scratched the surface.

When last heard from, Bourne was still at it. Although only a few weeks earlier he had said there was a "high incidence of marijuana use" among members of the White House staff, in an interview with the Associated Press on September 20, 1978, he declared that "I have no acquaintance of anyone in the White House using drugs." Clearly, Bourne seems to have considerable difficulty distinguishing between truth and fiction.

Bourne's behavior with regard to marijuana is significant not only for what it reveals about Bourne himself but also for what it reveals about the requirements for success as an American psychopolitician today. A generation ago, one had to lie about civil commitment—insisting that by depriving a person of his personal liberty, the psychiatrist was curing him of mental illness. Now one has to lie about psychoactive drugs—insisting that by depriving the whole American people of their liberty to take certain drugs, the psychiatrist is curing the nation of the collective illness of drug abuse.

Ostensibly, agencies of the United States government concerned with drug abuse are entrusted with safeguarding our health; actually, they lie to us about the true pharmacological effects of certain ideologically contaminated drugs, and they poison certain prohibited substances officially deemed dangerous to discourage their use. Marijuana, say the drug prohibitionists, is a poisonous weed; why then make it more poisonous by spraying it with toxic chemicals? Heroin, even the drug prohibitionists admit, is an excellent painkiller, especially for people dying of cancer; why then outlaw its use, even by prescription? Illicit drugs are prohibited, claim the drug abuseologists, because they are dangerous and addictive; why then do White House staff members use them? One could go on and on.

President and Mrs. Carter's unquestioning support of drug prohibition, like its support by their predecessors, is bad enough. Their support of Bourne and their response to the Bourne affair is worse. It incriminates them as agents in what can only be called an attempt to cover up Bourne's apparent violations of law and those of other White House staff members. Consider the following:

—On July 20, 1978, at a news conference held only hours after Bourne's resignation, Carter was asked about the paraquat spraying of Mexican marijuana. He made it clear that he supported the idea of making marijuana poisonous: "My understanding is that American money is not used to purchase paraquat . . . My preference is that marijuana not be grown nor smoked."

—Another questioner persisted, pointing out that $14 million a year is being channeled into supporting the paraquat spraying in Mexico. Replied Carter: "I favor this relationship with Mexico . . . Because of the work of Dr. Bourne and the officials of the DEA . . . we've mounted a very successful campaign . . . I favor this program very strongly."

—When asked directly about the Bourne affair, Carter replied: "I would prefer not to answer that question." This answer was seized upon by William Safire to castigate his colleagues in the media for not pressing the President harder on this issue. Bourne, asserted Safire, "will neither be missed nor prosecuted—there will be no 'Pillgate.' This 'unfortunate occurrence' is significant mainly in what it reveals of the Magnolia Mafia when confronted with an arrest for lawbreaking in its midst."

—On July 24, at a luncheon meeting with editors and reporters for the *New York Times,* Mrs. Carter declared: "There's not a drug problem at the White House, and everybody knows that. If there was, it would have been exposed long before now." That assertion by Rosalynn Carter and Peter Bourne's parting shot charging that White House staffers "often smoke marijuana" and "sometimes use cocaine" are incompatible. One person or the other is either mistaken or lying.

—The most revealing and self-incriminating of Carter's reactions to the Bourne affair was his warning to White House employees, issued on July 24, to obey the drug laws "or to seek employment elsewhere." That warning, repeated verbatim twice, is astonishingly obtuse and extremely offensive to anyone with a sense of fair play. I will remark on it at greater length.

Most violations of the drug laws are felonies; that is, they are considered to be serious crimes punishable—and, as everyone knows, often punished— by long prison sentences. Suppose, then, that a presidential assistant claimed, and that there was evidence for suspecting, that White House staff members spent their weekends embezzling public funds or burglarizing gas stations. Would it be an adequate and proper response for the President to ignore charges and suspicions of such crimes and to issue a warning that those on his staff who commit them in the future will have to "seek employment elsewhere?"

The accumulated evidence of Carter's reactions to the Bourne affair, and especially his warning to future drug-law violators in the White House, reveals Carter's utter blindness to the fundamental principle of individual liberty under the rule of law upon which the very republic of which he is president rests. Like Bourne, Carter displays the character of an oriental despot masquerading as an American populist. Bourne and Carter know that many Americans are in jail for doing no more than what Bourne allegedly had done and what Bourne insists that other White House staffers have done and are doing. They also know that the American taxpayer has been bilked of dollars to wage a holy war against "drug abuse." But do these men respect their own drug laws? Do they grasp the immense practical and symbolic significance of such laws for the hearts and minds and behavior of ordinary Americans? Not at all. Bourne's behavior in effect screams this message: "I make drug laws, and I break drug laws. You peasants obey them." Carter's behavior, in turn, announces: "I promote drug laws in the abstract, and I have them enforced against people I don't know. But my friends at the White House—well, they are in a different class. If they break the law [and get caught], then I ask them to get a job elsewhere."

Bourne's high jinks with drugs and deceptions seem not to have bestirred most of our lawmakers. However, at least one, Congressman Robert H. Michel of Illinois, has called for an investigation. "If Bourne knows who has been breaking the law in the White House," said Michel in a speech before the House of Representatives on September 7, 1978, "he has a moral and legal obligation to say who it is. If he does not know, he should be exposed as one who recklessly smeared the reputation of high-level officials and former associates. President Carter has neither asked Bourne to provide evidence of his charges nor demanded that he apologize."

Congressman Michel's remarks about Bourne having "smeared" his former associates are well taken and yet they are bitterly ironic. I say that because the United States Congress has itself long been a party to the systematic smearing of such perfectly good and useful drugs as marijuana, cocaine, and heroin by labeling them "dangerous" and "without medical uses." That classification is political, not pharmacological. For decades, congressmen and senators have been deliberately not interested in the truth about drugs. Why should they now be any more interested in the truth or falsehood of declarations delivered by a doctor whose very office symbolized, and continues to symbolize, America's institutionalized political mendacities about drugs?

There was a time when a surgeon who left a sponge in his patient's abdomen could not be sued successfully for the simple reason that, to win such a malpractice suit, it was necessary for another surgeon to testify against his colleague. And no surgeon would do that. So the courts began to apply in such cases the doctrine of *res ipsa loquitur* ("the thing speaks for itself"). I submit that Bourne's behavior and the Carters' behavior also speak for themselves.

The Romans, of course, understood all this. They had a proverb that declared: *"Quod licet Jovi, non licet bovi"* ("What is permitted to Jove, is not permitted to a cow"). Psychiatrists have also understood that this principle governed the making of psychiatric diagnoses and the enforcement of mental health laws, though they were usually willing to admit it only at cocktail parties. The psychiatric presidency—under Jimmy Carter, Rosalynn Carter, and Peter Bourne—is teaching the American people that the same principle applies to their beloved drug laws as well. Let us hope the students are paying attention.

The Protocols of the
Learned Experts on Heroin

The children of each generation are taught to want what they are taught they must not have.

—R. G. Collingwood (1939)

Why did the forgery of Janet Cooke's ugly story, "8-Year-Old Heroin Addict Lives for a Fix" go undetected at the *Washington Post?* Why did it win a Pulitzer Prize? Although these are two quite unrelated questions, the same answer fits both. I believe that this fabrication went undetected and won a Pulitzer Prize because it purported to prove, once more, that heroin is our deadliest enemy.

Religious and medical propaganda to the contrary notwithstanding, I hold some simple truths to be self-evident. One of these truths is that just as the dead do not rise from the grave, so drugs do not commit crimes. The dead remain dead. Drugs are inert chemicals that have no effect on human beings who choose not to use them. No one has to smoke cigarettes, and no one has to shoot heroin. People smoke cigarettes because they want to, and they shoot heroin because they want to. Furthermore, so far as the connection between heroin and crime is concerned, I contend that, the propaganda of the anti-drug crusaders to the contrary notwithstanding, this truth is also self-evident: people under the influence of a powerful central-nervous-system depressant drug, such as heroin, are less rather than more likely to commit crimes than are people who are not under the influence of such a drug; on the other hand, people who live in a society in which the use of certain drugs is popular, in which the sale of those drugs is prohibited, and in which the drug-prohibitions are not enforced, are indeed more likely to commit crimes than they would be in the absence of those conditions. However, since no one is so blind as the man who does not want to see, these truths are quite powerless against popular mythologies, as the *New York Times'* editorial comment on the Cooke affair illustrates. Under the title "The Pulitzer Lie" (April 17, 1981), the editors of the *Times* emphasize their

---

Reprinted, with permission, from the *Libertarian Review,* July 1981, pp. 14-17.

puzzlement:

> We do not know what possessed Janet Cooke to invent an interview with an imaginary 8-year-old drug addict who aspired to grow up to be a heroin pusher in the nation's capital. Nor do we know why the *Washington Post* was so quick to claim the protection of the First Amendment when city authorities sought help in locating children so obviously needing help. We do not know why this contested tale was then pushed for journalism's highest honor, or why the Pulitzer Prize judges jumped the entry from one category to another to bestow the award.

Although I do not want to sound arrogant, I believe that I know the answer to these questions. Indeed, I believe that the editors of the *Times* know it too, albeit they do not want to admit it, or, as Freud has put it, they repress it. And the repressed, as Freud observed, invariably returns.

In this case, the repressed appears in another editorial only a few inches above "The Pulitzer Lie." In that comment, entitled "To Fight Crime, Fight Drugs," the editors admonish the Reagan administration for its insufficient zeal in fighting the drug menace. "The East Coast is currently swamped with heroin," we are informed. "In New York, drug-related robberies and burglaries have more than doubled in three years." But I am afraid that just as Janet Cooke's story about "Jimmy" was not true, so the *New York Times'* editorial about "drug-related crimes" is also not true. The crimes in question are not "drug-related" but "drug-prohibition-related," which is not the same thing.

It is sad how quickly people have forgotten that when Nelson Rockefeller ran for governor, his principal campaign strategy consisted in placing full-page advertisements in the newspapers showing the arm of a young black male injecting heroin. In the accompanying caption Rockefeller pledged to free the people of New York state from this "plague" and the crime it "causes."

People seem also to have forgotten that only a few months ago Governor Hugh Carey offered this "truth" to explain why so many thugs stole so many gold chains in New York City. "The epidemic of gold-chain snatching in the city," declared Carey, "is the result of a Russian design to wreck America by flooding the nation with deadly heroin." If the Russians "were using nerve gas on us," the Governor continued, "we'd certainly call out the troops. This is more insidious than nerve gas. Nerve gas passes off. This doesn't. It kills. I'm not overstating the case."

In love and war all is supposed to be fair. The love of saving people from the Devil and the war on Evil have indeed always been regarded as ample justifications for fabricating strategic lies. Let us face it: Cooke's story was *not* a "weird and atypical hoax," as the *Post* characterized it in hindsight. On the contrary, it was typical anti-drug propaganda, virtually indistinguishable from the standard pharmacomythological tales with which "professionals" and the media have been deluging the American public for the past two decades. If Cooke's story had been "weird and atypical," the editors of the *Post* would have displayed more skepticism toward it and the Pulitzer Prize judges would not have gone out of their way to honor it.

The adjective invariably used to describe the images that Cooke evoked is "shocking." Were a reporter to paint a similarly shocking picture today about, say, Jews poisoning wells or black men raping white women, no respectable newspaper would print the story, nor would it win any prizes. That Janet Cooke's concoction was published and that it won the coveted Pulitzer Prize thus signifies that she tapped a vital artery in America's body politic, a vessel nourishing our most sacred fears and prejudices. There is much evidence to support this view.

First, we have learned that, at the Pulitzer Prize board, one of the most enthusiastic defenders of Cooke's article was an editor from the *Washington Star* who, according to the *Times,* maintained that the piece deserved the prize because it "'had done a great service' by alerting Washington residents to the problems of juvenile drug addiction." Then, there is the reaction of *Post* staffers to it, both before and after its exposure as a fabrication. According to *Time* magazine, the editors at the *Post* "were comforted by letters from readers who claimed they knew Jimmy or children like him." At the *Post,* City Editor Milton Coleman was "very frankly surprised" that the police had not located Jimmy, and was so impressed by the piece that "he wanted another story on young addicts."

After the hoax was exposed, *Post* Executive Editor Benjamin Bradlee revealed that the *Post* can dish it out better than it can take it. In an ironic inversion of the Watergate scenario, in a front-page interview in the *Detroit Free Press,* Bradlee incriminated himself by "obstructing" not justice (since no crime had been committed), but what may be even more important, truth (since a lie had been published). Asked "Have you talked to Cooke recently? What happens to her?" Bradlee replied:

> Well, I talked to her mother and father, but I haven't talked to her since early this morning. We're going to take care of her. We're going to see that she has professional help. We've talked to professional help about her, and we're going to get it for her and pay for it.

But Janet Cooke is neither a child nor an incompetent mental patient. Why talk to her parents? Why talk to "professional help"? Why call psychiatrists "professional help"? Why pay for the psychiatric treatment of a former *Post* employee who "resigns" to avoid being fired? I object to Bradlee's imposing an "insanity plea" on Cooke. Janet Cooke is a liar, not a lunatic, and Bradlee's casual categorization of her as a mental patient only serves to further diminish his own, and the *Post*'s, credibility.

More recently than most people care to admit, multitudes in the West celebrated their collective revulsion against what they then considered to be evil incarnate, the Jew, and its carrier, "International Zionism," through the mythopoesis of "The Protocols of the Learned Elders of Zion." Today, multitudes in the West celebrate their collective revulsion against what they now consider to be evil incarnate, heroin, and its carrier, the "pusher," through the mythopoesis of what could be called "The Protocols of the Learned Experts on Heroin." The Nazis did not have to invent new lies about Jews. Janet Cooke did not have to invent new lies about drugs.

The infamous "Protocols of the Learned Elders of Zion" was purported to be a true account of a conspiratorial plan for Jewish world conquest, drafted at a secret meeting of the first Zionist Congress in Basel, Switzerland, in 1897. The story was first published in the Russian newspaper *Znamia* ("The Banner") in 1903 and was quickly translated into German, French, English, and other western languages. The spurious character of this document was not revealed until 1921. Subsequently, it was established that the "Protocols" were commissioned by the Russian secret police. The full story of the forgery, at least so far as it could be uncovered, was not told until 1942.

We may not know it, or may not want to know it, but we live in an age in which we are deluged with a similar sort of allegedly true, but actually spurious, propaganda—about "drugs." One such example must suffice here.

Early in January 1968, Raymond P. Shafer, then the governor of Pennsylvania and subsequently the chairman of President Nixon's Marijuana Commission, announced to the press that six college students stared at the sun while under the influence of LSD and were blinded as a result. The story was all over the country. Less than two weeks later, the *New York Times* reported that "The Governor, who yesterday told a news conference that he was convinced the report was true, said his investigators discovered this morning that the story was 'a fabrication' by Dr. Norman Yoder [Commissioner of the Office of the Blind] . . . He said Dr. Yoder, who was unavailable for comment, had admitted the hoax." What happened as a result of this disclosure? Nothing. Dr. Yoder and his lies were disposed of by the method characteristic of our age. Pennsylvania Attorney General William C. Sennet diagnosed Yoder as "sick" and attributed his fabrication to "his concern over illegal LSD use by children." Janet Cooke and the *Washington Post* were no doubt similarly concerned over heroin use by children.

At this point, it is necessary to focus on, and to expose, the key role that the imagery of helpless children—cared for by good people and corrupted by evil people—plays in the rhetoric of scapegoating. Gathering under this banner, the drug-mongers lost no time defending the morality of anti-heroin mendacity, even before the clamor over the nonexistent "Jimmy" had died down. For example, William Buckley (who really should know better), pleaded that we "go easy" on Janet Cooke because the "the story of an 8-year-old addicted to heroin is, in our wretched times, far from unlikely." No doubt, the idea of the menace of children as drug-abusers seems "far from unlikely" to Buckley, just as the idea of the menace of children as self-abusers (masturbators) must have seemed far from unlikely to his father or grandfather. It is regrettable, however, that Buckley's boundless fear and loathing of heroin drive him to almost glorifying Janet Cooke by comparing her well-intentioned deception to the demonic deeds of the "pusher." "As one member of the white majority," writes Buckley, "I'd prefer the company of a black newspaperwoman who fabricated a story centered on a mythic *but entirely plausible little victim* [emphasis added] of drugs, to the company of the relatively untroubled black (or white) drug pushers who ride around in their Cadillacs sowing their poison."

But what has driving Cadillacs got to do with the morality of using heroin? Is murder more wicked if the killer leaves the scene in a Cadillac than if he leaves it on foot? If providing people with heroin is a grave wrong, as Mr. Buckley clearly believes it is, then giving it away gratis is at least as wicked as is selling it for a high price. In fact, Buckley is using cheap anti-capitalist rhetoric to whip up hatred against a scapegoat. Moreover, it is implicit in Buckley's argument that selling heroin is very bad, but selling cigarettes is not so bad or not bad at all. Surely, it is unimaginable that Buckley would employ his anti-Cadillac rhetoric against the American tobacco barons and the "pushers" who distribute their toxic products.

Buckley's foregoing remarks articulate what is now considered to be the received truth about heroin. A lead letter in the *New York Times* by Don Russakoff—identified as the President of the Therapeutic Communities of America—illustrates further that the American "experts" know everything about "narcotics" that isn't so. Lamenting that the Cooke story proved to be false, Russakoff actually praises the *Post* for publishing it. "Tragically," he writes, "many other stories about pre-teen narcotic addicts never reach the front page, although they are indisputably true." But none of those stories is indisputably true. And even it they were, it would not follow—except as a leap of faith—that prohibiting the use of certain selected "dangerous drugs" is the correct social policy for dealing with the problem.

Revealingly, Russakoff, like Buckley, also bases his argument on a propagandistic use of the imagery of the child as drug victim. "Not long ago," he writes, "at one of our professional conferences, a physician described the case of a 6-year-old child who had overdosed on 'angel dust.'" And what is that supposed to prove? That perhaps that physician too was a liar? That some parents neglect their children? That we should prohibit vacations in the Alps lest children overdose on poisonous mushrooms—or fall off the cliffs? Buckley and Russakoff are not presenting evidence or offering argument; they are whipping up mindless passion in the people against a scapegoat. Cooke may have written a false story and the *Post* may have been misled into publishing it. But the Satanic threat remains and the vigilance of the vigilantes is now more justified than ever. "The *Times, Washington Post,* and many other responsible publications," concludes Russakoff, "have reported often on the worsening drug epidemic. It is real, not imaginary. And a high proportion of its victims are children. *Small children."* (Emphasis added).

As I suggested some time ago, the contemporary American attitude toward "dangerous drugs" is best understood in religious-mythological terms—that is, as the "ritual expulsion of evil" incarnated in a scapegoat. In the Yom Kippur ceremony, the scapegoat is a goat. In Christian anti-Semitism, it is the Jew. In contemporary America, it is heroin (and other illicit drugs). Once people accept something—an animal, a person, a people, a drug—as a scapegoat which incarnates Evil, they ipso facto consider destroying the scapegoat as Good. Consider, in this connection, the following:

—Formerly, Christians feared the Jews because they allegedly poisoned wells; accordingly, the Jews were savagely persecuted. Today, Americans fear heroin because it allegedly poisons people, especially young people; accordingly, heroin and heroin "pushers" are savagely persecuted. In fact, the Jews did not poison any wells, and heroin does not poison anyone. (The difficulty the contemporary reader has in seeing the difference between heroin poisoning someone and a person poisoning himself with heroin is a major symptom of the success of the anti-drug propaganda.)

—People who believe in a scapegoat do not want to understand it, they want to destroy it. When people regard Jews as Christ-killers or vermin, they do not want to understand Jews, they want a society free of Jews ("Judenfrei"). Similarly, when people regard heroin as a "killer drug" or as a worthless "poison," they do not want to understand heroin, they want a society free of heroin.

Perhaps deep in her soul Janet Cooke actually believed that "The Protocols of the Learned Experts on Heroin" were true, and perhaps she simply wanted to support their admonitory tale by adding to it a fresh chapter of her own. Let us not forget that, in the past, many devout persons had dramatic encounters with devils and saints, and no one called them liars; and that, in our own day, many "devout" persons have dramatic encounters with heroin pushers and cured addicts, and no one calls them liars. Janet Cooke told a rousing good tale, as a good writer should. She inflamed the public passion against the Enemy, as a good rhetorician is supposed to. To expect that her story should also be true—when hardly anyone else's about "drugs" is—seems almost unfair.

Concerning Janet Cooke's mythic hero, Jimmy, one more reflection is in order. Some people in Washington actually believed that they knew him. Cooke herself maintained for as long as she could that Jimmy was real. Obviously, there was virtually no way of proving that Jimmy did not exist. All this made Cooke's denial or admission of the forgery exquisitely important. Which leads to my final observation—namely, that it seems quite possible that had Janet Cooke not lied about her academic credentials, her lies about heroin (for which the mythic Jimmy was, after all, only a vehicle) would probably have gone down America's collective gullet of gullibility just as smoothly as have all the other lies about heroin now passing as the received truth.

There is a moral to this story and it is this. No doubt unwittingly, Janet Cooke has done us a favor. She has held up a mirror in which we can catch a glimpse of a prevailing popular delusion. In the future, when people will worship at other shrines, they will scoff at our drug mythology just as we now scoff at the blood and race mythologies of our fathers and grandfathers.

Will we ever learn one of history's more obvious lessons—to be especially on guard against those who lie to us by appealing to the welfare of children? How many Jews were murdered to save Christian children from being turned into matzo? The ritual murder of people has always been preceded by the ritual murder of the truth—and, indeed, by the ritual murder of language itself.

Purifying America

Jack Abbott, Norman Mailer's famous murderer friend, is released from jail and kills again. He receives an eighteen-year prison sentence. At the same time, the Supreme Court upholds the forty-year prison sentence of a man convicted of possessing and selling nine ounces of marijuana. These two crimes and punishments dramatize the consequences of taking seriously the proposition that this nation's "number-one" crime problem is "drugs." However stupid and ugly that idea might seem to some of us, the fact is that it has fueled the great anti-drug crusade our nation has waged for the past several decades.

Instead of questioning the absurdity and futility of this unwinnable war—our second since World War II—we steadily escalate the conflict. Declaring that narcotics trafficking is "the nation's most serious crime problem," Attorney General William French Smith announced, on January 21, 1982, that the director of the Federal Bureau of Investigation will take over efforts to combat it. At a news conference Smith said that he had given the bureau concurrent jurisdiction with the Drug Enforcement Administration, "bringing the full resources of the FBI to bear on the problem of domestic drug trafficking." The stubborn American fantasy that "drugs" are a "crime problem," soluble by means of draconian laws compassionately administered, was thus given another shot in the arm.

What the two widely different books under review here have in common is that each tells us a good deal about the phenomenon now called, rather stupidly, "drug abuse." As nearly everyone must know by now, during much of his career as a performer, Elvis Presley used a variety of psychoactive drugs. How did Presley procure these drugs? He got them quasi-legally, by prescriptions from doctors; they were delivered to him, through his servants, by pharmacists. I say quasi-legally, because from the very first step of Presley's drug-procurement program the whole affair was a fraud. Many of the prescriptions were made out in the names of people in Presley's entourage, or in his wife's or daughter's name, and the drugs were then transferred to and used by him. This itself was a violation of the drug laws. But these laws were never intended to control people like Elvis Presley, as we shall see.

Review of *Elvis*, by Albert Goldman, and *Flowers in the Blood: The Story of Opium*, by Dean Latimer and Jeff Golderg, *Inquiry*, April 12, 1982, pp. 26-30. Reprinted with permission.

What drugs did Presley use? Mainly Quaalude, Placidyl (recently in the news in connection with Supreme Court Justice William Rehnquist), Demerol, Dilaudid, Dexedrine, and Biphetamine. Pills and tablets Presley took orally, liquids intramuscularly. This was very important for him. As Albert Goldman tells us in his brilliant, biting book *Elvis,* Presley "never takes a shot in the mainline. He associates intravenous injections with the despised character of the 'junkie,' a type he would like to see rounded up en masse and committed to lifelong imprisonment in concentration camps." If this seems like a delicious bit of hypocrisy, wait—there is more, much more.

The popular image of Presley—that when he was not making music, he was making love or counting his money—could not be more false. During much of his career, Presley's main interest in life was drugs: getting drugs, taking drugs, lying about drugs, and, above all else, participating in the American Holy War against drugs. Believe it or not, Presley was actually a fanatic drug-prohibitionist who believed that "drugs" were a "Communist conspiracy" against America. Goldman relates how Presley met and became infatuated with a narcotics agent named John O'Grady, and how, when listening to O'Grady's drug-busting tales, "he would sigh wistfully and say, 'Man, I wish I could be an undercover narcotics detective!'"

Presley's ambition to play a publicly recognized part in this purification program—America's latest and perhaps most hypocritical ever—was fulfilled in 1970, when President Richard Nixon appointed him as an agent of the Bureau of Narcotics and Dangerous Drugs. Presley treasured the gold-and-blue enamel shield symbolizing his achieving this lofty position and always kept it with him, in the same case in which he kept his illegally prescribed pills. The Swiftian irony of the meeting between these two clowns whom all the world mistook for kings is marvelously captured by Goldman:

> Richard Nixon was poised to launch at that very moment a mighty new crusade against drugs. He planned to label drug abuse "America's Number One Problem." Not content with just denouncing drugs and beefing up the federal drug budget, Nixon was already planning to set up a drug superagency, modeled along the lines of the FBI and the CIA, called the Drug Enforcement Agency. The cost of this new secret police force would be staggering. By Fiscal Year 1974, Nixon would have raised the drug law enforcement budget 1100 percent above what it was when he took office in 1968. . . . Now, just as he is to sound the clarion call to the nation . . . along comes one of the greatest heroes of American youth, Elvis Presley, America's Number One Entertainer, proposing to talk to the Number One American about America's Number One Problem! . . . This was an opportunity for a real summit!

When Elvis walked into the Oval Office, he was "high as a kite," says Goldman. Then Presley gave a little speech:

> Elvis's rap began with the advocacy of himself as "living proof that America is the land of opportunity." Overnight he had gone from truck driver to superstar.

. . . Now, he explained, his greatest concern was the youth of America, who had been seduced into drugs and immorality by the "filthy, unkempt appearance and suggestive music of the Beatles."

Having received "a BNDD badge and a complete set of credentials" as a drug agent, Presley set himself to purifying America. Goldman quotes an FBI memo of a meeting between Presley and an assistant director of the bureau according to which Presley volunteered "to make such information [i.e., information about fellow performers] available to the bureau on a confidential basis whenever it came to his attention." Adds Goldman: "Slashing through the bureaucratic gobbledygook you could sum it all up in one line: Elvis offered to work as an *informer.*"

Presley's massive illegal drug use was known, of course, to the narcotics agents, who chose, however, to look the other way when it came to dealing with this superstar. Indeed, since the good old days of Prohibition, antidrug laws have been the perfect weapon for discriminating tyrannization. With it, the narcs could endear themselves to those in power, not only by letting VIPs have all the drugs they wanted, but also by ruining the lives of their enemies (and of defenseless scapegoats, of course).

Actually, antidrug laws are rarely invoked against VIPs; and when they are—for example, against Hollywood personalities—the defendants are usually treated very leniently. In some cases, the selective enforcement of the drug laws goes further still. Senator Joseph McCarthy, for example, was not only unmolested for his addiction to morphine but was supplied the drug personally by Harry Anslinger, the head of the Federal Bureau of Narcotics. Contrast this with the fate of Roger Davis, whose forty-year prison sentence for possession and distribution of nine ounces of marijuana, worth about $200, was mentioned earlier; and more generally, with the fate of countless lower- and middle-class Americans prosecuted and convicted under the drug laws.

While Presley was never indicted for any violation of the drug laws (or for his flagrant violations of the gun laws), after he died his doctor, George Nichopolous, was indicted on the charge of "criminally overprescribing" sedatives, stimulants, and painkillers. Although the prosecution proved that Nichopolous prescribed "31,000 amphetamines, sedatives, and painkillers" over the last two-and-one-half years of the singer's life, the physician was acquitted of all charges by the jury. Why? Because, according to the *New York Times,* the jury "unanimously concluded that the doctor had made a good-faith effort to help . . . that he was a 'good Samaritan' who got into trouble only because he helped desperate patients that other doctors shunned." Perhaps in our scientific age people are prepared to believe nonsense as bad as our forebears ever believed in the Age of Faith. Or perhaps the jury did not really accept that explanation and was merely unwilling to implement our nation's beloved drug laws. (Had Nichopolous been found guilty on all the counts charged, he could have received a prison sentence of 140 years.)

It should be added here that Elvis Presley was not the first, and will probably not be the last, famous American to wage war on drugs while high on them. Another was John Kennedy, upon whose drug use and sordid relationship with his supplier, Dr. Max Jacobson, Eddie Fisher's recent autobiography (*Eddie,* Harper & Row) throws some fresh light. That Kennedy had been—what would have been called, had he not been president—a "junkie" has been known for some time. The details of that story, such as we have them, emerged after Kennedy was dead and sanctified, and his supplier was defrocked and satanized. In 1972 even the *New York Times* considered it fit to print that:

> in 1961 [Jacobson] went with the president to Vienna for the summit meeting with Khrushchev and . . . gave the president injections there. . . . Once, when Dr. Jacobson was in the audience for the Boston tryout of Mr. [Alan Jay] Lerner's *On a Clear Day,* he turned to Mrs. Burton Lane, the wife of the musical's composer, and made a boast that many persons say he often makes. As Mrs. Lane recalled it, Dr. Jacobson pointed to his tie clip, a PT-109 insignia, and said, "Do you know where I got this? I worked with the Kennedys. I traveled with the Kennedys. I treated the Kennedys. Jack Kennedy. Jacqueline Kennedy. They never could have made it without me. . . ." Jacqueline Kennedy Onassis confirmed through a spokesman that she had been treated by Dr. Jacobson but declined to elaborate.

On many of his visits to shoot up Kennedy, Jacobson took Fisher with him. Although Kennedy was high on speed and on Jacobson, some of the people around him were less enthusiastic about the unorthodox (to say the least) treatments the doctor was dispensing. Fisher's recollection of that situation is summed up in this vignette:

> But once I heard him [Kennedy] say, "I don't care if there is panther piss in there, as long as it makes me feel good." Max never told anyone exactly what was in the formulas. If asked, he would say with exasperation, "If I tell you, are you going to know?" You weren't supposed to question God. He even refused to let White House doctors analyze the injections he gave the president.

Fisher then adds this revealing glimpse into the Kennedy-Jacobson relationship: "I saw Kennedy offer him a five-hundred-dollar bill after one of his treatments, but Max shook his head and said, 'If I cannot serve the president of the country I live in, then I am not worth anything.'" Despite the fact that $500 is now worth only a small fraction of what it was worth twenty years ago, ironically the government has withdrawn $500 bills from circulation. Why? Because they are considered to aid the "traffic" in illegal drugs.

That alleged liberals and opponents of drug laws can be just as wrong-headed in their own way as conservatives and born-again crusaders is amply illustrated by Dean Latimer and Jeff Goldberg's *Flowers in the Blood*. These authors, who are professional writers, have produced a well-written book setting forth the history of opium use, in which they do not disguise their hostility to the scapegoating of drugs and drug users. Unfortunately, the story they tell is not particularly new. And the way they tell it is seriously damaged by their credulous embracing of medicomythological "explanations" of opiate addiction.

The book begins with an introduction by William Burroughs, in which he states that "the recent discovery of opium receptors in the brain, and the body's own painkiller endorphin, suggests that there is a preaddiction metabolism related to endorphin deficiency. The addict needs to supplement a vital substance insufficiently produced in his body much as the diabetic needs insulin."

But the idea that an endorphin deficiency plays a causative role in opiate addiction is no more than an unconfirmed hypothesis. Moreover, the analogy to diabetes is grossly misleading: The uncorrected insulin deficiency of the diabetic is fatal, whereas the (alleged) uncorrected endorphin deficiency of the opiate addict is not. I, for one, doubt that endorphins have anything to do with addiction to opiates. The similarities between the uses of opiates, barbiturates, cocaine, marijuana, alcohol, and nicotine make the endorphin-deficiency hypothesis rather unpersuasive. Do cigarette addicts smoke because they lack an "endonicotine"? Do people use cocaine because they lack an "endococaine"? Do people eat too many sweets because they lack an "endocarbohydrate"?

There is worse to come. Burroughs writes, and Latimer and Goldberg presumably agree, that "methadone maintenance was the first glimmer of sanity in the antidrug hysteria that gripped America in the fifties and sixties. . . ." But was methadone, as Burroughs asserts, the "first glimmer of sanity" in this period, or was it, as I would contend, one of the more grotesque symptoms of this very hysteria? It seems to me that our whole attitude toward drugs and drug controls will depend on how we approach this subject: whether with the assumption that certain drugs are so irresistibly tempting that their availability and use ought to be strictly controlled by the state; or with the assumption that the use of various drugs represents but one class of temptations among many, and that coping competently with such temptations is the duty of men, women, and children who value self-control and want to live in a free society.

Like Burroughs, Latimer and Goldberg eagerly prostrate themselves before the idols of modern pharmacomythology. "One can only marvel," they write in a worshipful tone, "at this vision of body and mind as a vastly complex chemical equation, interacting uniquely with the chemicals in plants like the opium poppy. We've been linked symbiotically, on a molecular level, man and poppy, endorphin and opium, since the first days of creation." This may be poetic, but scientific it is not.

How confused even "liberal" opponents of our drug laws are is sadly illustrated by Latimer and Goldberg's conclusions. "The inescapable conclusion of all this furious effort," they write, "may well be that there is no universal cure after all, and that the most efficacious solution to the opiate addiction problem is simply to give addicts opiates." What is there left to say? Taking opium on one's own is an addiction and a problem; getting it from the government is a cure and a solution. Such is the intensity of the prevailing religious fervor concerning drugs. Finally, Latimer and Goldberg's casual use of the knee-jerk anti-capitalist, antidrug jargon—referring, for example, to people who sell heroin as "heroin magnates" and to their financial rewards as "profiteering"—illustrates a powerful rhetorical consensus between right and left.

Libertarians—especially if they are rationalists and skeptics about fashionable pharmacomythologies—are now the only identifiable group of people that reject this humbug. For the realist about religion, there are no gods; and for the realist about drugs, there are no "dangerous" drugs. (I am taking for granted here that we all know that virtually all biologically active chemicals *may be* dangerous.) But deities and drugs are indispensable symbols for most people, which they have no intention of giving up. And if people confuse symbols with what they symbolize—well, that merely proves that they are human.

In the final analysis, all the current hullabaloo about drugs seems to me to come down to man's age-old passion to push his fellow man around, and to do so, to boot, in such a way as to make his victim look like the devil while making himself look like a saint. In an important sense, this is what mankind's great passion plays of purification—the religious persecutions and wars, the crusades and the witch hunts, communism and nazism—have been about. And this is what our contemporary persecutions of drugs, drug users, and drug suppliers are all about.

These purificatory rituals have been inspired and sustained by two dominant justificatory images: God and Health. For the religious zealot, God's will justifies all manner of human bestiality; for the medical zealot, Health plays the same role. In the name of loving God, we hate; in the name of protecting Health, we ruin lives. When these justificatory claims are combined with our most hypocritical claim of all—the need to Protect The Child—then, truly, all hell breaks loose and the wise know it is time to get out of the way of people running amok to do good.

Still, the reader would be mistaken if he thought that we Americans believed that using opium is always wrong. We only believe that it is wrong for Asians to grow the poppy that is the source of opium and for Europeans to ship its alkaloids to us. What is right, thank heaven, is for our farsighted government to stockpile opium for a "national emergency." Our health planners have already got some 70,000 pounds of it secreted away and plan to add 60,000 more pounds to it. The picture is clear enough: So long as we are free and are not dying, opium is *verboten;* after we shall be fatally irradiated in a nuclear holocaust, however, the government will give us all the opium we'll need for a narcotized death. That seems to me like a high price to pay for regaining our inalienable right to opium—but we seem quite ready to pay it.

The War Against Drugs

In 1980, crime and violence, long endemic to New York City, erupted in a new epidemic. Singly and in packs, hoodlums rampaged through the subways and the commuter trains, ripping gold chains off the necks of women. A typical newspaper story described one such public mass-robbery as follows: "Seconds after a packed Amtrak passenger train collided with a freight train last night, a wave of chain-snatching broke out at the scene. Gold chains and purses were ripped from commuters in a second passenger train, which screeched to a halt behind the Amtrak wreck near Dobbs Ferry."[1]

The public was horrified. The police were helpless. Although (New York State) Governor Hugh Carey could offer neither protection for the public nor compensation for the victims, he could—and did—offer an explanation for this mayhem. "The epidemic of gold-snatching in the city," he declared, "is the result of a Russian design to wreck America by flooding the nation with deadly heroin. In the streets, you know what's going on. Women are afraid to walk with a chain around their neck. Why? Somebody's grabbing that chain to get enough money for a fix." If the Russians "were using nerve gas on us," the Governor continued, "we'd certainly call out the troops. This is more insidious than nerve gas. Nerve gas passes off. This doesn't. It kills. I'm not overstating the case." Governor Carey made these remarks at a press conference in New York City, on September 25, 1980, announcing his plan to create a new commission to fight the drug menace.[2] He will name it "The Citizens Action to Combat Heroin."[2]

When Governor Carey spoke these words, the American war against "dangerous drugs"—especially heroin—had been going on for more than a quarter of a century. The political rhetoric about "drug abuse," the medical mendacity about "drug rehabilitation," the legislative prohibition of "illicit drugs," and the judicial persecution of drug users ("addicts") and drug sellers ("pushers"), aided and abetted by the popular media intoxicated with a blind faith in a holy war against unholy drugs—all this had been going on for much longer than the First and Second World Wars combined; much longer than Prohibition, or Nazism, or the war in Vietnam. Still, America's war against "dangerous drugs"—which has spread to Europe, to Australia, to Japan—shows no signs of letting up. There is no light at the end of the

Reprinted, with permission, from the *Journal of Drug Issues,* vol. 12, Winter, 1982, pp. 115-22.

tunnel.

Just what is this war about? Ostensibly, it is a war against "dangerous drugs." But drugs are the products of human inventiveness and technology; they are material objects, like buttons or baseball bats. How can human beings wage a war against such *things?* One would have to be blind—and deaf and dumb to boot—not to see and hear that this is a metaphorical war. But that cannot be the whole story. Millions upon millions of well-educated and intelligent Americans now believe that "drugs" are a danger to America— just as fifty years ago millions upon millions of well-educated and intelligent Germans believed that "Jews" were a danger to Germany. If history teaches us anything at all, it teaches us that human beings have a powerful need to form groups, and that the sacrificial victimization of scapegoats is often an indispensable ingredient for maintaining social cohesion among the members of such groups. Perceived as the very embodiment of evil, the scapegoat's actual characteristics or behavior are thus impervious to rational analysis. Since the scapegoat *is* evil, the good citizen's task is not to understand him (or her, or it), but to hate him and to rid the community of him. The German saying *Verstehen ist verboten* ("To understand is forbidden") applies quite literally to this situation: Attempts to analyze and grasp such a ritual purga- tion of society of its scapegoats is perceived as disloyalty to, or even an attack on, the "compact majority" and its best interests.

It seems to me that the American war against "dangerous drugs" repre- sents merely a new variation in humanity's age-old passion to "purge" itself of its "impurities" by staging vast dramas of scapegoat-persecutions.[3] In the past, we have witnessed religious or "holy" wars waged against people who professed the wrong faith—such as the witch-hunts. More recently, we have witnessed racial or "eugenic" wars, waged against people who possessed the wrong genetic makeup—such as Nazism. Now we are witnessing a medical or "therapeutic" war—waged against people who use the wrong drugs.

Like all spectacular scapegoat-persecutions, the war against "drugs" is enacted on the classic model of Saint George slaying the dragon. Thus we witness an endless succession of politicians riding forth on the backs of their faithful steed—the law-abiding, tax-paying citizens—promising to slay the phantom-enemy. Governor Carey, the *New York Times* informs us, is now "calling for an all-out offensive against what he believes to be a Russian- inspired flood of heroin in the nation. It is the root cause of crime and is destroying an entire generation of youth, particularly among the poor."[4]

While the American "war" against drugs resembles Nazism, Governor Carey's recent call for more vigorous action against heroin invites compari- son with Adolf Hitler's call for more vigorous action against the Jews during the closing years of the Second World War. In each case, we are faced with a self-intoxicated politican projecting an image of himself as the protector of his people. In each case, the people are indeed gravely endangered—but not by the threat from which the politician promises protection: then, the people killing Germans were not Jews, but Allied soldiers; now the people robbing, maiming, and killing Americans are not Russian "drug pushers," (or American "drug pushers," for that matter), but young Americans taking advantage of an absurd system of crime-controls. Furthermore, in each case, the deceitful and vainglorious scapegoat-monger is actually quite unable to protect the people from the dangers that, in large part, he himself (together with his fellow politicians) has helped to create and unleash on them. Obviously, for anyone not in the grips of the scapegoater's ideology, each exhortation—whether it be Hitler's against the Jews toward the end of the Second World War or Carey's against "drugs" today—is nothing but propaganda of the cheapest sort. To appreciate the historical context in which Carey offered his remarks, I cite below a few comments about the war against drugs that appeared in the American press during the 1960s and 1970s:

1966. C. W. Sandman, Jr., chairman of the New Jersey Narcotic Drug Study Commission, declares: "LSD is the greatest threat facing the country today . . . more dangerous than the Vietnam War."[5]

1967. The New York State Narcotics Addiction Control Commission, proposed by Governor Nelson Rockefeller, goes into effect. Rockefeller hails it as "the start of an unending war."[6]

1971. President Richard Nixon declares that "America's Public Enemy No. 1 is drug abuse." He creates a "Special Action Office of Drug Abuse Prevention."[7]

1972. Myles G. Ambrose, Special Assistant Attorney General of the United States, declares: "As of 1960, the Bureau of Narcotics estimated that we had somewhere in the neighborhood of 55,000 heroin addicts. . . , they estimate now the figure to be 550,000 addicts."[8]

1973. A public opinion poll reveals that 67 percent of the adults interviewed "support the proposal of New York Governor Nelson Rockefeller that all sellers of hard drugs be given life imprisonment without the possibility of parole." A typical comment: "The seller of drugs is not human . . ." Many authorities propose the death penalty for "drug trafficking."[9]

These excerpts barely hint at the duration and magnitude of the war against drugs that forms the backdrop against which Governor Carey's incredible intemperance—that no one challenged or criticized—must be seen. The scope of that war is perhaps best illustrated by the unbridled legislative enthusiasm and the vast sums that have supported it. [10]

For example, in 1965, when President Lyndon Johnson sought legislation imposing tight federal controls over "pep pills" and "goof balls," the bill cleared the House by a unanimous vote, 402 to 0.[11] In October, 1970, the Senate passed, again by a unanimous vote, 54 to 0, "a major narcotics crackdown bill hailed as a keystone in President Nixon's anticrime program. Added to the bill were strong new measures for the treatment and rehabilitation of drug abusers."[12] In 1971, the Senate approved, by a unanimous vote of 92 to 0, a "$1 billion-plus bill to mount the nation's first all-out, co-ordinated attack on the insidious menace of drug abuse." Fifteen months later, in February 1972, the House voted 380 to 0 for a $411 million, three-year program to combat drug abuse. And in March, 1972, the House voted, 366 to 0, to authorize a $1 billion three-year federal attack on drug abuse.[13]

The resemblance, once again, between the unanimity with which German society's leaders formerly supported "protective" measures against Jews and with which the American society's leaders now support such measures against "drugs" and "drug abusers" is both obvious and ominous.

Fifty years ago, Adolf Hitler incited the German people against the Jews—by "explaining" the various ways in which the Jews were "dangerous" to the Germans individually and to Germany as a nation. Millions of Germans—among them the leaders in science, in medicine, in law, in the media—believed in the reality of the "dangerous Jews." Indeed, they more than believed in it: they loved the imagery of that racial myth, they felt exhilarated by the increased self-esteem and solidarity it gave them, and they were thrilled by the prospect of "cleansing" the nation of its "racial impurities." Today, hardly anyone in Germany believes the myth of the "dangerous Jew"—a change in point of view that surely had nothing to do with more research on, or fresh scientific discoveries about, the problem of "dangerous Jews."

Mutatis mutandis, every American president since John F. Kennedy—and countless other American politicians, especially Governor Nelson Rockefeller (who was elected to four terms largely on the basis of his anti-drug propaganda)—have incited the American people against "dangerous drugs"—by "explaining" the various ways in which such drugs threaten Americans individually and the United States as a nation. Millions of Americans—among them the leaders in science, in medicine, in law, in the media—believe in the reality of "dangerous drugs." Indeed, they more than believe in it: they love the imagery of this pharmacological myth, they feel exhilarated by the increased self-esteem and solidarity it gives them, and they are thrilled by the prospect of "ridding" the nation of its sinister "mind-altering drugs."

Of course, in the end, the hematomythological quest to make Germany *Judenfrei* (free of Jews) proved to be extremely costly and self-destructive for the Germans. The pharmacomythological quest to make America free of heroin is proving to be similarly costly and self-destructive for us. For example, a recent study of crime in Miami "concluded that 239 heroin addicts were known to be responsible for an incredible total of 80,000 criminal offenses." Another study "showed that over an 11-year period 243 addicts accounted for an estimated 473,000 crimes."[14] Today, Germans know that the Nazis lied about the Jews—that Jews were scapegoats deliberately sacrificed for the greater glory of the National Socialist State. But hardly anyone in America now seems to know, or to acknowledge, that the "drug educators" lie about drugs—that "dangerous drugs" (and those who use and sell them) are deliberately sacrificed for the greater glory of the Therapeutic State.

Looking back to the 1930s, a young person in Germany today might wonder in what way the Jews were a danger to the Reich, as Nazi propaganda had it. What did Jewish doctors and lawyers, or shopkeepers and students in Germany do that was so different from what their non-Jewish counterparts did? And if the German Jews were such a grave danger to the Reich in 1933, why were German Jews not a danger to Germany in, say, 1913 or 1893? Why were Jews not a danger to England or America? I trust that these questions will be heard as they are intended—rhetorical queries whose purpose is to show that certain political appeals to the "dangerousness" of particular persons or things have no basis in facts and are not supposed to have any. Instead, their purpose is to unite people against a common enemy and to mobilize them to wage a "holy war" against that enemy.

As the Nazis declared the Jews to be "Public Enemy Number One" in Germany, so American presidents and politicians have declared "drugs" to be "Public Enemy Number One" in the United States. But let us ask: In what ways are drugs a danger to Americans individually or to the United States as a nation? What do the officially persecuted drugs—especially, heroin, cocaine, and marijuana—do that is so different from what other drugs do? If these drugs are such a grave danger to Americans in 1980, why were they not a danger to them in, say, 1940 or 1900? [15] These, too, are rhetorical questions. Anyone who reflects on these matters must realize that our culturally accepted drugs—in particular, alcohol, tobacco, and "mind-altering" drugs legitimated as "psychotherapeutic"—pose a much graver threat, and cause much more demonstrable harm, to people than do the prohibited (and so-called) "dangerous drugs."

There are, of course, complex religious, historical, and economic reasons (which I cannot discuss here) that play a part in determining which drugs people use and which they avoid. But regardless of such cultural-historical determinants, and regardless of the pharmacological properties of the "dangerous drugs" in question, one simple fact remains—namely, that no one has to ingest, inject, or smoke any of these drugs unless he or she wants to do so. This simple fact compels one to see the "drug problem" in a totally different light than that in which it is now officially portrayed. The official line is that "dangerous drugs" pose an "external" threat to people—that is, a threat like a natural disaster, such as an erupting volcano or a hurricane. The inference drawn from this image is that it is the duty of a modern scientifically enlightened state to protect its citizens from such dangers, and it is the duty of the citizens to submit to the protections so imposed on them for the benefit of the community as a whole.

But "dangerous drugs" pose no such threat. Obviously no drug poses a threat to anyone who chooses to leave it alone.[16] In short, the danger posed by so-called "dangerous drugs" is quite unlike that posed by hurricanes or plagues, but is rather like the danger posed (to some people) by, say, eating pork or masturbating. What I mean is that certain threats—so-called natural disasters, in particular—strike us down as "passive victims," as it were; whereas certain other threats—for example, "forbidden" foods or sexual acts—strike us down as "active victims," only if we succumb to their temptation. Thus, an Orthodox Jew may be tempted to get a ham sandwich and a Catholic may be tempted to use artificial contraception—but that does not make most of us view pork products or birth-control devices as "dangers" from which the state should protect us. On the contrary, we believe that free access to such foods and devices is our right (or "constitutional right," as Americans put it). It is in such a way, and in such a way only, that so-called "dangerous drugs" are dangerous.

In actuality—that is, at the present time, and especially in the United States—the so-called "drug problem" has several distinct dimensions: First, there is the problem posed by the *pharmacological properties* of the drugs in question. This problem is technical: all new scientific or practical inventions offer us not only certain solutions for old problems, but also create new problems for us. Drugs are no exception. Secondly, there is the problem posed by the *temptation* which certain drugs present—especially those believed to possess the power to "give" pleasure. This problem is moral and psychological: some drugs offer us certain new temptations that we must learn to resist or enjoy in moderation. They, too, are no exception. Thirdly, there is the problem posed by the *prohibition* of certain drugs. This problem is partly political and economic, and partly moral and psychological. Drug-prohibition and persecution constitutes a type of scapegoating, as discussed earlier. In addition, the prohibition itself generates certain otherwise unavailable economic and existential options: for example, it offers "meaning" and "jobs" to many people, especially youngsters and unemployable persons; it also offers an opportunity to ambitious but untalented individuals for easily dramatizing their lives and aggrandizing their individuality by defying certain modern "medical" taboos.

The role of defiance in so-called "drug-abuse" is, indeed, quite obvious. It is clearly displayed in the contemporary counterculture's righteous rejection of conventional or legal drugs and its passionate embrace of the use of unconventional or illegal drugs. The perennial confrontation between authority and autonomy, the permanent tension between behavior based on submission to coercion and the free choice of one's own course in life—these basic themes of human morality and psychology are now enacted on a stage on which the principal props are drugs and laws against drugs. The following tragedy—typical of countless similar stories reported in the press—is especially revealing:

A young couple about to be sentenced on drug charges horrified a packed courtroom when they swallowed cyanide and fell dying to the floor. After the probation judge refused to grant probation, William Melton, 27, put a white powder in his mouth and collapsed seconds later. His wife, Tracey Lee, 21, walked over to her husband and patted him softly on the head [and then put some cyanide powder in her own mouth]. . . They died in a local hospital. "It was crazy. It was as if they were going to the gas chamber. . . ," said court clerk Howard Smith. "They weren't even going to get a long sentence." Melton had been convicted of possessing marijuana and cocaine and his wife was convicted of possession of marijuana, cocaine, and LSD.[17]

It does not matter how transparently clear such power-games are. If people want to deny the conflict between self-control and being coerced, they will deny it. And having denied it, they will, if they want to, convince themselves that "their problem" is historically novel and that it is a matter of disease and treatment. So "enlightened," they can even manage to not see that they are merely re-enacting the biblical parable of the Fall. Did Eve, tempted by the Serpent, seduce Adam, who then lost control of himself and succumbed to evil? Or did Adam, facing a choice between obedience to the authority of God and the challenge of his own destiny, choose self-control? Or did Adam and Eve suffer from "substance abuse"?

How, then, shall we view the situation of the so-called drug abuser or drug addict? As a stupid, sick, and helpless child—who, tempted by pushers, peers, and the pleasures of drugs, succumbs to the lure and loses control of himself? Or as a person in control of himself—who, like Adam, chooses the forbidden fruit as a way of pitting himself against authority?

There is no empirical or scientific way of choosing between these two answers, of deciding which is right and which is wrong. The questions frame two different moral perspectives, and the answers define two different moral strategies. If we side with authority and wish to repress the individual, we shall treat him *as if* he were helpless, the innocent victim of overwhelming temptation; and we shall then "protect" him from further temptation—by treating him as a child or mental patient. If we side with the individual and wish to refute the legitimacy and reject the power of any authority to infantilize or "diagnose" him, we shall treat him *as if* he were in command of himself, the executor of responsible decisions; and we shall then demand that he respect others as he respects himself—by treating him as an adult, a free and rational person.

Notes

1. "It's a Chain Reaction as Snatchers Go Wild," *New York Post,* November 8, 1980, p. 5.

2. A. Greenspan, "Gold-Chain Grabbers? Carey Blames Soviet Heroin-War Strategy," *New York Post,* September 26, 1980, p. 10.

3. See T. S. Szasz, *Manufacture of Madness,* Harper & Row, New York, 1970, and *Ceremonial Chemistry,* Doubleday, Garden City, N.Y., 1974.

4. R. J. Meislin, "A New Carefree Carey Roils Political Waters," *New York Times,* October 27, 1980, pp. B1-B4.

5. Szasz, *Ceremonial Chemistry,* p. 205.

6. Ibid.

7. Ibid., p. 209.

8. Ibid., p. 210.

9. Ibid., p. 212.

10. For additional examples of other "Wars Against Drugs" since the seventeenth century, see: Szasz, *Ceremonial Chemistry,* pp. 185-212.

11. See Szasz, *The Theology of Medicine,* Harper/Colophon, New York, 1977, pp. 29-48.

12. See Szasz, *The Theology of Medicine,* pp. 29-44.

13. See Note 11.

14. Jack Anderson, "Security Lax for Drug Stockpiles," *Syracuse Post-Standard,* November 20, 1980, p. A5.

15. Cocaine and marijuana have, of course, been around for a very long time. Heroin (diacetymorphine) was first synthesized in 1898, and was immediately hailed as a "safe preparation free from addiction-forming properties" (A. Montagu, "The Long Search for Euphoria," *Reflections I* [May-June, 1966] p. 68.) The treatment of heroin addiction with methadone, which is an even more potent narcotic than heroin, proves that history does repeat itself.

16. To be sure, drugs can be used to *poison other people* and, in that way, do constitute a danger. But the contemporary anti-drug ideology and the policies it inspires are motivated not by the threat of using drugs for *poisoning others,* but by the threat of using them for *"self-poisoning."* It is astonishing, in this connection, how profoundly unaware people are of the similarities—medically as well as morally—between the behavior that used to be called "self-abuse" (forbidden sexual self-stimulation) and the behavior that is now called "drug abuse" (self-medication with forbidden chemicals). See Szasz, *Sex by Prescription* (Doubleday, Garden City, N.Y., 1980).

17. "Drug Pair Beat Court Forever—Cyanide," *New York Post,* November 8, 1980, p. 4.

Coerced Treatment for Addicts

The answer to the question, "Should alcohol and/or drug abusers be legally coerced into treatment?" depends on the kind of society we value. If we want to foster the development of self-reliant individuals living responsible lives in a politically free society, then the answer is no. On the other hand, if our "ideal" society is composed of child-like individuals, submissive to authority—especially medical authority—living under an authoritarian-paternalistic political system, then the answer is yes.

The political philosophy of classical liberalism emphasizes—as would I—that bodily and mental self-ownership is one of our most fundamental rights. Simply put, this means that so long as we do not directly injure others, we can do with our bodies and minds what we please. Adhering to this philosophy does not imply turning a blind eye to what may be medically undesirable behaviors, such as eating too much or too little, using toxic drugs, or otherwise "abusing" one's body or mind. It implies only rejecting *state-imposed coercion* as a legitimate interference with such acts.

As a physician, teacher, and practical person, I also believe in the wisdom of the proverb that "you can lead a horse to water, but you can't make it drink." In the modern world, it is axiomatic that the proper medical treatment of adults, including the imparting of therapeutically-relevant information to them, depends upon and requires their active, voluntary cooperation. In non-psychiatric medical specialties—for example, in ophthalmology, dermatology, hematology, rheumatology, nephrology, orthopedic or plastic surgery—the idea of treating a person against his will borders on the absurd. Moreover, authorities on medical ethics keep telling us that competent adults have an unqualified right to reject unwanted treatment.

As I see it, the idea of legally coercing the treatment of alcohol or drug abusers is not only morally objectionable, it is also impractical. Consider some of the difficulties with it.

What constitutes drug abuse? Using heroin once is now so defined, but habitually smoking cigarettes is not. Eating one marijuana cookie is now so defined, but habitually ingesting too much food is not. The point is that when physicians accept the legitimacy of legally-coerced treatment for "drug

First published as "Point/Counterpoint: Should Alcohol and/or Drug Abusers Be Legally Coerced into Treatment?" *U.S. Journal of Drug and Alcohol Dependence* 7 (June 1983), p. 7. Reprinted with permission.

abusers," they cease to be independent healers and thinkers and become, instead, apologists and agents of a coercive state apparatus. As a result, although their interventions may be defined as "treatments" by the "drug abuseologists," and the governments that pay them, such doctors will be despised as torturers by the "patients" whose welfare they ostensibly protect and serve.

There are other problems as well. How does one treat a person who "abuses" alcohol or drugs, but who manages capably and is satisfied with his own way of life? First of all, one must find him by stealth and detain him by force. This can be done. There is a long psychiatric history of doing so. But what does that history teach us? It teaches us that although it is possible to detoxify a person's body of certain chemicals, it is not possible—without his cooperation—to change his behavior as a free agent. The very concept of "abusing" alcohol or drugs implies a persistent pattern of actions on the part of the abuser—what used to be called a "bad habit." And habits, whether bad or good (a judgment that lies in the eyes of the beholder), can be broken only by the habituated person himself.

More than half a century ago, Karl Jaspers, the great German psychiatrist-turned-philosopher, warned us about the hopelessness of coerced treatment. "Rational treatment," he wrote, "is not really an attainable goal as regards the large majority of mental patients . . . Admission to a hospital often takes place against the will of the patient, and therefore the psychiatrist finds himself in a different relation to this patient than other doctors. He tries . . . to deliberately emphasize his purely medical approach to the patient, but the latter in many cases is quite convinced that he is well and resists these medical efforts."

To me, there is something astonishing about the arrogance of physicians who enthusiastically endorse the principles and practices of legally-coerced "treatment," especially for conditions that are diseases only in a metaphoric sense, such as alcohol or drug abuse. But perhaps Hegel was right when he said that we learn from history that we don't learn from history. In the past, when people were obsessed with religion, they believed that the "true faith" justified depriving others of liberty. Now, when people are obsessed with medicine, they believe that "scientific treatment" justifies depriving others of liberty. But if we reject coercion in the name of salvation, why should we accept coercion in the name of treatment? And if we accept such coercion, do we not become—knowingly or otherwise—true believers in our own blind and bigoted brand of "therapeutic" despotism?

VII
SEX

The Abortionist as Fall Guy

The recent trial of Dr. William Waddill, the California obstetrician accused of strangling the supposedly live baby he delivered in the course of a saline abortion, has helped once more to dramatize the dilemmas of abortion. The contemporary arguments for and against abortion have been articulated ad nauseam. I shall not rehash them. Instead, I shall focus upon a very practical aspect of the abortion controversy that is persistently ignored in contemporary considerations of the problem. This glaring omission reveals a grave inconsistency on the part of the anti-abortionists, rendering their moral position untenable.

The question of when the fetus becomes a "person"—at the moment of fertilization, at the time of quickening, after 28 weeks of gestation, at the time of delivery, or at some other point—is a matter on which biologists and ethicists may and do have honest differences of opinion. Regardless of such differences, however, I submit that abortion is always and necessarily, an act of killing. The question, therefore, is: What sort of killing is it? Justifiable or not? If abortion is justifiable killing as it is now considered to be (until an ambiguously late stage of pregnancy), then, of course, it falls outside the purview of the criminal law.

However, the anti-abortionists assert that abortion is a species of unjustified killing that should therefore be prohibited and punished by the criminal law. If that is the basic premise on which their position rests, then that position is untenable. The reason is this. If abortion is the killing of a human being or "person," then it is surely the quintessence of first-degree murder. What "murder" is more deliberately planned and executed than an abortion? Furthermore, if abortion is murder, then its chief architect and beneficiary is clearly the pregnant woman, the abortionist playing merely the role of an accomplice. (The eminently possible development of an effective chemical abortifacient, which the pregnant woman could administer to herself, would make him superfluous.) Accordingly, criminal laws against abortion penalizing the abortionist but not his client are as absurd and immoral as would be criminal laws against premeditated murder penalizing hired assassins but not those who hire them. Yet all modern anti-abortion laws are precisely of this type: They single out the physician for prosecution and punishment, and close

Reprinted, with permission, from *Inquiry*, July 24, 1978, pp. 4-5.

their eyes to the complicity of the "patient" in the prohibited act. Therein lies the inconsistency of the anti-abortionist: They advocate, and propose that the country reembrace, laws that define abortion as a crime and treat the abortionist as the only criminal in the case.

The Waddill case illustrates the absurdities into which out inattention to such considerations have led us. The facts are as follows. In February 1977, Mary Weaver, an 18-year-old pregnant, unwed high-school senior, sought an abortion at the Huntington Beach Free Clinic. Her request was denied because she was judged to be 28 weeks pregnant. Ms. Weaver and her father, the principal of the high school she attended, then turned for help to Dr. William Waddill, an associate of her family doctor. Ms. Weaver told Dr. Waddill that she was 20 to 22 weeks pregnant. Her father also asked Dr. Waddill to abort the baby. On March 2, 1977, Dr. Waddill did a saline abortion, as a result of which Ms. Weaver delivered a baby judged to be 31 weeks old.

The rest of the facts are disputed. Some witnesses claim that the baby had a heartbeat and was breathing, and that Dr. Waddill strangled it. Dr. Waddill claims that the baby was born dead. Dr. Waddill was indicted for murder. In May 1978, his three-month trial ended with a deadlocked jury and a mistrial. (On June 2, a California judge ordered that Dr. Waddill be retried, the new trial to be November 27.) Ms. Weaver was never charged with any crime whatsoever. In fact, she is suing Dr. Waddill (and the hospital where the abortion was performed) for the modest sum of $17 million, charging "negligence, assault and battery, and wrongful death."

Here is epitomized the hitherto repressed dimension of abortion. Clearly, Ms. Weaver is the moral agent primarily responsible for her abortion. Dr. Waddill performed the service for which he and Ms. Weaver had contracted, but is nevertheless sued by her. Inasmuch as Ms. Weaver had sought out Dr. Waddill to enlist his aid in killing the fetus and is now suing him partly for having deprived her of a live baby, her chances of winning her suit are probably quite good. I say that because there is a precedent now for settling medical tort litigation on such Alice-in-Wonderland principles of fairness and contract.

This precedent is the much-publicized case of Mr. Kenneth Donaldson. Donaldson, it should be recalled, was confined as an involuntary mental patient. Claiming to be a Christian Scientist, he asked his physicians to refrain from treating him with electroshock and drugs. The physicians honored his request. After Donaldson managed to obtain his release, he sued the hospital director for depriving him of his "right to treatment"—and, with the help of the American Civil Liberties Union, won an out-of-court settlement. In my critique of this case in *Psychiatric Slavery*, I compared Donaldson's legal posture to "that of a Catholic woman who refuses an abortion and then sues the doctors" for not aborting the fetus. In the Weaver case, the same argument is turned around 180 degrees: a woman requests an abortion and then sues for not having been delivered of a live infant.

Kenneth Donaldson's and Mary Weaver's suits are, of course, but two of the "symptoms" of the moral malignancy endemic to our age—that is, our refusal to treat patients and physicians as *equally* responsible moral agents. One might of course argue, with Oliver Wendell Holmes, that "The life of the law has not been logic; it has been experience." Unfortunately, that has been all too true. But can we, as members of a free society, afford even to debate a law whose life is the brazen illogic of punishing the accomplices to a crime, but not the masterminds who plan, contract for, and chiefly benefit from it?

The anti-abortionists are irrefutably right in asserting that the fetus is alive, that pregnancy is not a disease, and that abortion is not a treatment. An abortion is the fulfillment of a contract—between a pregnant woman and an abortionist—for killing a fetus. The contract originates with the "patient" and is executed by the physician. In earlier times, women who deliberately aborted their babies were prosecuted and punished. However, by the end of the eighteenth century, laws decreeing the punishment of such women, like the laws decreeing the punishment of suicides, were no longer enforced. American anti-abortion laws were always aimed against the "illegal abortionist," not against the woman who sought his services.*

No one would deny that the moral agent motivating the act of abortion is the pregnant woman. If that act is deemed unjustified and is declared illegal, then it follows that the main culprit is the pregnant woman. At the same time, it is abundantly clear that most people in modern Western societies—even those passionately opposed to abortion—are unwilling to punish the person most responsible for it. I submit, therefore, that until such time as the American people are willing to have the state prosecute and punish women who have, with premeditation, contracted for the violation of anti-abortion laws, such laws will continue to diminish rather than increase the human dignity which pro-abortionists and anti-abortionists alike supposedly cherish.

---

*The history of the status of abortion in Catholic theology and of the sanctions against it in ecclesiastic law is exceedingly complex. The act was most severely punished by the bull *Effraenatam* of Pope Sixtus V, issued on October 29, 1588. It decreed that all abortions be treated as murder, and it explicitly included the pregnant woman as a party sharing fully in the guilt for the act. However, few women guilty of abortion were so treated. The effort to control abortion by means of the criminal law began only in the nineteenth century. In practice, anti-abortion laws, like the anti-prostitution and anti-alcohol laws that followed them, singled out the seller for prosecution, treating the buyers as if they were the innocent "victims" of an irresistible temptation to purchase an overwhelmingly desirable, albeit forbidden, service or product.

Male Women, Female Men

Is Renée Richards, née Richard Raskind, a man or a woman? Raskind-Richards claims to be fighting for what he-she defines as a civil rights issue—a step "in the social evolution of transsexuality," whatever that might be. I disagree. Men calling themselves women and competing with real women in women's tennis tournaments is not my idea of advancing civil rights, the dignity of human sexuality, or anything else for that matter—save the rights of males to impersonate women and of females to impersonate men. As a defender of civil rights, and especially of the rights of persons persecuted by psychiatrists, I believe that males and females should have a right to impersonate each other but, to paraphrase John Stuart Mill, I believe that that right should stop where it begins to infringe on the rights of others—in this case, real men and real women.

Since modern psychiatrically-imbued sex research and the journalism it has captivated have, like God at Babel, confused our tongue, we must first clarify our terms. We must first agree that two and two make four. As Raskind, Raskind-Richards was married and fathered a child. He-she is quoted as saying that "Ever since I was an infant, I always wanted to be a girl. I used to go to bed at night and pray, 'I wish I were a girl.'" Since female children are girls, they do not go to bed praying to be girls; and female adults do not, as a rule, father children. On the basis of the evidence, then, we are justified in concluding that Raskind-Richards is a male.

Being male (or female) is a biological condition, just as having blond hair or dark skin is a biological condition. That is the first "two" in our frighteningly simple equation of two plus two equals four. The other "two" is the concept of manhood or womanhood as social roles and performances. Being a man means dressing, walking, talking, working, in short, acting like a man, whatever that means in any particular culture. When a male acts like a man, he is a real or genuine man. I am not saying that these things are good or bad; only that they are lexical facts.

We must be clear about elementary distinctions because, unless we make them, we cannot grasp the nature of the impersonations of sex roles. For it follows that if a female acting like a woman is a real woman, then a male acting like a woman is a fake or impersonated woman.

Reprinted, with permission, from the *New Republic*, October 9, 1976, pp. 8-9.

I submit, then, that Raskind-Richards is a fake—that is, male—woman. He-she is no more a woman than a bogus Renoir is a Renoir. He-she may look like a woman, act like a woman, claim to be a woman, but he-she is, in fact, a man who pretends to be a woman.

There are many ways men can pretend to be women, and vice versa. Such impersonations may be achieved by means of dress, mechanical prostheses, the use of hormones, and surgical alterations of the body, especially the genitals and breasts. The medical and mechanical methods are important only from the point of view of their effectiveness in enabling doctors and "transsexuals" to produce better imitations of men or women; they are not important from the point of view of enabling us to distinguish between masculinity and femininity as biological conditions and as social roles.

I have, as I stated before, no objection to individuals assuming control over their bio-social destinies and remaking themselves into persons at variance with their biological gender. Indeed, in a society that values individual self-determination, people should be allowed to make such a choice, just as elderly people should be allowed to enlist the services of a plastic surgeon to give them a more youthful appearance. But we do not pretend that a 65-year-old man rejuvenated by plastic surgery and looking like a 45-year-old is in fact 45 years old. And who among us would support such a man's claim to a right not to be compulsorily retired because, in contrast to his plastically unreconstructed age-mates, he is a "trans-chronological"?

Thanks to medical technology, we can now make men to look like women, and old men to look like young men. It seems to me arbitrary and unjust, however, to make fiction rather than fact our standard for judging the economic, legal, and political status of female-looking men, but not of youthful-looking elderly persons, or of mature-looking children, or of the many others who would also prefer to be categorized by the appearance rather than the reality of their identity.

Male and Female
Created He Them

In the old days, when I was a medical student, if a man wanted to have his penis amputated, my psychiatric teachers said he suffered from schizophrenia, locked him up in an insane asylum, and threw away the key. Now, when I am a professor, my psychiatric colleagues say he is a "transsexual," my urological colleagues refashion his penis into a perineal cavity they call a "vagina," and *Time* magazine puts him on its cover and calls him "her." Anyone who doubts this is progress is considered to be ignorant of the discoveries of modern psychiatric sexology, a political reactionary, a sexual bigot, or something equally unflattering.

Like much of the medical-psychiatric mendacity characteristic of our day, the official definition of "transsexualism" as a disease comes down to the strategic abuse of language—epitomized by confusing and equating biological phenomena with social roles (in the present case, chromosomal sexual identity with acting as a man or a woman). Although there are connections between these concepts and facts, neither one "causes" or "determines" the other.

Since "transsexualism" involves, is indeed virtually synonymous with, extensive surgical alterations of the "normal" human body, we might ask what would happen, say, to a man who went to an orthopedic surgeon, told him that he felt like a right-handed person trapped in an ambidextrous body, and asked the doctor to cut off his perfectly healthy left arm? What would happen to a man who went to a urologist, told him that he felt like a Christian trapped in a Jewish body, and asked him to recover the glans of his penis with foreskin? (Such an operation may be alluded to in I Corinthians, 7: 17-18.)

"But," the medically informed reader might object, "isn't transsexualism a disease? Isn't it—in the grandly deceptive phrase of the American psychiatric establishment used to characterize all 'mental diseases'—'just like any other illness'?" No, it is not. The transsexual male is indistinguishable from other males, save by his desire to be a woman. ("He is a woman trapped in a man's body" is the standard rhetorical form of this claim.) If such a desire

Review of *The Transsexual Empire: The Making of the She-Male*, by Janice G. Raymond, *New York Times Book Review*, June 10, 1979, pp. 11 & 39. Reprinted with permission.

qualifies as a disease, transforming the desiring agent into a "transsexual"—then the old person who wants to be young is a "trans-chronological," the poor person who wants to be rich is a "trans-economical," and so on.

Such hypothetical claims and the requests for "therapy" based on them (together with our cognitive and medical responses to them) frame, in my opinion, the proper background against which our contemporary beliefs and practices concerning "transsexualism" and transsexual "therapy" ought to be viewed.

Clearly, not all desires are authenticated in our society as diseases. Why the desire for a change in sex roles is so authenticated is analyzed with great sensitivity and skill by Janice Raymond in *The Transsexual Empire*. Arguing that "medicine and psychology . . . function as secular religions in the area of transsexualism" (p. 21), she demonstrates that this "condition" is now accepted as a disease because advances in the technology of sex-conversion surgery have made certain alterations in the human genitals possible, and because such operations re-articulate and re-inforce traditional patriarchal sex-role expectations and stereotypes. Ostensibly, the "transsexers" (from psychologists to urologists) are curing a disease; actually, they engage in the religious and political shaping and controlling of "masculine" and "feminine" behavior. Raymond's development and documentation of this thesis is flawless. Her book is an important achievement.

The claim that males can be transformed, by means of hormones and surgery, into females, and vice versa, is, of course, a lie. ("She-males" are fabricated in much greater numbers than "he-females.") Chromosomal sex is fixed. And so are one's historical experiences of growing up and living as boy or girl, man or woman. What, then, can be achieved by means of "transsexual therapy"? The language in which the reply is framed is crucial—and can never be neutral. The transsexual propagandists claim to transform "women trapped in men's bodies" into "real" women and want them to be accepted socially as females (say, in professional tennis). Critics of transsexualism say that such a person is a "male-to-constructed-female" (Raymond's term), or a fake female, or a castrated male transvestite who wears not only feminine clothing but also feminine-looking body parts. Raymond quotes a Casablanca surgeon, who has operated on over 700 American men, characterizing the transsexual transformation as follows: "I don't change men into women. I transform male genitals into genitals that have a female aspect. All the rest is in the patient's mind."

Not quite. Some of the rest is in society's "mind." For the fact is that Renée Richards was endorsed by Billie Jean King as a real woman and was accepted by the authorities monitoring women's professional tennis as a "real woman." This authentication of a "constructed female" as a real female stands in dramatic contrast to the standard rules of Olympic competition in which the contestants' bodily contours count for nothing, their sexual identity being based solely on their chromosomal makeup.

Raymond has correctly seized on transsexualism as an emblem of modern society's unremitting—though increasingly concealed—anti-feminism. And she correctly emphasizes that "the terminology of transsexualism disguises the reality . . . that transsexuals 'prove' they are transsexuals by conforming to the canons of the medical-psychiatric institution that evaluates them on the basis of their being able to pass as stereotypically masculine or feminine, and that ultimately grants surgery on this basis" (p. 13). The "transsexual empire" is thus a veritable Trojan Horse in the battle between the sexes, helping men to seduce unsuspecting women, or women who ought to know better, to join forces with their oppressors.

Still, why should anyone (especially feminist women) object to men wanting to become women? Isn't imitation the highest form of flattery? Precisely herein lies the "liberal" sexologists' betrayal of human dignity and integrity: they support the (male) transsexual's claim that he wants to be a woman—when what he wants is to be a caricature of the male definition of "feminity." What makes transsexual surgery a male-supremacist obscenity is the fact that transsexing surgeons do not perform the operation on all comers (just for the money) but insist that the client prove that he can "pass" as a woman. That is as if Catholic priests were willing to convert only those Jews who could prove their Christianity by socially appropriate acts of anti-Semitism. Janice Raymond's analysis is bitterly correct. The very existence of the "transsexual empire" is evidence of the persistence of our deep-seated religious and cultural prejudices against women.

The war between the sexes is a part of our human heritage. It's no use denying it. If that war will ever end, it will be not because of a phony armistice arranged by doctors, but because men, women, and children, will place personal dignity before social sex-role identity.

The Rapist as Patient

The most striking thing about the past century of medical history is the paradox that as our diagnostic and therapeutic technology has taken giant steps forward, our common understanding and legal articulation of what constitutes disease and treatment have taken giant steps backward. That is why the optimist sees modern medicine as a glass half-full of achievements: he emphasizes, correctly, that we can now detect and treat diseases better than we ever could before in human history. It is also why the pessimist sees modern medicine as a glass half-empty of common sense: he emphasizes, correctly, that we are now more confused about demarcating the categories of illness and treatment than we were centuries ago.

Both the medical optimist and the medical pessimist are right, because each looks at a different aspect of medicine: the optimist at its technology, the pessimist at its philosophy. Having to choose between these is a Hobson's choice. For what good is diagnostic and therapeutic technology if we lack understanding of what needs, and constitutes, "fixing"? And what good is a clear and coherent understanding of disease if we lack the means to treat it?

The two fundamental aspects of medicine are thus at odds with each other. As a healing art, medicine ought to serve human ends by humane means. As a biomedical technology, medicine has presented physicians with a temptation they have not been able to resist—that of serving themselves by defining as desirable that which is merely dramatic or difficult. When the fake diagnoses of psychopathology and the fake treatments of psychotherapy are added to the picture, the result is an invasion of common sense by a plethora of new "medical" illnesses and interventions, as the following vignettes illustrate.

On January 14, 1978, a federal judge in Detroit ordered the Aetna Insurance Company to pay $12,000 to a convicted rapist. Why? Because the rapist, Paul D. Duffy, 36, was "confined for more than five years for medical treatment as a sexual psychopath." The facts are briefly as follows.

In December 1966, Duffy confessed to a charge of rape and was ordered confined at the Ionia State Hospital in Michigan by a Macomb County Circuit Court. Michigan then had a criminal sexual-psychopath law which empowered courts to commit "mentally ill sex offenders" to state institutions

---

Reprinted, with permission, from *Inquiry*, June 26, 1978, pp. 3-4.

for treatment rather than to prison for punishment. (That act was repealed in 1968.) In 1972, Duffy was released, another proof of the miraculous healing powers of modern psychiatry. He returned to his job at a Chrysler assembly plant, only to be arrested again, on another rape charge, in 1974. A Wayne County Circuit Court then sentenced him to a term of 35 to 50 years at Jackson Prison. Duffy's suit against the Aetna Insurance Company, with which he had a health policy, was based on the claim that his first confinement was due to his "illness." Attorneys for the insurance company argued that it was due to his "crime." According to U.S. District Judge James P. Churchill, who decided the case, the issue was: "Was he [Duffy] disabled? . . . Forget that what he did was repulsive and sexual and that he's serving nearly a life sentence." Duffy, the judge said, was considered sick and "his illness required him to be confined. The law merely recognized that."

Rape is a form of violence—one person, the rapist, violating another person, the victim. Two things follow from this: first, that rape is a criminal act; second, that it is—must be, by definition—desired by the rapist. We deny these facts at great peril to our moral and political integrity.

Adultery is not a form of violence. Although the act betokens a violation of the moral contract between the adulterous person and his or her marital partner, the sexual act itself is consensual. Two things follow from this: first, that the act is not a crime (or, if it is, the statutes prohibiting it are dead-letter laws); second, that the act is—must be, by definition—desired by the adulterer. Hence, if adultery, too, were an illness, then adulterers (if "disabled" by their sexual activities) should, like rapists, be eligible for "medical disability" compensation. But who says adultery is an illness? Psychiatrists do!

On December 18, 1977, in a newspaper story headlined "Adultery linked to 'success depression,'" Arthur J. Snider, *Chicago Daily News* science editor, reported on this fresh psychiatric discovery. The discoverer of adultery as a disease was identified as Dr. Morton L. Kurland, a Palm Springs, California psychiatrist, among whose clients are "a large number of middle-aged women who are upset over their husbands' sudden adulterous behavior." Don't get Dr. Kurland or Mr. Snider wrong: the women who are "upset" are not sick; their husbands who are "adulterous" are. How does Dr. Kurland know this? By asserting that the men in question have not *chosen* to be unfaithful to their wives, but have been *caused* to be unfaithful. "In almost all cases, the cause is depression," says Dr. Kurland. "But rather than look upon their problem as a depression, the men project it onto their sexual life and their marriages. The extramarital love affair is an attempt at self-cure." Dr. Kurland does not say whether the costs of such love affairs should be deductible medical expenses. More on that shortly.

Because many of the men seen by Dr. Kurland, and another psychiatrist Snider quotes, are very successful, the experts have decided that these men "had unfulfilled and frustrated needs of dependence as children," which "caused" their depression in middle age, which in turn "caused" their "promiscuity." Dr. Maurice J. Martin of the Mayo Clinic calls such "success depression" the "meal ticket syndrome"—illustrating, I suppose, the first rule of psychodynamics: "When in doubt, give it a name." Snider reports that in Dr. Martin's view, "Middle-aged promiscuity due to depression may severely tax the strength of the marriage. The wife must be understanding and tolerant of the symptoms. This requires recognition and treatment of the problem." Since the "disease" of "success depression" and its characteristic symptom "adultery" are extremely common, I assume that Drs. Kurland and Martin will be appropriately rewarded for their important medical discovery.

Although psychiatrists are among the leading contenders in the race to confuse the categories of disease and treatment, they are by no means the only serious competitors. Other physicians, lawyers, legislators, and judges are also doing their best.

In the January 1978 issue of the *Physician's Financial Letter,* one item was the answer to this question: "Is face lifting a deductible medical expense?" Here is the answer, almost in its entirety: "Does the fact that personal rather than medical considerations motivate a face lifting operation bar a medical expense deduction for its costs? The Internal Revenue Service rules it does not. A woman paid fees for plastic surgery that improved her personal appearance. . . . The operation was not recommended by a physician. The IRS says the deduction is allowed because the operation affected a structure of the human body, and the law specifically allows for fees paid for the purpose of affecting any structure or function of the body."

As I wrote some time ago, if a man cuts off his own penis, he is schizophrenic; but if he can get a urologist to cut it off, he is a transsexual. Furthermore, as the next two examples illustrate, amputation of the healthy penis is not only a "treatment" for which the state must pay, but, if successful, it also produces a compensable "disability."

On April 21, 1978, the *San Francisco Chronicle* reported the California State Court of Appeals' decision that the state "must pay for sex change operations for two welfare recipients." Declared the court: "We do not believe, by the wildest stretch of the imagination, that such surgery can reasonably and logically be characterized as cosmetic"—an opinion that surely says more about the judges' lack of imagination than about transsexual therapy. Both cases involved persons who were born male. One of the "patients," identified as "G.B.," was described as "an adult male transsexual who had not been helped by psychotherapy and needs radical surgery for sex conversion."

The following case illustrates the outcome of a medically, psychiatrically, and surgically successful "treatment" for "transsexualism." In March 1971, Paul Monroe Grossman, a music teacher in the Bernards Township (N.J.) school system, underwent a sex-change operation. Five months later, with his name changed to Paula Miriam Grossman, he/she was fired from his/her job. On February 17, 1978, the Appellate Division of the New Jersey State

Superior Court ruled that Grossman was entitled to a disability pension. The 3-0 decision held that "the transsexual, Paula M. Grossman, was obviously incapacitated within the eligibility definitions of the state pension laws, and therefore deserved the monthly pension from the statewide Teachers' Pension and Annuity Fund." The court did not dispute Grossman's claim that "she was mentally and physically fit to perform her duties." Instead, the court noted that "no school district will employ her because of her transsexual status." "I'm delighted that I won," Grossman told the *New York Times*. "It's a victory in the sense that if the state decides to disable anybody for any reason, then they're going to have to pay for it."

The Erewhonian and Orwellian dimensions of disease and disability are here nicely developed. Was Grossman sick before the transsexual operation? Is he/she sick now? If so, what is the origin of his/her illness—the transsexual "treatment" or the dismissal from employment?

Enough. Rape is now an illness. Adultery is now the symptom of an illness. Amputating a man's genitals and giving him hormones to help him impersonate a woman is now a treatment. Although medically successful, transsexual therapy may nevertheless lead to a "disability" that is now compensable.

At the same time, some of the interventions that were treatments a century ago are now crimes. In 1878, selling an alcoholic tincture of opium was the paradigm of free enterprise in chemotherapy, and ingesting it the paradigm of medical treatment. In 1978, selling heroin is a crime often punished more severely than first-degree murder; ingesting it is a disease considered more important and more serious than diphtheria, polio, or even syphilis.

Had we lived in 1878, each day would have brought us fresh examples of the tragedy of the impotence of medicine: children dying of diphtheria, adults of diabetes. Now, each day brings us fresh examples of the tragedy of the imbecility of medicine: rape and adultery classified as diseases, "genital reconstruction" and cosmetic surgery classified as treatments. Then, the tragic loss was the death of individuals; today, it is the "death" of language and the undermining of the economic and legal fabric of the whole society.

Voyeurism as Science

Thy Neighbor's Wife is an amusing book. Perhaps it could have been more than that, but it isn't. The basic trouble with it is that although Talese knows all there is to know about sex, he just doesn't understand what it's all about. He says that he wrote *Thy Neighbor's Wife* because he wanted to produce a "work that would reflect the social and sexual trends of the entire nation. . . ." and he characterizes the "tone" of his report as "non-judgmental." His tone is, of course, anything but nonjudgmental: He likes those who advocate the free expression of sexual images and impulses and dislikes those who advocate sexual censorship and restraint.

Human sexual behavior, like all human behavior, has a biological base, but, unlike animal sexual behavior, human sexual behavior is inexorably a cultural product. The "naturalizers" of human sexuality—à la Hugh Hefner and William Masters—tell us that because sex is a "natural function" it is good, and a good society ought to allow the greatest possible scope for its expression. Talese, who has been completely taken in by the notion that contemporary Americans are the beneficiaries of a vastly successful revolution, believes this attractive, but absurd, proposition.

The situation, I am afraid, is a bit more complicated. Actually, what Talese's own "research" has revealed is that never before have so many Americans masturbated and copulated so much and enjoyed it so little. Why else would they need books instructing them about the *joys* of sex? Even the Victorians—not to mention our more remote ancestors—took it for granted that sex was pleasurable.

Anyone who writes about the sex lives of certain persons—especially if they are real, identified individuals—runs the risk of offending good taste, and Talese is no exception. I am (I believe) no prude, but I found this book to be morally distasteful. When the author includes, as Talese does, revelations about his own sexual experiences, one wonders what he hopes to achieve by means of that extra flourish of exhibitionism. In an odd last chapter, in which Talese refers to himself in the third person, he offers us some clues about what went wrong with this book.

For five hundred pages Talese tells us sexual stories—mainly about men

---

Review of *Thy Neighbor's Wife,* by Gay Talese, *Inquiry,* June 9, and 23, 1980, pp. 15-16. Reprinted with permission.

masturbating themselves to the visual paraphernalia supplied by the modern sex merchants and about men being masturbated by women in massage parlors (establishments that seem to hold a special fascination for Talese). Finally—calling himself "Talese," as if, like Hugh Hefner and Alex Comfort, he were one of the characters of his own book, which indeed he is—on page 522 Talese notes plaintively that although his sexual fieldwork seemed to entail much erotic activity, "his allegedly ideal assignment was frequently less pleasurable than other people believed." I believe him. Then comes what might be his quintessential self-revelation. "And what bothered him [Talese] even more," he writes, "was that after three years of research and many months of pondering behind his typewriter, he had been unable to write a single word. He did not even know how to begin the book. Nor how to organize the material. Nor what he hoped to say about sex that had not already been said in dozens of other recently published works written by marriage therapists, social historians, and talk-show celebrities."

After six more years of "research" and pondering, Talese still had nothing to say about sex—but produced a book on the subject nevertheless. And that is what's wrong with *Thy Neighbor's Wife*. Discounting that defect, it's not a bad book. Certainly, it's not as dull as are the typical productions of modern sex therapists. And it is, in a way, informative. Not about sex, but about people—especially their weaknesses. Consider some of the revelations:

—One of John Kennedy's campaign workers who in 1960 "thought that she had gained a White House job because of her intelligence and idealism, was disappointed to discover that what Kennedy and a few of his men found most desirable about her was her body."

—During a weekend when President Kennedy and his staff were in Palm Beach, the President's mother attended a party with an escort that *Time* magazine's Washington correspondent Hugh Sidey had overheard being referred to as her "gigolo." A confidential memo from Sidey to the staff of *Time* magazine found its way to the desk of Attorney General Robert Kennedy, who bullied Sidey with threats of suing for slander.

—At Esalen, famed for its encounter group therapy, massage was being "administered in the nude by attractive suntanned masseuses and masseurs to oilslick patrons of the California spa. . . ."

—In a New York massage parlor ". . . there were Orthodox rabbis who covered their penises with condoms or plastic sandwich baggies so that they could be masturbated *without* fleshly contact."

—In California, at one of the country's most pretentious sex centers, Dr. Alex Comfort, biologist and best-selling author, "was unabashedly drawn to the sight of sexually engaged couples. . . . [W]ith the least amount of encouragement—after he had deposited his cigar is a safe place—he would join a friendly clutch of bodies and contribute to the merriment."

According to the dust jacket, *Thy Neighbor's Wife* "is about the men and women who shaped our sexual revolution." However, Talese's book certainly does not support the idea that there has been a sexual revolution in America. It supports only the impression that a few men (and women and their pathetic followers), who were sex-starved as adolescents and young adults, embraced uninhibited sexual behavior as "the answer" to what human life is—and should be—all about. As previously people worshipped gods, power, fame, or celibacy, so these Timothy Learys of sex worship mastur-bation and copulation engaged in as often as possible and with as many partners (perhaps of both sexes) as possible. Which, of course, is just plain silly. The least amount of careful reflection could warn anyone about the promises of the pansexual utopians: Why should a lot of "good" sex be any more important for a good life—and that, after all, remains even the sexual-ists' goal—than, say, a lot of "good" food, drink, or drugs?

The naiveté that informs much of Talese's commentary is surprising. For example, Talese refers to ours as "this Freudian age" in which "Ameri-cans were opening up, acknowledging their needs . . ." as if these observations were self-evidently true. I am not sure that we have good reasons for believ-ing that Americans, en masse, are engaging in much more sex now than they did, say, in the antebellum South. But never mind the weakness of that generalization. Consider rather the shallowness—indeed, the absurdity—of characterizing a therapeutic ideology of sexual salvation through masturba-tion (and unrestricted copulation for sensual pleasure) as "Freudian." To his dying day (in 1939), Freud maintained that masturbation was a dangerous and damaging practice—a view that even contemporary psychoanalysts more often support than oppose. In fact, Freud called masturbation "the one major habit, the 'primal addiction'" for which other addictions, such as to alcohol or morphine, are mere "substitutes." Furthermore, in his definitive *Introductory Lectures on Psycho-Analysis,* Freud defined the psychoanalytic criterion for a "perversion" as "the abandonment of the reproduction func-tion. . . . We actually describe a sexual activity as perverse if it has given up the aim of reproduction and pursues the attainment of pleasure as an aim independent of it." Believing that Freud and psychoanalysis favor sexual freedom and pleasure is like believing that Lenin and communism favor economic freedom and pleasure. That many people believe these things proves not that they are true beliefs—but only that those who hold them are true believers.

Taken as a serious work on human sexuality, *Thy Neighbor's Wife* has other major shortcomings: It is mainly about male sexuality, which it treats in an unabashedly macho style; it says virtually nothing about homosexuality; and it falls flat-faced for the view that sex is a medical concern. After working as a nonsalaried manager at a New York massage parlor, Talese "began to see the masseuse as a kind of unlicensed therapist. Just as thousands of people each day paid psychiatrists money to be heard, so these massage men paid money to be touched." But his "research" has stupefied, not enlightened him.

For human beings, sex, like life itself, can be a source of great joy or a heavy burden or both. Which it is, and why and how it is one or another— these are matters of the utmost complexity and delicacy. To assume that the maximal expression of the human sexual impulse is a good thing, as Talese and his "sexual revolutionaries" assume—is not very different from assuming that its minimal expression is a good thing, as the Church Fathers and other puritans assumed. Such inversions of values are dramatic and may be the source of great riches and power—but they are not very instructive, intellectually or morally.

The sad but simple fact is that the satisfaction of the sexual appetite is likely to be in conflict with the satisfaction of other human desires—not merely because some bigots seek to deprive us of harmless pleasures, but because all of mankind's major pursuits compete, as it were, with each other for the limited amount of attention and time that people can devote to such things. For example, intense cultivation of religion interferes with scientific pursuits; intense cultivation of athletics, with intellectual pursuits; and intense cultivation of family life, with professional pursuits. *Mutatis mutandis,* intense cultivation of sexual experiences may be gained only at the expense of sacrificing some other sources of satisfaction—and intense attachments to family, work, religion, and so forth are very likely to interfere with sexual pursuits and pleasures.

In what ways different people—men and women, young and old, of one religion or another or of none—ought to satisfy or curb their sexual appetites remains much the same problem for mankind that it has always been. Like Masters and Johnson's sexual recipes, Talese's sexual reportage pretends to give us answers without even knowing what the questions are.

The Case
Against Sex Education

"We actually describe a sexual activity as perverse if it has given up the aim of reproduction and pursues the attainment of pleasure as an aim independent of it." This opinion—that the aim of human sexuality should be the begetting of babies—was put forward, not by the Pope, but by the man widely regarded as the greatest sexual revolutionary of our century—Sigmund Freud.

William Masters and Virginia Johnson, the great sexual revolutionaries of our era, maintain the opposite view—namely, that the aim of human sexuality should be the procuring of pleasure. If a person doesn't derive pleasure from heterosexual or homosexual acts, then he or she suffers from "anorgasmia." If autoerotic acts are not pleasurable, then the person (who is always a woman) suffers from "masturbatory orgasmic inadequacy"—which Masters and Johnson define as follows: "A woman with masturbatory orgasmic inadequacy has not achieved orgasmic release by partner or self-stimulation in either homosexual or heterosexual experience. She can and does reach orgasmic expression during coital connection."

These two views highlight the procreational and recreational perspectives on sex. Which is correct or "true"? Which should sex educators teach? Obviously, the traditional Judeo-Christian sexual ethic, which Freud disguised and rationalized as "psychosexual health," and its inversion, which Masters and Johnson disguise and rationalize as "sexual adequacy," are mutually incompatible as moral prescriptions. Although the need for sexual expression can be very intense in human beings, the satisfaction of this need—unlike the satisfaction of the need for food, water, and sleep—is not essential for individual survival. Therein, in fact, lies the reason why the gratification and curbing of sexual desire serve such diverse purposes in various cultures and religions. And therein, too, lies the reason why so-called sex education, as presently practiced, is a mass of misinformation, misrepresentation, and outright fraud.

Actually, the term *sex education* conceals far more than it reveals. It conceals the specific social, educational, and economic policies used to implement sex education; the moral values secretly encouraged and discour-

---

Reprinted, with permission, from *Penthouse*, January 1981, pp. 124-25.

aged; and, last but not least, the problems that derive inexorably from involving the American public-school system—and hence the state and federal governments—in defining what constitutes education in human sexuality. The upshot is that many thoughtful and well-meaning persons now endorse sex education (especially in public schools) as a good thing. They should, instead, oppose it as one of the most deplorable consequences of the combination of liberal-statist politics with medicalized morals.

Engaging in certain sexual acts (as well as refraining from some or all such acts) serves important individual and social needs, such as the expression of love, the creation of families, pleasure, domination, torture, ritual, escape from boredom, companionship, monetary gain, self-definition, and the preservation of the group. The "proper" aim of human sexuality is thus a matter of cultural and moral convention. And the masturbatory therapy of Masters and Johnson is, quite simply, the inversion and medicalization of the cardinal sin of self-abuse of traditional Judaism and Christianity. How, then, can "sex education" be taught in American public schools without its violating the beliefs of either the religionists or the sexologists—not to mention all the rest of us?

To be sure, teaching evolution has also offended some religious sensibilities. But that problem pales in comparison with the problems posed by sex education. How the solar system, the earth, and mankind arose were matters of religious mythologizing long before they became subjects for scientific theorizing. But cosmological and evolutionary processes are not things that we, as individual human beings, *do*; we can only observe, reflect, and speculate about them. But "sex" is at once something we *are* and something we *do*. Accordingly, sex education could be instruction in the anatomy and physiology of the sexual organs or about the facts of reproduction, fertility, contraception, abortion, or venereal disease. Or it could be instruction about approved and disapproved sexual practices, the dangers of teenage pregnancy, and the threat of the population explosion.

Clearly, only the purely biological aspects of sexuality are a matter of science. And biology has always been, and should be, taught in schools. But biology is an insignificant element in sex education, which is concerned with human sexual *behavior*. And human sexual behavior is never morally neutral; it is either good or bad. For example, as recently as 1939, a U.S. Public Health Service manual admonished that "masturbation . . . is destructive because it breaks down self-confidence and self-control." Today a Planned Parenthood pamphlet aimed at teenagers advises that "if the [sexual] feeling and tension bother you, you can masturbate. Masturbation cannot hurt you, and it will make you more relaxed."

The basic presumption about sex education—the attribution that has made it possible to mobilize popular opinion and political support for it—is the same misleading claim that underlies many social policies in modern technological societies: namely, that the matter at hand is a *health problem*.

As the Moonies chant their mantras, so sex educators chant phrases like "sex is a health entity." Who can be against health? Only a madman—or a "right-winger," which, in the rhetoric of Mary Calderone, the founder of SIECUS (the Sex Information and Education Council of the United States), comes to much the same thing. Calderone, the Joan of Arc of the sex-education movement, never tires of claiming sex for health, as is evident in this statement: "Fundamentally, sex has always been preempted by the religions, and everybody has kept hands off. By putting it into the area of health, where it scientifically belongs, by recognizing its role in physical, mental, and social well-being, we immediately freed it for objective, less emotional study." Calderone's objectivity is illustrated by her identifying the opponents of sex education as antiscientific fascists. "Sex education," she has declared, "is the best issue the right wing has discovered in years, and they're exploiting it for all it's worth." This is perhaps the most colossal example of guilt by association since the days of Joe McCarthy. Calderone's logic implies that because the "right wing" is against sex education, sex education must be a good thing and we should be for it. By that logic, because the Klu Klux Klan is against communism, we should be for it.

The sex educators have thus managed to convince many people that, in opposition to the bigoted "right-wingers" who stand for sexual repression, they stand for sexual liberation. Ironically, that claim, too, is an utter falsehood, indeed. Mary Calderone has characterized herself as the very opposite of a sexually liberated person. "What kind of sexual persons would we like our children, grandchildren, great-grandchildren, to become?" she asks. And she answers: "We would hope that they are *not* to be: furtive, leering, guilt-ridden, pathetic, compulsive, joyless. In other words, not like ourselves!" It seems only fair to take Calderone at her own word and to conclude that her self-characterization is correct. That conclusion is also consistent with her insistence, at a lecture, that she is "not suggesting the distribution of . . . contraceptive information to teenagers." Taken literally and seriously, this means that Calderone believes that even 19-year-old married adults should be denied access to contraceptive information. That is sex *education?*

Still, we might ask: Have the sex educators abused their mandate, or is the idea of providing sex education in the public schools inherently faulty? The evidence—which I have set forth in detail in my book *Sex by Prescription* and summarize in what follows—points in the latter direction.

It would be possible, of course, to teach students the presently known facts about the biology of sex. But doing so would constitute "biology education," not "sex education." What sex educators want is not to impart information but to influence behavior. Sex education *is* teaching morality. Christian sex theorists have thus stigmatized sexual pleasure as a sin and glorified chastity as a virtue. Modern medical sex theorists are doing the same sort of thing: they are stigmatizing lack of sexual pleasure as a disease ("anorgasmia") and glorifying copulation as a treatment ("surrogate sex therapy"). But the fact is that sex is neither inherently sinful or sick, virtuous or therapeutic. Sexual ignorance can be replaced by sexual information. Sexual values can be replaced only by other sexual values.

In addition, sex education—not as an idealized abstraction but as a practical reality—suffers from another fatal flaw, related to its context rather than its content. Because the public-school system is a tax-supported institution that possesses subtle, and not-so-subtle, powers to coerce parents as well as children, it carries in its bosom the danger of politicizing whatever it touches. The risk of thus corrupting education becomes a reality as we move from the hard natural sciences toward the soft social sciences—reaching its apogee with sex education. Thus, the basic trouble with sex education is that it replaces biology and ethics with a particular sexual ideology—which is neither that of the Christian fundamentalists nor that of the readers of *Penthouse,* but is rather that of the "healthy sex as mental hygiene" of the ever-meddling, liberal-statist social worker. In short, it is precisely because sex education in the public school is inexorably a political matter that its proponents find it necessary to deny its moral dimensions and to affirm its medical pretensions.

The propaganda of the sex education lobby and its uncritical acceptance by the leading opinion-makers of our society have made it appear that anyone who opposes sex education is against both sex and education. But that is simply not true. Because all public education is an affair of the state, the advocates of sex education support, above all else, an expansion of the scope and power of state intervention in our personal lives. In a world where we are increasingly controlled by the state, the last thing we need is to have the state program our sex lives for us, too.

The Sadness of Sex

Until recently, the word "sex" meant gender. Its colloquial but now quite conventional use, as in "having sex," appears to be a post–World War II development. The change in the word "sex" from a noun denoting gender to a term denoting a class of human actions (or "events"?) signals an important cultural transformation. When sex became something one "had," like lunch or dinner, what was obscured was precisely what sexual revolutionaries wanted to obscure, namely *valuation*. When a man says that he has had lunch, that does not tell us whether he ate cottage cheese or his wife's pet canary.

This new sexual semantic has doubtless helped to counteract traditional anti-erotic prejudice, and that may be a good thing. However, as with most good things, this one has a bad side as well, namely, that speaking of "having sex" obscures the fact that a moral agent is engaged in some sort of action based on a choice. Such choices and actions are susceptible of being judged right or wrong—or morally indifferent—according to various ethical or religious standards. The attempt to deny this truth about the human condition is the cardinal manifestation of the bad faith on which all "scientific" sex education and sex therapy rest.

Today, one of the most ardent toilers in the vineyards of scientific sex education is Mary Calderone. First as president of the Planned Parenthood Federation of America, then as founder of the Sex Information and Education Council of the United States (SIECUS), and now as the senior author of a "family book about sexuality," Calderone has been crusading for "sexual sanity."

Although Mary Calderone is a leader in the field of so-called sex education, this seems to be her first full-length testimony to her beliefs. It illustrates the truism that if only people are allowed to talk enough, or to write enough, they will give themselves away. Mary Calderone's testimony in this book is every bit as self-incriminating as was Jean Harris's in court. Her aim, she asserts, is to "bring you [us] up-to-date on important *facts* science has discovered about how people develop into sexual persons." (Emphasis added.) These "facts," moreover, she credulously believes to have been discovered by

---

Review of *The Family Book About Sexuality*, by Mary S. Calderone, M.D., and Eric W. Johnson, *Inquiry*, April 27, 1981, pp. 22–24. Reprinted with permission.

"scientists at major universities only over the past ten to fifteen years." However, what Calderone calls a fact is, as we shall see, more often than not, a rule.

This "family book" insistently disavows any intention of categorizing sexual behaviors as normal or abnormal, healthy or pathological—let alone as good or bad. It is, the authors emphasize, "almost impossible correctly to apply the word *normal* to sexuality." Yet Calderone's whole career as a sexologist has been devoted to, in her own words, "establish[ing] man's sexuality as a health entity." In 1969, at a meeting appropriately cosponsored by one of her favorite organizations, the American Psychiatric Association, Calderone asserted that her aim was to medicalize sexuality: "At the outset this author must emphasize that she writes . . . as a physician specializing in the point of view of public health and preventive medicine." In other words, Calderone is someone who insists on approaching sexual behavior as a physician and public health specialist, yet eschews the concept of pathology and denies the legitimacy of diagnosis.

This pervasive inconsistency may be the source of Calderone's incessantly repeated claim that she is a truthful person: In fact, whenever she clearly asserts something, she is likely, somewhere else, to assert its opposite as well. Thus, in her 1969 paper, she wrote: "One might therefore postulate that the adult society shows many symptoms of dis-ease regarding sex and sexuality, and this requires intensive therapy and that the incoming generations of *susceptibles,* the children from birth upward, should be accorded an education for knowledge and attitudes that would immunize them against the sexual dis-ease observable in their elders." (Emphasis added.) Then, in referring to the founding of SIECUS, she proudly acknowledged that "In actuality, its primary mission is to develop a valid and viable ideology about human sexuality." (The term "ideology" usually refers to a political or social program, one characterized by dogma and militancy.)

Jimmy Carter, the born-again Baptist, assured us that he would never lie to us. Mary Calderone, the professional Friend, affects the same style of unctuous self-righteousness. Twice, in the preface, the authors—this book is written with Eric W. Johnson, identified on the dust jacket as "a leading sex educator"—tell us that they are both "members of the Religious Society of Friends, or Quakers."

Why this emphasis? Because, as the authors explain, their faith informs what they write: "As Quakers, our moral values depend on our belief in the infinite worth of each human being." But then, perhaps inspired by Jimmy Carter, they assert that "The things we say in this book about sex and sexuality will be truths, as nearly as we can determine them." That their ability to determine the truth is so slight as to be imperceptible, I shall soon try to demonstrate. Before doing so, however, I want to list the principal standard the authors set for themselves. They write:

We describe rather than advocate. We try to explain all sides of a subject on which serious professionals in the field disagree; we do not advocate any specific position on an issue other than to indicate, when possible, where most workers, researchers, therapists, and religious counselors in the field of human sexuality tend to agree.

Calderone and Johnson's claim that they "describe rather than advocate" is totally inconsistent with what they write. Since virtually every other sentence in their book is prescriptive rather than descriptive, one hardly knows which statement to select to illustrate that their posture is consistently advocatory. For example, in the paragraph that follows the one in which they first claim to "describe rather than advocate," they write: "Any irresponsible use of sex is likely to damage individuals and society; therefore, such irresponsibility is, in the deepest sense, immoral." Calderone and Johnson thus advocate "responsible sex"—without, of course, ever specifying what that is.

Oddly enough, the greatest concentration of disguised propaganda occurs where one might expect the most facts to appear—namely, in a glossary at the end of the book. "Arranged alphabetically, the items in this Encyclopedia"—that is, what, inanely, they call their glossary—"will help you to find out immediately what you need to know." For example:

Adultery. The historic and legal term for sexual intercourse between a married person and someone who is not his or her wife or husband. The term preferred today is extramarital sexual intercourse.

Preferred by whom? Certainly not by the Pope. Note the attempts to remove moral valuation from the term and hence the act, and the pretense that such devaluation is not a moral act by a moral agent.

Breasts. Two milk-producing organs on a woman's chest. . . . [After twelve more lines of such enlightening information, Calderone and Johnson conclude:] Preoccupation with breast size on the part of both women and men is unfortunate, since it is unconnected with the meaningful aspects of relationships between them, sexual or otherwise. See also Nursing.

Real killjoys, aren't they? The size—and, more generally the appearance—of the female breast has no "meaningful connection" with erotic pleasure? If that's what Calderone and Johnson call telling the truth, one wonders how they would know that or when they are lying. A *real* encyclopedia, the *Encyclopedia Britannica,* throws some light on why these authors indulge in these antimammary exhortations in their "Encyclopedia." In the discussion of the beliefs and practices of Quakers, the *Encyclopedia Britannica* notes that "There was [in the Quaker code], an objection to anything that excited rather than calmed the senses." So sexy breasts are a no-no. Anything that's sexually exciting is a no-no. Still, the authors staunchly maintain that their statements are "descriptive":

Variant sexual behavior (or sexual variance). The preferred term for sexual behavior that is not engaged in by most people. The term *variant* is simply descriptive, whereas terms like "perverted," "unnatural," or "abnormal" are judgmental.

Incredibly, Calderone and Johnson seem to be utterly oblivious of the fact that preferring a nonjudgmental term to a judgmental one is itself a judgment.

Although Calderone and Johnson claim to eschew value judgments about sexual conduct and seemingly approve most of the behaviors which until recently were regarded as sexual perversions, the fact is that they do have their own categories of approved and disapproved sexual acts. Indeed, undeterred by their earlier claim that it is "almost impossible correctly to apply the word *normal* to sexuality," the authors assert that

> There are, however, some aspects of sexuality that scientific researchers and sexologists might properly consider to be "abnormal," in the sense that it is not behavior usual to most people; rigid compulsiveness about cleanliness, for instance, with constant washing of hands or genitals; or compulsiveness about never appearing nude before a partner or about sexual intercourse always taking place in the dark.

In addition to these horrid sexual abnormalities, Calderone and Johnson regard "sexual dysfunctions" (à la Masters and Johnson) also as diseases—to be cured, of course, by sex therapists.

The intensity of Calderone and Johnson's desire to be and to appear to be sexual middle-of-the-roaders is best revealed in their embracing as right and true the prevailing psychiatric fashions on the subject. Thus in a 1973 interview in *The Humanist,* Calderone spoke in these terms: ". . . if a girl gets raped or if a child has a homosexual experience, people survive these things very well." In a mere seven years she has come a long way from such casual conjoining of rape with homosexuality, now affirming not only that homosexuality is not an illness, but that the prejudice against it is. The authors define "homophobia" as "a condition of being afraid of or despising homosexuality or homosexuals. A person suffering from this condition is *homophobic.*"

Sexual exhibitionism—in men, but not in women—is an illness too: "Exhibitionism is a truly compulsive act, for the man cannot help himself." I would love to know how Calderone and Johnson *know* this. But they are sure of it: "Parents should not overreact but simply explain that the man is a disturbed person."

What it is that sex educators such as Calderone and Johnson really peddle is their particular set of sexual prejudices and prescriptions. Although the notion of a "fact" is not as simple as it might seem, in this connection we can, and must, distinguish clearly between facts and rules. To state that tires, batteries, and engines, for example, are parts of a car is to observe a fact; to set the highway speed limit in the United States at 55 miles per hour is to make a rule. It is embarrassing to have to remind people of this distinction, but when it comes to discussing sex, it is apparently necessary to do so, for most of the claims of modern sex experts are premised on presenting rule making as fact finding.

The most obvious example of this is the way the old "prophylactic" anti-masturbation rule has been transformed into the modern "therapeutic" pro-masturbation rule. According to Calderone and Johnson, "Science today can say that masturbation is normal." It is hard to tell who is demonstrating more bad faith—the "expert" who endorses masturbation as a good thing because "science" tells her so, as does Mary Calderone, or the "expert" who endorses it because God tells her so, as does Ruth Carter Stapleton. "The Lord," wrote Stapleton in the *Atlanta Journal* more than two years ago, "wants us to experience whole, complete lives, and He offers this gift [masturbation] to each of us as we surrender to Him." Each of these mountebanks of masturbation is invoking a seemingly unimpeachable authority— the one "science," the other God—to support a particular sexual act as acceptable, good, or "therapeutic."

The more familiar one becomes with Mary Calderone's posturings as a sex educator, the more absurd and pathetic her act appears, especially the peculiar combination of naiveté and grandiosity that she brings to bear on the pains and pleasures of sex—a subject that is, after all, not exactly virgin territory. Somehow Calderone manages to believe that men and women were waiting to learn about sex until fifteen years ago, when she discovered the subject, and that since then some gigantic breakthroughs have occurred in the field, thanks largely to Masters and Johnson.

Clearly, Calderone has convinced herself that it is her calling—as a Quaker and as a doctor—to emancipate an erotically benighted humanity from its sexual ignorance. This pitiful conceit is rendered positively dangerous by her unshakable conviction that the proper way to bring about such enlightenment is by channeling "sexual information" through the coercive apparatus of the American public school system.

It is all too silly and depressing. The Moral Majoritarians at least treat sex as dirty but interesting; Calderone treats it as clean but insipid. If Alex Comfort is the high priest of the joy of sex, then Mary Calderone is surely the high priestess of its sadness.

Speaking About Sex

Contemporary intellectuals—especially if they happen to be sexologists—are likely to believe that sexual science and sexual rhetoric are distinct and separate matters. It is possible, of course, to make certain factual statements about sexual matters. Accounts concerning the anatomy, physiology, and pathology of the genital organs fall into this class. But typically this is not what sexual discourse is about; it is about adultery and abortion, teenage pregnancy and the prevention of venereal disease, erotic technique and orgasm. In short, sexual discourse is about sexual behavior. Since all human behavior affects other persons, and since sexual behavior affects other persons very powerfully, discourse about such behavior is bound to be rhetorical. Whether or not we agree with the thrust of one or another species of sexual rhetoric is, of course, an altogether different issue.

Ironically, the rhetorical nature of sexual discourse is recognized today only when it issues from religious authorities; such authorities do not pretend that their message is scientific or value-free. This is why the admonitions of such authorities are listened to respectfully and are then ignored as irrelevant.

Whereas the sexual rhetoric of the cleric is couched in terms of God's needs or a divine plan for the world, the sexual rhetoric of the clinician is couched in terms of the requirements for healthy living or nature's plan for the world. But how do doctors determine what is sexually healthy or unhealthy? The same way the divines determine what is sexually virtuous or wicked: by imagination and attribution. As religions differ, so do their divine schemes for the sexually proper behavior of men and women; as cultures differ, so do their scientific schemes for such behavior. Since, historically, the paradigmatic pathology of human sexuality is masturbation, I shall use the medical-sexological fantasies that have been fabricated around this simplest and most elementary of sexual acts to illustrate the rhetorical character of sexual-pathological and sexual-therapeutic discourse.

A hundred years ago the belief that masturbation caused disease was unquestioned and unquestionable medical dogma. How could that be, when we know that masturbation cannot have any such effect? The answer is as

---

First published as "Speaking About Sex: Sexual Pathology and Sexual Therapy as Rhetoric," *Syracuse Scholar* 3 (Fall, 1982), pp. 15-19. Reprinted with permission.

simple as it is important. The belief in the pathogenic powers of masturbation rested on the lack of a clear distinction between distress and disease, just as the belief in its therapeutic powers now rests on exactly the same ground.[1]

Instead of rehashing the legend of masturbatory insanity, [2] I shall cite some passages by a physician from a typical medical period piece of 1879, illustrative of the sexological discourse characteristic of that era. The essay, with its tantalizing title, offers what is purported to be a typical case of the syndrome caused by masturbation and cured by morphine. Obviously I selected this example from the vast literature on self-abuse and opium therapy because the delusions embraced in it stand in such deliciously ironic contrast to the delusions embraced in the contemporary literature on self-pleasuring and drug abuse.

> The patient, a youth of about 14 years old, was led to my office by his father. His sight was so far lost that he could not walk unguided, and he presented a striking picture of anaemia and mental weakness. It was with great difficulty I discovered that he had contracted the habit of masturbation, and this was only accomplished by his own confession. The patient promised to discontinue the habit. . . . Ophthalmoscopic examination showed that the loss of sight was of cerebral origin, the retinae and optic papillae being healthy.[3]

Determined to prove the specificity of morphine as a therapeutic agent for this disease, Dr. B. A. Pope first treated the patient with injections of strychnine. After ten days, he says, the patient's

> general condition was but little improved, and I determined to give up this method of treatment as a failure. I now decided to make trial of such nervous agents as might give most promise of benefit, commencing with opium. . . . This treatment was commenced by the injection daily of 1-16 of a grain of the sulphate of morphia into the arm. After ten days the dose was increased to 1-12 of a grain. . . . At the end of a month the patient was dismissed from treatment the picture of health, having fattened very much and losing every type of anaemia and mental imbecility. There was a marked improvement in the sight after the first dose of medicine. . . . At the end of a week he could read ordinary print. . . . At the end of three weeks, his sight was perfect, though he could only see the fingers at six inches from the eyes when first seen.[4]

Rather than dismiss this report, which we might be tempted to do, let us try to make use of it. Actually it offers a splendid opportunity for inverting the usual approach to the study of sexual pathology and sexual therapy: Instead of studying the so-called patient, let us study the doctor; instead of studying the patient's alleged disease, let us study the doctor's discourse; instead of studying the patient's alleged recovery, let us study the doctor's remedy.

On the face of it, the case history is a caricature. The patient is a pubertal boy brought to the doctor by his father. Presumably, the father has been warned throughout his life that self-abuse causes weakness, blindness, and madness, and he has duly transmitted this warning to his son. The boy reaches puberty—and, presto, he presents a textbook case of masturbatory insanity.

So father and son repair to the doctor. The doctor, sharp diagnostician that he is, quickly makes the correct diagnosis and corroborates it by establishing its cause. Then he examines the patient. What does he find? Perfectly normal eyegrounds. But is that what he says? No. He says that "ophthalmoscopic examination showed that the loss of sight was of cerebral origin. . . ." Ophthalmoscopic examination cannot, of course, show any such thing. We could call the doctor's statement a lie, or we could call it a mistake, or we could call it rhetoric. The point is that the whole story is a morality tale.

Although the doctrine of masturbatory insanity may seem quaint to us today, the fact is that Sigmund Freud, who supposedly revolutionized our sexual morality, never wavered in his belief of its validity. Actually Freud borrowed the doctrine, refined it to suit his purposes, and then used it as one of the centerpieces in his theory of the "sexual causation" of what he called the neuroses. Freud's first comments on masturbation appeared in 1894, fifteen years after Pope published the paper from which I quoted. This is what Freud then said about it: "Neurasthenia develops whenever . . . normal coition, carried out in the most favorable conditions, is replaced by masturbation or spontaneous emission."[5]

It was a stroke of genius to make spontaneous seminal emissions (in plain English, wet dreams) the cause of disease. It was, to be sure, the genius of the rhetorician rather than that of the researcher; but clearly it was a brilliant move in the medical mystification of sex. By 1898, masturbation was one of the pillars on which Freud's so-called theory of the sexual etiology of the neuroses rested:

> Neurasthenia can always be traced back to a condition of the nervous system such as acquired by excessive masturbation or arises spontaneously from frequent emissions. . . . So far as the theory of the sexual aetiology of neurasthenia is concerned, there are no negative cases.[6]

This rhetoric of sexual pathology obviously did a lot more good for Freud than for his patients. Indeed, the emphasis Freud placed on the pathogenic powers not only of masturbation but of all departures from conventional, genital, heterosexual intercourse aimed at procreation cannot be overemphasized—as the following statement illustrates:

> On the other hand, the abandonment of the reproductive function is the common feature of all perversions. We actually describe a sexual activity as perverse if it has given up the aim of reproduction and pursues the attainment of pleasure as an aim independent of it.[7]

Freud's rhetoric here is similar to that of Pope John Paul II, the main difference being that Freud uses clinical jargon and the pope uses clerical jargon.

Having illustrated the rhetorical character of the notion of masturbatory pathology, I would like to discuss briefly the rhetorical character of its inverted version. The proposition that masturbation is *therapeutic* rather than pathogenic constitutes the backbone of contemporary "scientific" sex therapy and sex education. Among sex therapists, Masters and Johnson have developed and deployed this rhetoric most successfully.

In contrast to the debased and debasing language of the earlier anti-masturbators, Masters and Johnson refer to sexual self-stimulation in exalted and exalting terms. The masturbating male, for example, has a "penis unencumbered by vaginal containment,"[8] while the masturbating female is in the happy position of being unhindered by "the psychic distractions of a coital partner."[9]

Armed with such rhetoric, Masters and Johnson are ready to replace the centerpiece of the old sexological ideology, masturbatory insanity, with the centerpiece of the new one, masturbatory sanity. How do they accomplish this goal? By claiming to have discovered a new disease, which they call "masturbatory orgasmic inadequacy." I shall quote their own definition of it:

A woman with masturbatory orgasmic inadequacy has not achieved orgasmic release by partner or self-stimulation in either homosexual or heterosexual experience. She can and does reach orgasmic expression during coital connection.[10]

Masters and Johnson are just as distressed about this disease whose etiology (not masturbating) they have discovered as Freud was by the diseases whose etiology (masturbating) he had discovered. But Masters and Johnson are much more successful as therapists than Freud was: Out of eleven patients diagnosed to be suffering from masturbatory orgasmic inadequacy, they cured ten.

There is no need, at this point, to further belabor how sex educators have deployed, and continue to deploy, one or another of these rhetorical stratagems. In 1939 a Public Health Service manual admonished that "masturbation . . . is destructive because it breaks down self-confidence and self-control."[11] Today a Planned Parenthood pamphlet advises that "masturbation cannot hurt you and it will make you more relaxed."[12] The old anti-masturbatory rhetoric was presented and promoted as if it represented the results of clinical judgments or scientific discoveries, which is exactly the way the new pro-masturbatory rhetoric is touted.

The scientific discoveries of the born-again sexologists are, moreover, supported by the theological revelations granted to some born-again Christians. To Mary Calderone and Eric Johnson, two leading sex educators,

"Science today can say that masturbation is normal."[13] While science speaks to these scientists, God speaks to others—for example, to former President Carter's sister. Says Ruth Carter Stapleton, a famous faith healer, "The Lord wants us to experience whole, complete lives, and He offers this gift [masturbation] to each of us as we surrender to Him."[14] Persons who refuse to surrender to Mrs. Stapleton's God are presumably doomed to unrelieved suffering from the ravages of masturbatory orgasmic inadequacy.

I would like to conclude with a few lines from Mark Twain's long-suppressed satire on self-abuse, offered when the belief in the pathogenic powers of masturbation was at its height. In 1879, the same year that Dr. Pope published his paper on curing masturbation with morphine, Twain delivered a brief, humorous speech before a small gathering of American expatriates in Paris. Entitled "Some Remarks on the Science of Onanism," his talk was considered so scandalous that it did not see print until eighty-five years later. Here, in part, is what Mark Twain said:

> Homer, in the second book of the Iliad, says with fine enthusiasm, "Give me masturbation or give me death!". . . Cetewayo, the Zulu hero, remarked, "A jerk in the hand is worth two in the bush." The immortal Franklin has said, "Masturbation is the mother of invention." He also said, "Masturbation is the best policy". . . Michelangelo said to Pope Julius II, "Self-negation is noble, self-culture is beneficent, self-possession is manly, but to the truly grand and inspiring soul they are poor and tame compared to self-abuse."[15]

Mark Twain was jesting. But he knew that masturbation, despite the belief of doctors, scientists, and the public, was not pathogenic. Today, professionals and increasing numbers of lay persons earnestly believe exactly the opposite: that masturbation is therapeutic. I have tried to show that both views are mistaken and misleading. Sexual behavior, of which masturbation is a simple and simplified paradigm, is sexual behavior. Like any behavior, it may be judged to be good, bad, or indifferent. Conflating and confusing such judgments with diagnoses and treatments is unworthy of the human intellect.

Notes

1. T. S. Szasz, *Sex by Prescription* (Garden City, N.Y.: Doubleday, 1980), chaps. 2-4.

2. See T. S. Szasz, *The Manufacture of Madness* (New York: Harper & Row, 1970), chap. 11.

3. B. A. Pope, "Opium as a tonic and alterative; with remarks upon the hypodermic use of the sulphate of morphia, and its use in the debility and amorosis consequent upon onanism," *New Orleans Medical and Surgical Journal*, n.s., 6 (1879): 724-725.

4. Ibid., p. 725.

5. Sigmund Freud, "On the grounds for detaching a particular syndrome from neurasthenia under the description 'anxiety neurosis'" (1894), in *The Standard Edition of the Complete Psychological Works of Sigmund Freud*, 24 vols. (London: Hogarth Press, 1953-74), 2:109.

6. Freud, "Sexuality in the aetiology of the neuroses" (1898), in *Standard Edition,* 3:268-269.

7. Freud, *Introductory Lectures on Psychoanalysis* (1916-1917), in *Standard Edition,* 16:316.

8. W. H. Masters and V. E. Johnson, *Human Sexual Response* (Boston: Little, Brown, 1966), p. 213.

9. Ibid., p. 65.

10. W. H. Masters and V. E. Johnston, *Human Sexual Inadequacy* (Boston: Little, Brown, 1970), p. 240.

11. B. C. Gruenberg and J. L. Kaukonen, *High Schools and Sex Education,* U.S. Public Health Service, Educational Publication No. 7 (Washington, D.C., 1939), p. 67.

12. Quoted in J. Kasun, "Turning Children into Sex Experts," *Public Interest,* Spring 1979, pp. 3-4.

13. M. S. Calderone and E. W. Johnson, *The Family Book About Sexuality* (New York: Harper & Row, 1981), p. 112.

14. R. C. Stapleton, "God Gave Man a Variety of 'Gifts'," *Atlanta Journal,* January 23, 1979, p. 9.

15. Mark Twain, "Some Remarks on the Science of Onanism," in *The Mammoth Cod: An Address to the Stomach Club* (Waukesha, Wisc.: Maledicta Press, 1976), p. 23.

EPILOGUE

There are several reasons why a person may call something by a wrong name—that is, by a name others consider to be wrong.

A young or uneducated person may call a whale a fish. He does so because the whale looks like a fish. If given the proper explanation, he will understand that a whale is not a fish and why it is not a fish.

A man may call his wife "Honey." He does so because he likes her and has learned how to express an endearment by means of a conventional metaphor. He knows he is using the word "honey" metaphorically, and everyone else knows it too. No one confuses a human being with the substance secreted by bees.

A man may call bread and wine the body and blood of Jesus. He does so, typically, because he is a Roman Catholic priest saying Mass and the bread and wine in question are the ritually consecrated elements of the Eucharist. The priest knows the Eucharist is bread and wine, his parishioners know it, everyone knows it. But for the priest to say so would constitute utterly inappropriate behavior; in the past, it would have been called "heresy." For his parishioners to say so would be a grave offense against their religious community. For anyone else to say so—especially for a non-Catholic addressing Catholics—would be in very poor taste, to put it mildly. In short, there are times when educated people knowingly use metaphoric language but pretend or insist—often for reasons obvious to outsiders—that their metaphoric statement be interpreted literally. And there are times when other people seemingly go along with such usage out of deference to custom.

The sort of misnaming, or literal intepretation of a metaphor, that characterizes the Catholic description of the Eucharist often occurs in a secular version in mass movements. Such speech patterns are emblematic of the loyalty the speakers are expected to exhibit toward the leader. In *Chinese Shadows,* a classic account of life in Communist China, Simon Leys relates how Maoists did not dare

> to trust their own senses, to see for themselves the objective reality, but instead waited for the official version of what happened before they uttered an opinion. If necessary, if such are the instructions, they will not waiver in proclaiming that the deer is a horse, like the sycophants of Ch'in.[1]

In a footnote, Leys explains this reference to the sychophants of Ch'in as follows:

> A Chinese proverbial saying: the scheming prime minister of the second Ch'in emperor (3rd century, B.C.), trying to determine who among courtiers were his followers, pretended that a deer presented in court was actually a horse. All those who insisted it was a deer were later eradicated.

Many psychiatrists would like to treat those who defy their authority—by insisting that behavior is behavior, that homelessness is homelessness, that crime is crime—the same way.

When people now speak of mental illness, they may engage in any of these types of misnamings. However, as a rule, the misnaming of troubling or troublesome behavior as "mental illness" is not due to ignorance or error, but serves powerful ideological and economic interests. Hence it would be naive to believe that it can always be easily corrected by arguments based on reason and evidence. On the contrary, it seems that, like virtue, understanding mental illness is its own reward.

Note

1. Simon Leys (pseudonym for Pierre Ryckmans), *Chinese Shadows* (New York: Penguin, 1978), p. 11.

INDEX